"A worthwhile addition to any collection."—*Choice*

"Verburgh examines how we age and takes a valuable look at ethical issues surrounding the prevention of aging."—*Library Journal*

"Why do we grow old? In *The Longevity Code,* Kris Verburgh tackles this age-old question and arrives at some startling conclusions—with practical suggestions for how to slow down our biological clock."
—**David Ludwig, MD, PhD,** Harvard Medical School, author of the #1 *New York Times* bestseller *Always Hungry?: Conquer Cravings, Retrain Your Fat Cells, and Lose Weight Permanently*

"A brilliant and important book. Dr. Kris Verburgh, like no other, is able to represent the complex relationships between nutrition and aging. . . . Recommended for anyone who wants to know what to eat in order to age as healthily as possible."
—**Hanno Pijl, MD, PhD,** endocrinologist and professor of diabetology at Leiden University Medical Centre, Netherlands

"Informative, fascinating, and inspiring. . . . Based on current knowledge, *The Longevity Code* clearly describes how we ourselves can delay the unwelcome symptoms of aging and presents an extraordinary preview of what the future will bring."
—**William Cortvriendt, MD,** author of *Living a Century or More* and *Total Health Reset*

"*The Longevity Code* summarizes current scientific knowledge of the topic, dispels common and persistent fallacies, and offers perspectives on the future. It does all this in easy-to-read and understandable language."
—**Emmy Van Kerkhove,** emeritus professor of physiology, Faculty of Medicine and Life Sciences and the Centre for Environmental Sciences, Hasselt University, Belgium

THE LONGEVITY CODE

Slow Down the Aging Process *and* Live Well for Longer

SECRETS FROM THE LEADING EDGE OF SCIENCE

KRIS VERBURGH, MD

THE EXPERIMENT

NEW YORK

The Library of Congress has cataloged the earlier edition as follows:

Names: Verburgh, Kris, 1986-
Title: The longevity code : secrets to living well for longer from the front lines of science / Kris Verburgh.
Other titles: Veroudering Vertragen. English
Description: New York : The Experiment, [2018] | Originally published in
    Dutch as: Veroudering Vertragen (Amsterdam : Prometheus/Bert Bakker,
    2015). | Includes bibliographical references and index.
Identifiers: LCCN 2017025679 (print) | LCCN 2017029381 (ebook) | ISBN
    9781615194254 (ebook) | ISBN 9781615194131 (cloth)
Subjects: LCSH: Longevity. | Aging--Prevention. | Life spans (Biology)
Classification: LCC RA776.75 .V4613 2018 (ebook) | LCC RA776.75 (print) | DDC
    613.2--dc23
LC record available at https://lccn.loc.gov/2017029381

ISBN 978-1-61519-497-1
Ebook ISBN 978-1-61519-425-4

Translation by Tina Vonhof
Cover design by Beth Bugler
Text design by Sarah Smith
Author photograph by Michel Porro/Contour/Getty Images

Manufactured in the United States of America

First paperback printing December 2019
10 9 8 7 6 5 4 3 2 1

CONTENTS

PREFACE

We live in a strange world. A world in which people are mortal. A world in which most life-forms age and die. There are a few exceptions: organisms that do not age, that are immortal, or that can even become younger. But for the large majority of everything that walks, crawls, swims, or flies on this earth, mortality is an integral part of existence. That is strange, because from a biological viewpoint there is no reason why aging and mortality should exist. For centuries biologists have addressed the question of why something as strange as aging exists. As we shall see, aging is not simply the result of what is generally thought to be "inevitable wear and tear," nor is aging meant to combat "overpopulation," whereby "older animals must make room for younger animals."

In this book we will discuss why some organisms age very rapidly and other organisms can grow hundreds or thousands of years old or not age at all. In the second part of the book we will talk about what happens in our body that makes us age. Once we have a better understanding of why we age, we will also be better able to figure out how we can slow down the aging process. That is what the third part of this book is about. We will see that certain foods, interventions, and substances can slow down the rate at which we age. The problem in the West is that we are consuming too many foods that accelerate aging and cause obesity as well. It is not a coincidence that overweight people are at risk of all kinds of aging-related diseases, such as heart attack, dementia, and diabetes. We will also see that the epidemic of obesity is not simply a matter of "too many calories" and "too little exercise," as is often claimed.

Then we will focus on therapies that are currently being developed to slow down aging or that are already in use to treat certain rare diseases that bear similarities with aging. Not only can these therapies drastically slow down the aging process but they could even reverse it. Reversing aging means making people younger, such as by erasing wrinkles, making blood vessels elastic again, and curing aging-related diseases, such as heart failure and Alzheimer's disease. We will see that this is not impossible. To the contrary, many scientists are amazed by how easy it is to reprogram a body into a more youthful state. In the final part of this book we will discuss the great social revolutions that are rapidly approaching due to the fact that we will be living longer and longer. Current life expectancy increases by six hours every day, and in a relatively near future, when technologies become available to drastically slow down the aging process and even reverse it, we must consider a scenario in which people can stay healthy and young for a very long time. Even without these new technologies we know that the first person who will reach the age of 135 has already been born. Some scientists even suggest that the first person to reach the age of 1,000 has also already been born.

Regardless of whether the latter will turn out to be true, one thing is certain: Our increasing knowledge will enable us to transform disease, life, and death. This future is closer than we think, and therefore we need a plan—a plan that will enable us to benefit from this future revolution as much as possible, so that we have a greater chance of enjoying the fruits of these new developments. This book is intended to serve as a guideline for that plan. First, however, we need to understand why something as strange as aging exists to begin with.

A brief note: This book contains references to scientific studies. The references are added to serve as an introduction for those readers who want to delve deeper into the matter. Every claim I make in this book is based not only on the references mentioned in this book but on my training as a medical doctor, my research, thousands of other scientific studies, books, articles, lectures, and conversations with experts in their fields.

INTRODUCTION

Why do we have to die? This is one of the most important questions one can ask. It is, after all, the question why our existence is finite. Although the answer is very interesting, misunderstandings surrounding it abound. One reason for this is because the question can be answered in two ways: *why* we age, and *what* causes aging. The *why* examines why aging exists in the first place; why does it occur in nature? The *what* looks at exactly what takes place in the body that causes it to age.

Let's look first at why aging exists. At first glance, aging is a very strange thing. First nature allows you to exist: You are born from a fertilized egg cell that divides many times until there are 40,000 billion cells, which together form your body. The complexity of that body is amazing; it consists of more than 250 different kinds of cells (liver cells, muscle cells, eye cells, stomach cells, etc.) that work closely together to form a body, which contains as many cells as there are stars in 400 galaxies (a galaxy on average contains 100 billion stars).

That is not all, however. After it is born, that body will then amass dozens of years of experiences and memories. It will learn to walk, to bring a spoonful of porridge to its mouth without spilling, to talk, play soccer, solve math problems, dance, drive a car, and play bingo. That body will store a treasure trove of memories and knowledge, enough to fill an entire library with sounds, images, and smells. Then nature abandons that same body, which has finally built up all these cells, knowledge, experiences, and memories, and leaves it to wither and die.

Of the 150,000 people who die every day, 100,000 die of old age. Each human being who dies is a microcosm of billions of cells, experiences, and memories that implodes and is lost forever. Why? Would it not be much more efficient for nature not to allow people to age, but to continually repair and maintain them, so they would stay young and fit forever? That is very well possible. As we shall see, not a single law of nature forbids immortality. But Mother Nature does exactly the opposite: She allows bodies to age and die, only to replace them with newborn bodies. That is much less efficient and it costs a lot more time and energy. After all, she has to start from scratch every time: A baby has to grow and learn for many years, only to age and die. It would take much less time and energy to keep a body young and fit for centuries than to replace it each time with a newborn child. Mother Nature is the greatest squanderer that exists: After building a very complex body, she abandons that body and lets it age and die. It is ultimately thrown away. Nature has thrown out quite a few bodies—roughly more than 150 billion of them: all the people who ever lived and are now dead.

In other words, on the face of it aging and mortality are not logical at all. It is strange that aging exists. For centuries biologists have wondered about this. Not until the twentieth century did they finally find an answer. That answer is not self-evident. It is not true that we grow old because we wear out. Furthermore, the answer nicely explains why some animal species age hardly at all, whereas others age and die very rapidly.

In short, the *why* of aging inquires why aging occurs everywhere, or almost everywhere, in nature. The *what* of aging, on the other hand, tries to explain what causes us to age: what mechanisms are at work in our body that slowly but definitely cause that body to age, so that in the end we succumb to these aging processes, most often in the form of a heart attack, stroke, cancer, pneumonia, or dementia. If we can understand what causes us to age, we will be better able to understand what we can do about that aging process.

Let's start with the why of aging. It is an extremely interesting story about elephants, bats, cancer, strange brain diseases, and sex. A lot of sex actually, because reproduction and life span are intricately intertwined.

SUMMARY

The **why** of aging explains **why aging occurs** in nature.

The **what** of aging explains the **processes** that take place in the body that cause it to age.

1

Why Do We Age?

Many people believe that we age because we wear out. After all, our body must work continuously, day in day out, for dozens of years, and that causes it wear and tear. When we leaf through a standard medical handbook, we indeed encounter numerous diseases that appear to be the result of wear. Take, for example, osteoarthritis, also called joint wear. Dozens of years of walking and lifting are thought to be responsible for the inevitable erosion of our joints. Another disease that appears to be due to wear is narrowing of the blood vessels (atherosclerosis) due to the passage of all kinds of sticky debris (certainly after a visit to a fast-food restaurant). Although you can slow down this buildup with healthy eating, it is deemed as an inevitable result of the passage of time. Or take dementia. Our brain consists of 86 billion brain cells that fire frantically at all times and will eventually suffer damage. In short, the constant working of our body causes it to wear, and aging is assumed to be the unavoidable result.

The interesting thing is that this is not really true. Aging is not simply a result of inevitable wear and tear. Take, for example, mice and bats. Both animal species have a very fast metabolism. *Metabolism* is a collective term for all the processes in the body that allow the body to function: the beating of the heart, the contracting of muscles, the breathing, and the firing of nerve signals. Since mice and bats have a comparable metabolism, one would expect that they also wear and age at the same rate. However, the average life span of a mouse is two years, whereas a bat can live to be 30 years old or more. Some bats have been found that were at least 40 years old. In short, although mice and bats both have a very fast metabolism, these two species do not wear at the same rate. That means that the joints, heart, and brain of the bat wear fifteen times more slowly than do those of a mouse. Obviously, nature has found a way to drastically slow down joint wear in bats, as well as the clogging of bats' blood vessels and aging of the bat brain. It appears, therefore, that wear and tear is not simply inevitable but something that to a large extent can be controlled by nature.

You could also look at hummingbirds. These little birds live on insects, spiders, and the nectar in flowers. A hummingbird can flap its wings a hundred times per second for many years, without developing osteoarthritis or joint wear. If people flapped their arms a hundred times per second, their joints would be worn down to the bone within a few hours. So hummingbirds can stave off the wearing out of their joints much better than humans. By flapping its wings a hundred times per second, a hummingbird can fly from flower to flower at over 30 miles per hour to suck out the nectar. A hummingbird therefore needs a superfast metabolism: Its heart can beat up to 1,200 times per minute, compared to the human heart, which typically beats about 70 times per minute. A hummingbird has a metabolism that is a 100 times faster than that of an elephant. An elephant lives, on average, for 55 years. If the metabolism of a hummingbird is a 100 times faster than that of an elephant, and if aging is merely a result of wear, one would expect a hummingbird to age 100 times faster than an elephant. In that case, the hummingbird would survive for only about six months (55 years divided by 100). However, a hummingbird can live to be twelve years old—at least twenty times older that what we would expect based on its metabolism or on wear and tear.

In short, aging is not simply a matter of inevitable wear and tear. Mother Nature can determine how fast an animal species wears and how long it can live. If she wants to, she can even arrange for living creatures or cells to simply not wear, or age, at all. We will come back to this later.

Making Room?

Thus, an initial misunderstanding about the why of aging has now been disproven. Another myth about aging is also a classic one. This myth originates with nineteenth-century German biologist August Weismann. According to Weismann, aging exists because this process allows older animals to make room for younger animals. There is, after all, only a limited supply of food and other resources available in nature. It is better to let an old animal—

which has already been damaged during its life by broken bones; poorly healed wounds; damaged senses, such as having lost an eye in a fight; diseases; or accidents—age and die to make room for younger animals that are still fit and healthy.

Intuitively this argument may seem logical, but it is not true. In the first place, why would nature prefer a brand-new animal to take the place of a damaged animal? From the point of view of energy, would it not be much more efficient to simply repair the damage to the existing animal? It takes less energy—in the form of nutrition and bodily processes—to allow a broken bone to heal properly or even let an arm or tail that was bitten off grow back—as some lizards do or worms that have been cut in half and form new worms—than to make a new young animal grow from a microscopically small fertilized egg cell. Mother Nature (read: the process of evolution) is very smart and a very good bookkeeper. In short, she could have designed better mechanisms to repair the damage to older animals instead of creating a completely new animal each time.

Another reason Weismann's explanation is wrong is that this theory of aging does not explain why we grow older in the first place! It is a circular argument, for Weismann argues that animals age because they need to make room for younger animals. But what if animals simply do not age at all? Then they would all stay young and fit and they would not have to make room for a new generation.

And finally, there is yet another important reason that Weismann's theory does not make sense: In nature most animals die before they can grow old; that is, most mice, tigers, and pheasants have perished from disease, violence, or deprivation long before they could reach the age of retirement. Why would older animals need to make room for younger ones when old age is so difficult to reach in nature?

In short, this theory did not square with the facts. In the decades following Weismann's theory, numerous scientists racked their brains about the why of aging. Finally, in the mid-twentieth century, some interesting explanations came to the fore.

Dying Before Growing Old

The reason we age is that our ancestors in prehistoric times usually died long before they had a chance to grow old. This becomes clear through an example.

Let's look at a mouse. As we have seen, in optimal circumstances, such as in captivity, a mouse has an average life span of two years. Imagine that this mouse is born with a mutation that allows it to grow twenty years old. Mutations are spontaneous changes in the genetic material (DNA) of the mouse that makes its body function differently and, as a result, it acquires a new characteristic. Since these are random changes, most mutations have negative consequences. Still, a mutation can accidentally have a positive consequence. Mutations appear spontaneously and are hereditary (for more information, check the glossary in the back of this book). Suppose that, thanks to this mutation or new characteristic, our lucky mouse can live twenty years instead of two. However, in nature this mutation would have no benefit, because the mouse would have been killed by predators or died as a result of famine or cold long before it could grow that old. More than 90 percent of mice in the wild die before they are one year old. In fact, most animals die precisely when they are fittest and healthiest. Only if you keep them in captivity, or if they are extremely lucky, will they ever have time to grow old.

Most mice in the wild are eaten or perish before their life span of two years is over. They die from *external causes*, such as disease, deprivation, or predators, not due to *internal causes*, such as aging. Since they die so early from external causes, it is not useful for them to be able to live much longer than two years, let alone to live for twenty years. That is why nature has made mice to live, on average, for no longer than two years. Now we have arrived at an important point: The average life span of an animal species, or the rate at which it ages, is determined by the average time that this animal species can survive in the wild. If an animal species, such as a mouse, frequently dies of external causes, it will also age faster and have a shorter life span. If an animal species can survive longer in the wild, it will age at a slower rate and have a longer life span, as is the case with turtles. That explains why a bat can live to be 30 years old. In contrast to mice, bats can fly, which is why they can evade danger much faster. Unlike mice, they do not have to live on the ground, where they can fall prey to cats and mouse traps. Thanks to their wings, bats can also cover longer distances and are better able to find food. Every mutation in the past that made it possible for a bat to live longer was useful, because bats are much better able than mice to flee from danger, find food, and survive.

Of course, you could ask whether a mutation that makes a mouse live for twenty years is really of no use: Suppose that a mouse is lucky enough to stay out of the claws of cats, church owls, diseases, and accidents for twenty years. In that case, this lucky mouse has been able to reproduce much longer and more prolifically, so that it has more offspring that inherit this mutation, enabling them all to live longer.

That could indeed be true if the mutation had no disadvantages but only advantages, such as the longer life span. But in nature there is always a trade-off. A mutation that gives the mouse a longer life span also consumes more energy. In all likelihood the mouse has to spend more energy on the mainte-nance of its body, to be able to age at a slower rate. But why would the mouse do that if it has a 90 percent chance to perish in the first year? This energy is better spent on finding a mate and reproducing as quickly as possible, rather than spending this energy on bodily maintenance for the infinitesimally small chance of living to be twenty years old.

What is true for mice is also true for people. Our life span, too, is deter-mined by the length of time that our ancestors could overcome dangers and survive in the wild. In prehistoric times humans often perished by around age 30 from disease, hunger, accidents, or violence. A mutation that allowed them to age at a slower rate and live longer (to 200 years, for example) was not useful, because before their third decade they usually had been eaten by a saber-toothed tiger or died from blood poisoning caused by a tooth abscess. That explains why we look healthy and fit up to age 30 and then we begin to see the first clear signs of aging: The first gray hairs appear, as well as crow's-feet around the eyes, and kidney function and muscle strength diminish. Nature expects that by then we have been eaten or killed in an accident. The human body is strong, however, so it can last for at least another 50 years before it has declined to such an extent that death follows. Compare it to a good watch that is no longer maintained: It takes many more years before it finally stops working.

We can look at aging as a kind of neglect by Mother Nature. Since in ancient times people usually died before age 30 from external causes, such as disease, hunger, or accidents, there was no reason to enable humans to live for hundreds of years. Or to be immortal. We are aging today because in prehistoric times staying young for a long time was a waste of effort.

These insights about the why of aging also explain the large differences in life span among various animal species. Turtles are the best-known example:

They can live to be 150 years or more. According to official sources, Adwaita, a turtle that died in 2006 in a zoo in India, was 150 years old, but there are also indications that it was at least 250 years old. Some sources claim Adwaita was one of the three turtles that had been presented in around 1750 as a gift to British general Robert Clive, who had conquered large parts of India in the name of the British Crown. Another well-known turtle was Tu'i Malila, which was recorded as the oldest ever. This turtle, thought to have been born in 1777, died in 1965 at the respectable age of 188.

It is difficult to determine how old turtles can really be, as they live much longer than their human keepers and their information is often lost over time. Nevertheless, an age of 250 does not seem exaggerated, since it takes more than 30 years before Aldabra turtles, such as Adwaita, are sexually mature. One guideline for biologists to estimate the life span of animals is to multiply by six the age at which they sexually mature. Humans on average become sexually mature at around age thirteen and live until age 78 (13 × 6). If we multiply by six the age at which Aldabra turtles sexually mature, we get a figure of around 200. That is a respectable age, but they can probably live even longer. Some researchers even think that several species of turtles do not age at all, or very little, because their fertility and mortality rate (risk of dying) remains constant. They refer to this as "negligible aging."[1] Normally, when an organisms ages, its mortality rate increases year after year. That is one definition of aging: The older you get, the weaker your body becomes and the more risk of dying you have. So animals for which the mortality rate remains constant year after year, and decade after decade, seem not to age, or age "negligibly." Some turtles, like Blanding's turtles, seem even to age backwards, meaning that they grow younger and younger as time goes by. Year after year, their mortality rate declines and their fertility increases. Biologists call this "negative aging." To date, only a few animal species are known to age negligibly or negatively, including certain species of turtles, some lobsters, and certain fish, such as the rougheye rockfish, which can live more than 200 years.

Adwaita did not die of old age but from an infection. Without this infection, this turtle might have been able to stroll around its zoo for many more decades. So why can turtles live to be so old? An important reason is their shield: Thanks to this armor they can protect themselves very well against predators. In a distant past, a mutation that gave them the ability to live longer could be useful; their shell enabled them to survive. It is therefore no coincidence that in nature, many armored animals, such as turtles and crustaceans, age more slowly and have a longer life span. The oldest known animal is in fact a crustacean. This honor goes to Ming, the mollusk, probably the most famous of the oldest animals in the world. Ming, fished up off the coast of Iceland, turned out to be 507 years old. Scientists determined this by carbon dating, a chemical method used to determine the age of organic matter, and by counting the growth rings of the shell. Ming was born in 1499, at the time of the Ming dynasty in China—hence its name. For five long centuries, this mollusk was safely tucked away in its shell, which provided good protection against the whims and hazards of nature. Some mussels can also grow very old, such as the freshwater pearl mussel, which can live to be 210 years old.[2]

There is also a mammal that shares an important characteristic with turtles, in the sense that it, too, can protect itself very well against predators, not via a shield but with spines, namely, the porcupine. The fact that you cannot pet porcupines has played an important role in their life span. A porcupine can become at least twenty years old, which is very long for a rodent living on the ground. The spines make most predators wisely decide to allow the porcupine to waddle away. On the Internet you can find all kinds of video clips in which a porcupine meets a group of lions, which for most rodents (and humans) ends in death. The lions try all kinds of ways to turn the porcupine onto its back, but they cannot get past the razor-sharp spines that it puts up every time a lion comes sniffing nearby. Finally, the lions take off without any dinner and the porcupine quietly shuffles on.

Like spines and shields, size can also provide protection. Large animals are much more difficult and dangerous for predators to attack. That is why large animal species, such as elephants and giraffes, often live longer than small animal species. African elephants can be 55 years old or more, and some Indian elephants can even be older than 80. It is no coincidence that the largest mammals in the world—whales—also have a very long life span. Scientists suspect that the bowhead whale can reach at least 200 years of age. In 2007, a bowhead whale was found to have a harpoon in its neck that had come from an American harpoon manufacturer in New Bedford, where it had been made around 1880. This shows that the whale had probably swum around with this harpoon in its neck for at least 127 years.

What also makes whales interesting is that they rarely have cancer, which is unusual in view of their large size. You would think that the larger the animal, the greater the risk of cancer. Large animals consist of many more cells than small animals do, and the more cells you have, the greater your risk of cancer. Cells divide, and in the process a mutation (a fault) can occur, when the DNA in the dividing cells is copied incorrectly. This can cause cancer when the mutation gives the cells new properties, such as uncontrolled growth. A blue whale has thousands more cells than a human does, since it can become more than 30 yards long and can weigh 200 tons. In theory, therefore, a blue whale has a thousands-of-times-greater risk of getting cancer than a human does, because one mutated cell is enough to develop cancer. This does not happen, however. Scientists call this Peto's paradox, named after the scientist who first reported it. Whales can protect themselves against cancer many times better than humans. This is one of the many examples to show that nature can prevent many so-called unavoidable diseases. Currently scientists are studying the DNA of whales to find out why they are so well protected against cancer.

Aside from body armor, such as shields or spines, and size, the ability to fly also makes an animal better able to deal with danger, which in turn causes that species to age more slowly. Animals with wings can flee quickly from danger, they can move over longer distances, and they are better able to find food. Pigeons can be at least 35 years of age, which is old for such small animals. The oldest seagull found to date was 49 years old; since it is difficult to keep track of the age of seagulls, it is quite likely that they can live to be much older than that. Parrots can even live to be 80 years old, and there are reasonably well-documented reports of parrots that were more than a 100 years old. That some species of birds can live so long is remarkable, certainly given that the metabolism of birds is five times as fast as that of humans and that their body temperature is up to seven degrees higher. If aging were only a matter of wear and tear or the speed of the metabolism, such birds as parrots would age several times faster than humans.

Conversely, birds that can no longer fly, or not fly very well and live on the ground, such as chickens, pheasants, and turkeys, grow old much faster. A chicken usually lives only seven years. There is no point for a bird that cannot fly to become 100 years old when it mostly gets eaten by a predator within a few years.

Wings were such a useful invention that nature reinvented them several times, for birds as well as insects (from delicate dragonflies to rotund bumblebees), fish (flying fish), and mammals (bats). Bats are interesting because they grow so old. The oldest bat ever found was at least 41 years old. But since it was found by chance, there may be many more undiscovered, much older bats. Bats developed not only wings but also echolocation, which enables them to navigate in the dark. Most birds are unable to do this and this gives bats an extra trump card. That explains why bats, in relation to their weight, have the highest score in terms of the life span of all mammals. It also explains why there are so many species of bats: more than 1,200— almost one quarter of the 5,400 species of all mammals.

Bats are one of the success stories among mammals. But even the ability to fly just a little can influence the speed at which an animal ages. Flying squirrels are rodents that have a large skin fold between their arms and bodies, so that they can glide from one branch to another. A regular squirrel can live to be seven years of age, but flying squirrels can live to be at least seventeen.

Besides flying, an ability to hide can also be a good survival strategy, making a mutation that allows an animal to live longer useful. As we have seen, small rodents that live aboveground, such as mice and rats, have a pathetically short life span, usually only a few years. But that is often not the case with animals that live underground. Take, for example, naked mole rats, small rodents that live in holes underground, well protected from predators. Naked mole rats have adjusted very well to life underground: They have no fur but a naked, wrinkly pink skin; they are half-blind; and they have large protruding incisors and strong paws for digging, making them look like a furless cross between a rat and a mole. They are also fairly insensitive to pain, which enables them to live and dig in holes without the protection of fur. Found in East Africa, they live in close-knit communities with a queen who, as the only female in the colony, reproduces with the help of a few chosen males.

Naked mole rats can live to be very old: In contrast to rodents of comparable size, they can reach not just three, but 30 years of age. That is ten times older than the average rodent. Furthermore, they are very resistant to cancer: No mole rats with cancer have ever been found thus far. Their long life span and protection against cancer raised the curiosity of scientists, who have worked on mapping the DNA of the naked mole rat for many years. That work is completed, and now scientists are trying to find indications as to why these animals age more slowly and why they are so resistant to cancer. We will discuss their findings later.

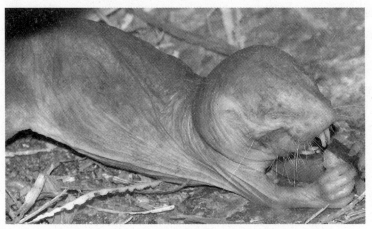

Naked mole rats look ugly, but they can live to be very old.

Just like naked mole rats, other animals like to nestle somewhere safely so they can survive longer. They do not nestle underground but below the skin. These are the parasites. Several parasites, from single-celled ones to six-foot tapeworms, can be thousands of times older than their cousins that live free in nature. They have evolved like this because they could safely hide in the gut, a muscle, or part of the lung of their warm, cozy host.

Apart from shields, spines, body size, wings, and hiding, intelligence as well as sociability can also enable a creature to survive better in nature; hence mutations that allow it to grow older can be useful. This is one of the reasons why humans have a significantly longer lifespan than many other mammals. Jeanne Calment, who attained 122 years of age, is the oldest known person ever to have lived. Mrs. Calment was born in February 1875 and died in 1997. She first saw the light of day in the year that the opera *Carmen* by Georges Bizet was written and one year before Alexander Graham Bell invented the telephone. She said that as a thirteen-year-old girl, she sold paint to Vincent van Gogh, who walked into her father's store in 1888. When she was 90, she signed a contract with a 47-year-old lawyer, who thought he had made the agreement of his life: He was to pay her a small sum of money monthly until her death, on the condition that he would get her apartment upon her death. But Mrs. Calment lived on, and following the lawyer's death of cancer at the age of 77, his widow had to continue to pay Mrs. Calment. Ultimately, Mrs. Calment earned a sum of money that was worth at least twice as much as her apartment. Of course, this woman is an exception: The average age of humans is about 80, which is still a lot compared to mammals of similar size.

Finally, the best way to evade predators is not by having wings, a shield, a colossal body, or a large brain, but by simply evading predators. That is what some opossums have accomplished. Opossums are small marsupials that live aboveground and therefore often become lunch for all kinds of predators. At a certain time, however, about 4,000 years ago, a few opossums floated across the water from mainland Georgia to Sapelo Island, where there are no predators. Any mutation that allowed the opossum to live longer (as well as its offspring that automatically inherited this mutation) was useful. They could not be eaten by predators at any time and, as a result, in barely 4,000 years the maximum life span of the island opossums had increased by 45 percent. These opossums, therefore, lived 45 percent longer than their relatives that stayed on the mainland. This, and other natural experiments, show that nature can quickly increase the life span of animals whenever the circumstances make it feasible.

We have seen that animal species have widely varying life spans. Since biologists like to order and classify things, they have mapped these life span variations and thereby developed the *longevity quotient*, or LQ. The LQ is a measure for the life span of an animal in relation to its size. Size is an important factor to take into consideration because, as we have seen, larger animal species generally live longer than smaller animal species do; just compare an elephant and a mouse.

The larger the LQ, the longer the animal lives. An LQ of 2 means that the animal lives twice as long as you would expect based on its size. The LQ of an elephant is 1. Indeed, you would expect that such a large animal would be able to reach the average age of about 60 years. A white-eared opossum has an LQ of 0.3. It is a small ground-dwelling rodent that is not too intelligent and is an easy prey for all kinds of predators. Chickens, mice, and rats also have a low LQ. Bats, naked mole rats, and humans rate high, due to their wings, digging front paws, and intelligence, respectively. Humans have an LQ of 4.2: That means that we live more than four times as long as you would expect us to, based on our size. The animal with the highest LQ is the Brandt's bat, which has an LQ of 9. We now know why: Wings and echolocation have allowed this bat to evolve to such an extent that it ages very slowly.

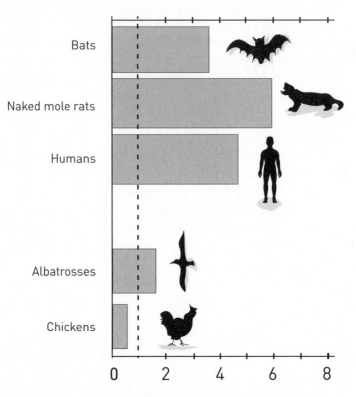

The LQ of various animal species. An LQ of 1 means that the animal lives as long as you would expect based on its body size. Humans, naked mole rats, and bats have an LQ that is several times higher. They live longer than you would expect them to, based on their size.

Young and Healthy, Old and Sick

For the first time, and not until the middle of the twentieth century, the points discussed here provided a good explanation of why old age exists. Around 1957, American biologist George Williams went one step further. Whereas we just saw that good mutations, or new characteristics, that can make us live longer are not useful because, in the wild, we cannot live long enough, Williams showed that bad mutations that accelerate the aging process can be useful at a younger age. Suppose that a boy is born with a mutation, or new characteristic, that makes him able to absorb more calcium from food. By absorbing more calcium he develops large, strong, calcium-rich bones. This mutation makes him a strong young man with bones that are more resistant to breaking. He is then able, for example, to better counter an attack from a saber-toothed tiger or survive a fall into a ravine. Thus, at first sight it is a good mutation. But this mutation also causes more calcium to circulate through the blood vessels, where it can then settle in the blood vessel walls and cause hardening of those vessels. After several decades this may put the man at greater risk of a heart attack. What was a good thing at a younger age (strong bones) may cause accelerated aging (hardening of the blood vessels and heart attack) at a later age.

This shows that fitness, strength, and strong bones at a young age potentially can cause you to die prematurely at a later age. Researchers have noted that some people who look large, strong, and husky may age faster and at age 50 already have a substantial potbelly, sagging skin, and narrowed blood vessels. Of course, we cannot generalize: Many people are strong and fit in their youth and also have a very long life. Furthermore, there are many other factors that play a role in life span, such as eating habits, exercise (which also makes us strong), smoking, and stress.

Nevertheless, in medical practice there are many examples of Williams' theory. Take, for example, Huntington's disease. This deadly neurological disease occurs when certain areas of the brain begin to die (from protein accumulation, as we shall see later on in this book). At first this affects mainly areas of the brain that are responsible for the execution and stream-lining of our movements. As a result, Huntington's patients begin to make involuntary, uncontrolled movements with their arms, legs, and sometimes their whole body. They twist their neck, grin, and sometimes make dance-like movements with their upper body, continuously and completely invol-untarily. The disease progresses relentlessly as the agglomeration, or piling up, of proteins expands into other areas of the brain, causing dementia. Often people die of pneumonia because they forget how to properly swallow their food and it gets into their lungs. This disease often begins at age 40 or 50. What makes it even worse is that it is hereditary. When a parent has Huntington's, each child has a 50 percent risk of also developing the disease. By investigating what type of mutation causes the disease, doctors can even fairly accurately predict at what age its symptoms will begin. This is a terri-fying verdict for the family to face.

Normally such a dreadful mutation would have been eliminated imme-diately by natural selection. That does not happen in this case because the disease does not appear at a young age but after most people have already had their offspring. Thus, there is no pressure on natural selection to eliminate this mutation. If a child would develop Huntington's, it would die before it could reproduce, so that the mutation would not be passed on and would automatically disappear. Adults with Huntington's have already had children and passed the mutation on to them, usually even before the disease manifests itself. That is why the disease continues to exist. It is of no concern to nature that someone gets such a terrible disease, as long as it happens later in life, after they have produced offspring. The same is true for aging: Nature does not care that you age and decline after you have produced children. Furthermore, nature may even have good reason to keep Huntington's disease around. One way or another, this mutation that causes a horrible disease in old age may have certain advantages at a younger age. Some studies, for example, show that Huntington's patients have higher fertility or a better immune system.

Thus, people may carry genes that accelerate aging or cause serious diseases, such as Huntington's, but that offer advantages at a younger age, for example higher fertility, stronger bones, a better immune system, or greater stamina. Another example is Alzheimer's disease and susceptibility to infections. Researchers have discovered that certain mutations can increase the risk of Alzheimer's. A certain mutation doubles a person's risk of developing Alzheimer's and shortens his or her life span by an average of six years. The bad news is that 25 percent of the population has this mutation. Worse yet: Three percent of the population has a mutation that multiplies the risk of Alzheimer's by a factor of nine. What researchers found, however, is that people with this mutation have less risk of becoming sick. Their immune system is stronger. This mutation must have been useful on the African savanna a hundred thousand years ago, when a gum infection or an injured foot could mean the end of you. A strong immune system fights bacteria rapidly and vigorously to stop them from growing into a large abscess or reaching your bloodstream and cause you to die from blood poisoning. In the Middle Ages, as well, such a mutation would have been very useful, since people at that time were living close together in cities without sanitation, greatly increasing the risk of infection. Researchers have discovered that, even today, children with this mutation who are living in slums are less sick. In prehistoric times, this mutation could be extremely useful because it reduced the risk of infection. Now the situation is different. In our society with its soap, Mr. Clean, and antibiotics, the chances of dying of infection are very slim. You can live long enough for this mutation to make its appearance and so have a greater risk of Alzheimer's disease and of heart attack as well. This is because a stronger immune system also releases more substances that trigger inflammation and can damage your own cells, including the cells that form the blood vessels and the brain. This general and continuous inflammation is like a low flame that sparks the aging process.

Other examples of these opposing forces are cancer and Alzheimer's disease. It has become clear that there is a reverse relationship between these two diseases: People with a higher risk of cancer often have a lower risk of Alzheimer's and the reverse is true as well. How is that possible? First, we need to keep in mind that cancer is not a typical disease of aging, although Alzheimer's is. The risk of cancer does increase with age, which makes many people think that it is an aging-related disease, just like Alzheimer's or heart and arterial disease. But at a certain age, when you are around age 75, the risk of cancer no longer increases, whereas the risk of typical aging-related diseases does keep increasing. That is strange. It seems as if at a certain time, the body begins to protect itself against cancer and that is indeed true. All our cells have a kind of built-in safety system that is activated when cells have been damaged. With too much damage (mutations), the cells run the risk of turning into cancer cells. When this security system is activated in a cell, the cell can no longer divide. That cell is put on nondividing status, you might say, and the cell cannot turn into an uncontrollably dividing cancer cell.

Thus, you are better protected against cancer if that security system is functioning well and it quickly prevents these cells from dividing. But these nondividing cells do have a disadvantage: They tend to swell and release all kinds of substances that can cause inflammation, which in turn makes the cells around them sick and causes them to age more rapidly. In short, in people who have a lower risk of cancer, this security system is functioning well, preventing mutated cells from dividing, but it increases the risk of aging-related diseases, such as Alzheimer's, because these nondividing cells poison their environment and fan inflammation. This is typical for the human body: It is difficult to outsmart it. There are balances that can become disturbed. Fortunately researchers are working hard on finding solutions, because cancer cells and aging do have one thing in common: growth and hyperstimulation. In addition, hormesis can also decrease the risk of cancer and slow down aging. We will come back to this later.

Sex and Aging

Now we know quite a bit about the why of aging. We know that aging exists because in the distant past we would die before we could grow very old. We also know that some mutations or characteristics that make us fit or fertile in our younger years can make us grow old faster in the years after our reproductive period is past. Regarding this latter point, there is an interesting fact about sex. Whereas before we were talking about mutations or characteristics that offered advantages at a young age but can be damaging at an older age, this point concerns in particular the *fertility* advantages of these mutations at a young age and how these can be harmful in old age. What it amounts to is that various mechanisms that stimulate reproduction when you are young can be harmful later on and accelerate the aging process. You could put it this way: There is an inverse relationship between reproduction and life span.

A good example is the Pacific salmon. These salmon are born upriver somewhere in Canada or the United States, and when sufficiently grown they swim downriver to the Pacific Ocean. They live there for several years until they return in large numbers to their place of birth, the river where they were born. This is easier said than done. The salmon have to swim many hundreds of miles upriver against the current, until they reach their birth river, where they mate and deposit their eggs. Then, in the following days, they die. How? To be able to make this demanding reproductive journey, the salmon pump themselves full of hormones (mainly cortisol). This gives the fish great strength and energy to accomplish this exhausting trip and the even more exhausting mating ritual. However, large doses of cortisol are harmful, as is the immense effort they have to make. In the process the salmon cause so much damage to their body that they die in droves in the rivers where they have deposited their eggs. They lose their life to reproduce just this once. The link between reproduction and mortality could not be more obvious than in this species: For them, sex means death. Reproduction and some hormones related to it, therefore, can shorten the life span.

There are also variations of this among mammals, such as, for example, Macleay's marsupial mouse, *Antechinus stuartii*. This small rodent lives in Australia. When the mating season approaches, the males produce large amounts of testosterone and cortisol, which makes them strong, muscular, irascible, wild, and aggressive. They need all that in the coming weeks to fight male rivals so as to mate with a female. In the days following all these fights and orgies, the males collapse and die, killed by wounds, ulcers (from stress and from the cortisol), and parasites that infect the mice because the cortisol has paralyzed their immune system. Biologists call this form of sex "big-bang reproduction" because salmon and Macleay's marsupial mice mate in a one-time, intense event and destroy themselves in the process. Since these animals often gather for this in large numbers, you could also call it "big gang bang reproduction," which covers it completely.

Fortunately, humans reproduce in less drastic ways. We do not have sex once in our lives and then die. Imagine that the groom would die after the wedding night and that everyone would consider that completely normal. We humans have sex many times in our lives. Nevertheless, it seems that even in animals that mate regularly, too much exposure to some sex hormones can shorten the life span.

A well-known experiment with fruit flies illustrates this. This was the first scientific experiment that could extend the life span of animals over many generations. It went as follows: Each time, researchers took the last-laid eggs to produce the next generation of fruit flies. First, the researchers took the eggs laid by the old fruit flies (45 days old): Only from these eggs did they grow new fruit flies. Then the researchers took the eggs of fruit flies laid at the age of 47 days, and so on. Through this intervention the fruit flies were forced to age more slowly, so that they could reproduce at an older age, since each time the last-laid eggs were selected for the next generation. Thus, the researchers managed to double the life span of the fruit flies over several generations. How did the fruit flies manage to live longer? This was possible because when the flies were young, they were less fertile. In this way, less energy was spent on reproduction, so that more energy could be spent on maintenance of the body (read: slower aging; later on in the experiment, the fertility of the long-lived fruit flies also increased, probably because by always taking the eggs of the oldest fruit flies, you not only select for lifespan but also for improved fertility).

Sex hormones show the link between sex and aging as well. Lab animals that receive testosterone die more quickly. The opposite is also true. There is an efficient way to reduce the amount of sex hormones in the body: castration. Castration is the removal of the sex glands, such as the testicles in men and the ovaries in women. In view of what we know about aging and sex, it should not surprise us that castrated animals live longer. If you castrate our Macleay's marsupial mouse mentioned earlier, he can live up to six months longer. That is not bad for a mouse that otherwise lives only one year. Veterinarians have long known that castrated cats and dogs live longer. It is the same for humans. Evidence of this can be found in old documents about eunuchs, men who were castrated at the court so that they could not be a threat to the wives of the emperor. In this procedure it was often not only the testicles but also the penis that was removed, so that the men had to urinate through a tiny hole. Documents show that eunuchs often lived longer than noncastrated men at the court. One study investigated the life history of 81 Korean eunuchs over several centuries in the past. It shows that eunuchs who were castrated before puberty lived an average of seventeen years longer than their contemporaries from the same social class. One eunuch is said to have been 109 years old.[3] Other research was done in the twentieth century in mentally handicapped men who were castrated on orders of their government. This research shows that the castrated men lived an average of fourteen years longer.[4] However, in this book we will discuss other, less drastic methods of living longer.

The role of sex in aging may also help us answer the following question: At what age do we actually begin to age? Many people think that we begin to age at around age 30. The first gray hairs may then appear, the skin becomes less elastic, and after a night on the town it becomes harder to get out of bed the next morning. However, this seems not to be the age at which we start to age. We do begin to show the signs of aging around our thirtieth year, but the aging process must begin earlier to allow these signs, such as gray hairs, to appear. Some argue that we begin to age immediately after birth, which is also not true. It appears that people start aging when they are around eleven years old. How did researchers come up with that? Because when we are eleven, our risk of dying is lowest and from age eleven on that risk begins to increase. In the West, babies have about a 1 in 1,000 risk of dying at birth. That risk decreases up to age eleven, when we have a risk of dying of 1 in 40,000. With such a young and healthy body we could on average live to be 1,200 years old, provided that our risk of dying remained constant. One person in a thousand could even reach an age of 10,000. Today, if this person were your grandfather, he would be able to tell you how he used to hunt mammoths. But such old grandfathers do not exist because from eleven years on the risk of dying increases.

That is what aging really means: your risk of dying, or mortality, which increases year after year because your body becomes weaker. Every eight years, you double your risk of dying. Someone who is 38 years old, therefore, has a twice greater risk of dying than someone who is 30. An 88-year-old has a twice greater risk of dying than someone who is 80. This doubling time applies to both men and women. That means that women age just as fast as men. Still, women on average live six years longer than men and there are at least four times as many women than men over the age of 100. How is that possible? Women are innately built better than men. Despite the fact that they age just as fast as men, their body is more robust, so that they can stand the test of time longer.

Another thing that shows that men are the weaker sex is that the risk of mortality is twice as high in men as in women. The risk is always higher in men but increases equally fast for men and women: It doubles every eight years, as we have seen. This difference in the risk of dying is due to the weaker construction of the male body and the fact that men take more risks. It is no coincidence that the risk of mortality in men is highest in the age group of eleven to 23. At that age, men have a three times higher risk of dying than women. Researchers sometimes describe that period as "testosterone dementia." This sex-specific form of reversible dementia is characterized by risky driving, bar fights, drug or alcohol abuse, and other macho behavior, which drastically increases the risk of mortality.

By studying the risk of mortality, researchers have been able to conclude that we begin to age from the time we are about eleven. That makes sense because you have to age about twenty years or so first for the first signs of aging, such as gray hair or crow's-feet, to appear at around age 30. It is no coincidence that we begin to age from age eleven on because it is around that time that puberty begins. Our body is pumped full of sex hormones that stimulate muscle growth, voice change, body hair, breasts, and maturation of the sex organs. In exchange for our capacity to reproduce, we begin to age drastically. We are a bit like the Pacific salmon, although our reproduction period is not just a few days, but several dozen years. In exchange for that, however, we shorten our life span from a generous 1,200 years to a mere 80. We exchange our (near) immortality for sex.

Thus, there is a clear link between reproduction and life span. The more energy you invest in reproduction, the faster you seem to age. Does that mean that having less sex would make you live longer? No, not really. Whether you have sex or not, your body continuously produces sex hormones and other substances that can influence your life span. You would have to surgically remove your reproductive organs, as in castration, to stop that. I do not think that many people are keen to do that, certainly in view of the side effects (infertility, decreased libido, hot flashes, and crying spells, in both men and women). Furthermore, all sex hormones are not made equal. We see that in particular too many *male* sex hormones, such as testosterone, can shorten the life span, whereas specific female sex hormones may even protect against some aging-related diseases. An example is estrogen. It is important to note that we are talking about *bioidentical* female hormones, not the synthetic hormones that are sometimes prescribed in postmenopausal hormone therapy.

In addition, the influence of sex on the life span is the result not only of circulating sex hormones but of thousands of years of evolution. Having less sex in your lifetime has no influence on the genes that determine your life span because you were born with these genes.

There is, however, a period in the life of a woman characterized not necessarily by less sex but by less reproduction, namely, menopause. This is the transition period in which a fertile woman becomes permanently infertile. Menopause is actually a remarkable phenomenon. First, it is rare; there are very few animals that have a menopause. Some animals, such as chimpanzees, have something akin to menopause, but it usually does not occur until very late in their life. What is the most remarkable is that women become infertile as a result of menopause, while they sometimes still have as much as half of their life ahead of them. Does nature not revolve around sex and reproduction? Is it then not strange that long-term infertility occurs in humans?

One popular theory states that infertile women can still be useful in nature after menopause, because they can keep caring for their children and grandchildren. Women are too useful, so that nature has decided to save them, by making sure that after a certain period they can no longer become pregnant because a pregnancy in later life would be too risky. In prehistoric times, women were at high risk of dying from infections and other complications during and after delivery. This applies especially to humans. Since humans walk upright, their pelvis is narrower in shape, so that babies cannot move through easily. As if a too-narrow pelvis were not enough, human babies have a large brain. Because giving birth is so risky for human females, nature may have decided that it is best if older women cannot become pregnant and instead use their knowledge and experience to help raise their grandchildren.

That may also be why people may live long enough to be grandparents. Since humans are very intelligent and social animals that can talk, they can very easily transfer knowledge. Older people, therefore, become very valuable; they have gathered a lot of life experience and are able to transfer it via language. When researchers studied the teeth of hundreds of ancient skeletons, which allowed them to determine their age, they discovered that about 40,000 years ago, there was a sudden increase in grandparents (the ratio of older people versus younger people increased exponentially). It may not be a coincidence that during that same period humans also made enormous cultural advances: Suddenly more complicated tools were developed, and more intricate body adornments and art appeared. Some scientists suspect that this happened because there were more grandparents who began to play an important role in the transfer of knowledge, and that at a certain point in time, this led to a cultural revolution.

Therefore, older people came to be an important asset. It was through them that the human species and our civilization could develop much faster and further. Today, the contrast could not be greater; instead of playing an important role as the sage elders of the tribe who had knowledge and experience to offer about climate, herbs, tools, and human relations, the role of older people in our society becomes ever less important. They are sent into retirement and dispatched to senior residences or resorts abroad. This is regrettable, since they contributed to the most important cultural leap forward the human species has ever made, about 40,000 years ago, when humans became really human. They deserve something more than a free bus pass.

Being a eunuch or a woman are all ways to have a long life span, but you can even become immortal by procreating in a different way. In nature, there are organisms that do not seem to age, that seem to be immortal. An example is the freshwater polyp. These little animals do not show any signs of aging when times passes, and this is again related to sex. These organisms seem to be immortal because they procreate in a different way from mortal mammals, such as humans. Scientists call this "sexless reproduction." Instead of a female egg cell and a male sperm cell that meet and merge via sex to create a new progeny, a freshwater polyp does not have to do any of that. It simply releases one of its cells, which then floats away and forms another polyp somewhere else. No fuss, no uninterested female partners, aggressive high-testosterone male rivals, or exhausting mating rituals: Simply release a cell and your reproduction job is finished.

Since a cell in the body of the freshwater polyp has the potential to create a brand-new polyp, these body cells may not grow older. Imagine that they would grow older and that, for example, a ten-year-old cell is released from a ten-year-old polyp. In that case, the polyp that grows from it would already be ten years old and all of its cells would also be ten years old. That is why the (stem) cells of the freshwater polyp may not grow older: Their cells must stay young and fresh, so that they in turn can form reproductive cells. Freshwater polyps stay young forever. The same is true for some jellyfish. *Turritopsis dohrnii* is a tiny jellyfish, measuring about one sixth of an inch (four millimeters), that floats around in most large oceans and does not age. It can even do the reverse. When the *Turritopsis* feels old and worn down, it can magically change its body into that of a young jellyfish. Biologists were amazed when they found out about this capacity. It turns the entire idea of the life cycle (you are born, you grow up, you grow old, and then you die) on its head. It is as if a butterfly became a caterpillar again or a chicken crawled back into its egg and then reappeared as a chick when circumstances were favorable. *Turritopsis* is sometimes called the "Benjamin Button of jellyfish," after the well-known story about a man who was born old and wrinkled but over time became younger again, to eventually die as a baby.

Freshwater polyps and jellyfish: These immortal organisms seem to be very distant from us. However, our body also contains cells that do not age and are immortal. Every one of us harbors cells that have lived for thousands of generations but have not become a day older. These are our reproductive cells—egg cells in women and sperm cells in men. These cells stay young. Reproductive cells cannot get older because then babies would be born old. Imagine that reproductive cells could get old: The reproductive cells of a 30-year-old mother and father would then be 30 years old. If they had a baby, the cells produced by these reproductive cells that form the baby would all be 30 years old right from the start. Once the baby formed by these 30-year-old cells becomes an adult and has a child (and his reproductive cells are also 30 years older), the cells of that offspring would be 60 years old, and so on. If reproductive cells could age, children would be born with wrinkles, or Alzheimer's disease, or have a heart attack at age two. But that does not happen: Babies look fresh and young and healthy. Nature does not allow egg cells and sperm cells to age, or more specifically, nature ensures that reproductive cells age very slowly and can rejuvenate themselves. Of course, it is not that one reproductive cell individually can live for thousands of years.

Reproductive cells continuously divide, just like skin cells, gut cells, and liver cells. But contrary to these body cells, reproductive cells do not age despite the fact that they divide. Biologists call this "the *immortal* germ line" versus the *mortal* body cells, such as the skin, gut, and liver cells (some people will note that egg cells and sperm cells do age, increasing the risk of birth defects, for example, especially when the mother is older, but the main point here is that reproductive cells can maintain and rejuvenate themselves, so that healthy babies are born at age zero, generation after generation, for hundreds of thousands of years).

In our own body, therefore, we carry cells with us that fool old age. For millions of years they have jumped from one generation to the next and remained young. Our body ages and dies but the immortal reproductive cells are passed on and continue to exist. If you think about it, you'll realize that all the cells that make up your body are in fact almost four billion years old, because the first life on earth appeared about 3.8 billion years ago in the form of single-celled organisms. Every cell in your body is the result of a previously dividing cell. These cells divided again and again, evolved and worked together to form countless organisms, from jellyfish to reptiles to humans. Each organism consists of cells that have been dividing continuously for billions of years. You originate from your mother's fertilized egg cell, which divided many times to form you, which originated from an egg cell of your grandmother, who was born from an egg cell of your great-grandmother, and so on. Each cell in your body originates from cells that have made countless divisions, for almost four billion years, from cells of distant single-celled, fishlike, reptile-like, apelike ancestors, and eventually created you. When you die, that chain will be broken for the first time in almost four billion years. The cells that form your body will disappear for good. Since each cell can start only from a previously existing cell, the billion-year relay race abruptly ends—unless you have reproduced. Then, at least one of your reproductive cells gets to participate in the race.

Once you realize that, you can understand how smart nature is: It managed to let life (in the form of cells) survive for billions of years, via countless cell divisions, which formed a profusion of organisms that populate earth, water, and sky. Because cells can continue to exist by continuously renewing themselves, there is no reason at all why an organism (which consists of a collection of cells) could not continue to exist forever.

In addition to reproductive cells, we can harbor other cells that are immortal, except you would not want to have those cells, because these are cancer cells.

An accumulation of cancer cells, or tumor, is made up of cancer cells that are immortal, in the sense that they can keep dividing without showing signs of aging. First, cancer cells form a small lump, somewhere in a lung of someone who smokes or in the skin of someone who has had too much sun. The cancer cells keep growing until they meet a blood vessel, and via the bloodstream they can then spread through the entire body, where they nestle in the bones, the liver, or the brain to create more tumors. In the long run, these tumors become so large that they constrict blood vessels, nerves, or areas of the brain, and the person dies. Cancer cells are cells that discovered how to become immortal. However, the drive for immortality is then punished, which shows how smart, but also dumb, evolution can be. To become a cancer cell, many very clever things need to happen. A cell must undergo hundreds of mutations, each time in specific genes (pieces of DNA) that regulate the growth, the metabolism, or the protein production of the cell. Cancer cells have all these mutations with which they outsmart the body. On the other hand, by continuously dividing and thinking only of themselves, the cancer cells ultimately destroy themselves by killing their host.

However, never underestimate the ingeniousness of nature or rather the process of evolution. In some animal species, cancer cells themselves have found an answer to this dilemma: They can transfer from one animal to another. These cancers are contagious. Their cells can be transmitted from a sick animal to a healthy one, which then also develops cancer. For instance, there is a certain cancer that forms tumors in and around the mouth of Tasmanian devils, doglike marsupials that are found in Tasmania, an island south of Australia. This fatal cancer begins with small tumors around the mouth and then spreads throughout the body. One Tasmanian devil transmits the tumor to another by biting or by sharing food, enabling the cancer cells to jump over from one animal to the other. This parasitic cancer causes a veritable massacre among the Tasmanian devils: More than 70 percent of these animals have already died from the disease. All kinds of conservation programs are in progress to prevent Tasmanian devils from becoming extinct.

Dogs are also known to develop a parasitic cancer that is sexually transmitted. Imagine that a cancer cell in a human person mutates and becomes contagious, such as via the skin (skin cancer), sneezing (lung cancer), or sexual contact (penile or vaginal cancer). Then you could become infected with cancer and there could even be a real cancer epidemic. Fortunately, the chance of this happening is very small.

The immortality of cancer cells led to the immortality of at least one person, albeit in an unusual way: Henrietta Lacks. This woman died in 1951 from cervical cancer, but part of her is still alive, you might say, because before she died medical researchers took some cells from her tumor and grew them in a culture dish. These cells keep multiplying without getting older. The immortal cancer cells were grown in ever larger quantities and distributed to laboratories around the world. Today, more of Lacks' cells have been spread across the world than the cells that originally formed her body. We can say that Henrietta Lacks has become immortal, albeit in a diffuse form, via her cells that are now alive all over the world. Her story shows that even normal body cells can become immortal.

Cancer cells, water polyps, rejuvenating jellyfish and our own reproductive cells. These examples show that no law of nature prohibits immortality or orders organisms to wear and age. The popular notion that aging is a matter of irreparable damage stems from the so-called machine myth. People tend to view the human body or any other organism as a machine that is subject to wear and eventually breaks down. But living beings are not machines. Contrary to machines, living beings can continuously rejuvenate and repair themselves. They do that by extracting energy from their environment (in the form of nutrients, light, and oxygen).

That also explains why immortality does not contradict the well-known second law of thermodynamics, which holds that disorder always increases. This law is often quoted to argue that aging is inevitable. The law holds that it is impossible to decrease the disorder in the universe. If you overturn your trash can, for example, the disorder in your room has increased. Of course, you can turn the trash can upright and put the contents back in, thinking that you have outsmarted the second law of thermodynamics, but that is impossible. It cost you energy (muscle strength, heart beats, breaths from your lungs) to tidy up your room, and all this energy (which is also released in the form of body heat and carbon dioxide gas when you breathe out) increases the disorder in the room and in the universe, even though you have turned the trash can back up.

According to the second law of thermodynamics, disorder is ever increasing. Everything becomes more disordered, everything wears down: Trash cans are upset, iron rusts and dissolves into the ground, drops of ink irretrievably spread in a glass of water, blood vessels clog up, and our cells become more and more disordered and damaged. However, you cannot quote the second law of thermodynamics when it comes to aging. The second law, after all, applies only to *closed systems*, where indeed the disorder always increases. A closed system is a completely closed environment that is not in contact with the outside world and in no way allows objects, heat, or gases to come in or go out. The universe can be viewed as a closed system (if we ignore the hypothetical black holes that make contact with other universes). Indeed, the disorder in this universe continuously increases, from upset trash cans to planets that evaporate in supernova explosions. But a body is not a closed system. It is an *open system* that is in continuous contact with the outside world. We breathe oxygen in and out, we eat food and drink liquids, we urinate, and we produce stools. In short, a stream of energy flows through people in the form of vegetables, meat, chocolate, oxygen, water, urine, sweat, and excrement. That stream makes it possible for us to continuously renew and repair ourselves. Thereby we decrease the disorder in our small open system, the body, but we still increase the disorder in the universe, a closed system, so that the second law of thermodynamics nicely remains valid.

Not only can life-forms rejuvenate and repair themselves to prevent decline but they can even make progress. Many organisms do not age during the first years of life, but they continuously get younger or better. Look at children: During the first ten years of their life they become stronger, smarter, and fitter. Their coordination improves, their speech becomes more refined, their immune system becomes stronger, and their brain gets better at processing information. Machines cannot do that, not in the foreseeable future, at least. Machines begin to wear down and deteriorate from the moment they were made. But as has been demonstrated in nature, living beings do not unavoidably wear down; some creatures or cells are virtually immortal. Thus, aging and mortality are not an inevitable law of nature but a biological process that various organisms are able to bypass.

Can human beings bypass this process? Before answering that question, we first need to know what causes aging. What processes take place in the body that make it slowly but definitely age? That is what we will discuss in the next chapter.

SUMMARY

Aging exists because

1. **Mutations** (new characteristics) that make organisms live longer are **not useful**, because the organism usually dies early due to **external causes**, such as violence, accidents, and hunger.

Example: More than 90 percent of mice die before the age of one year, so that a mutation that makes the mouse live to be twenty years old would not be useful and costs energy.

2. **Mutations** or characteristics that offer **advantages at a younger age** may be **disadvantageous at a later age**.
Example: Better calcium uptake may give you stronger bones when you are young but can increase calcification of the arteries at a later age, making you more susceptible to a heart attack.

3. **Greater fertility**, which is usually present at a younger age, may have disadvantages in later life.
Examples: Salmon die after reproduction and eunuchs live seventeen years longer on average because they have been castrated.

Some animals grow much older than others or age more slowly. Usually this is because these animals are **better protected** against external causes of death, such that any mutation that caused them to live longer was useful and became permanent. Examples are

• Armor and protection: turtles, shells, and porcupines

• Body size: elephants and whales

• Ability to fly: birds, bats, and flying squirrels

• Avoid predators: living underground, such as naked mole rats; opossums, which floated to an island without predators

• Intelligence: people, apes, and birds

Menopause and **grandparents** appeared because older people gradually became more **useful**: They could care for their offspring and pass on knowledge.

There is **no law of nature** that prohibits immortality. Examples of immortal organisms are

• Freshwater polyps

- The jellyfish *Turritopsis dohrnii*, which can rejuvenate itself

- Sperm and egg cells, which must stay young to be able to form young babies

- Cancer cells, which can divide indefinitely

Our own body is made of cells that have been dividing for almost **four billion years**.

2

What Causes Aging?

Aging has always fascinated people; it is, after all, the reason why our life ends. For thousands of years, our ancestors have wondered why they have lost some of their strength and vitality decade by decade. Various cultures have tried, each in its own way, to explain aging. According to the ancient Greeks, aging was the result of overheating: The heart produced a kind of heat—an inner fire that heated the entire body and kept it working. The lungs were there for cooling. The heating heart and cooling lungs kept each other in balance, but that balance was not perfect and slowly the body aged because of this. It dried up by too much heating of the heart and too little cooling by the lungs. According to the Greeks, it was better, therefore, not to live in a warm climate, because that increased the heating and drying up process even more. They believed sex and masturbation were not a good thing because the release of sperm, which contains moisture, also accelerated the drying process, explaining why men, who regularly release sperm, have a shorter life span than women—an accurate observation for those ancient Greeks.

In the following centuries, in Christian Europe, aging was viewed as a punishment by God for the fact that Eve, who was immortal, had taken a bite out of the apple from the Tree of Knowledge of Good and Evil. That made God angry and his ire had far-reaching consequences: Adam, Eve, and all their progeny would lose their immortality. From that moment on, humanity was condemned to mortality, old age, and death. In the sixteenth and seventeenth centuries, various theologians, and some scientists as well, added an extra spoonful of torment: Not only did we lose our immortality, we would age ever faster. Whereas an ancient biblical ancestor, such as

Methuselah, could reach the respectable age of 969 years, the age of the average seventeenth-century person was considerably less—only 40 years, or a little bit more if they were lucky and had a good constitution. People aged ever faster because the Great Flood had caused devastating damage to the earth. The Great Flood had torn open the earth's crust, thereby releasing toxic vapors and creating soggy swamps and dirty rivers. People must live in this unhealthy, irreparably damaged environment, which weakened them and shortened their life generation after generation, certainly compared to the ancient ancestors who could reach an age of almost 1,000.

As our knowledge developed, we came to different understandings. One of the first scientific theories that attempted to explain aging, was the *free radical theory* proposed by physician and scientist Denham Harman in the mid-twentieth century. Even today, this popular theory is often cited as the true explanation of aging, particularly in popular weeklies, TV shows, and advertisements for beauty products and dietary supplements. According to Harman, mitochondria (the energy generators in our cells—more about this later) create toxic substances called free radicals. These free radicals damage our cells and that is what causes us to age. However, as we will see, there are problems with this theory. For example, research has shown that lab animals that produce many free radicals actually live longer, and that such substances as antioxidants, which reduce free radicals, usually do not prolong life. In short, our aging is due to many things other than just free radicals. Harman's popular theory of aging is badly in need of revision.

Why do we age, then? In this chapter we will discuss several important causes, such as protein agglomeration, sugars, poorly functioning mitochondria, and shortening of our telomeres. It is interesting that proteins and carbohydrates (sugars) play a prominent role in aging. These nutrients form an important part of our diet, which implies that our diet can also play a significant role in slowing down the aging process. So let's focus first on these two nutrients.

Proteins and carbohydrates are also called macronutrients. Macronutrients are the sources from which we obtain our energy. The best-known macronutrients are proteins, carbohydrates, and fats. There is a fourth macronutrient in the sense that this nutrient can also be converted to energy, and that is alcohol. Too much alcohol can make you fat. These macronutrients, and particularly the quantities and the form in which they are consumed, play a crucial role in aging. We'll start with proteins and their role in the aging process.

Proteins

What do Alzheimer's disease, intestinal infarcts, supercentenarians, and some rare neurological diseases have in common? Proteins! Proteins are an important factor in aging. When we understand the role of proteins in the aging process, we can also figure out how we can slow it down—via our diet, among other things.

Proteins consist of thousands of atoms. Proteins have different, specific shapes. It is the specific shape that determines the type of protein. The body contains more than 20,000 different kinds of proteins. Since proteins are clusters of atoms, and since atoms are minuscule in size, proteins are also very small. The average diameter of a protein is about 10 nanometers (a nanometer is one millionth of a millimeter).

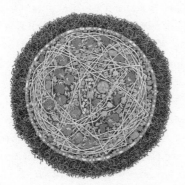

A cell—albeit a very small one— filled with all kinds of proteins. All these round and long structures are different types of proteins. (Source: David S. Goodsell, the Scripps Research Institute.)

The following figures show a few proteins in detail. Each little ball is an atom.

This protein is located perpendicular to the cell wall. It pumps sodium (atoms) from the cells. (Source: David S. Goodsell, the Scripps Research Institute.)

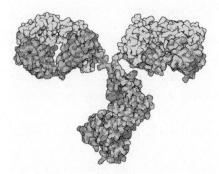

This protein is called an antibody. Antibodies attach themselves to the wall of unwanted intruders, such as bacteria and viruses, and damage them. Antibodies are produced by white blood cells and released into the bloodstream. (Source: David S. Goodsell, the Scripps Research Institute.)

Proteins have two functions: First, they are the building blocks of our cells. A cell contains millions of proteins that provide shape and structure to our cells. Just as wooden beams form the framework for a house, long rods of proteins form the specific shape of the cell. White blood cells can capture bacteria with their long, protruding arms because the arms contain a hinging framework of proteins that moves the arm of the white blood cell toward the bacteria. The cells that form our bronchia have long protrusions that wave back and forth to sweep up dust and mucus from the bronchia. The framework of these long protrusions is made up of proteins.

Second, proteins are also the workhorses of our cells. They perform almost all tasks in and around our cells: They break down substances such as drugs, alcohol, or food; they build up substances such as fats or hormones; they allow substances such as glucose or sodium to pass into and out of the cells; and they store or package other substances, like iron or vitamin B12. There is virtually nothing about our body that proteins are not involved in. Specific proteins in the cells of your stomach produce and secrete stomach acid. Other proteins located in the wall of nerve cells in your buttocks and back register pressure, which allows you to feel the chair in which you are sitting right now. Certain proteins in the cells of your eye register light, which allows you to read this book. Long protein strands in your muscles can shorten and contract them, so that you can turn over this page, but also dance, laugh, or walk. Proteins are the engines of life. The DNA in our cells contains the instructions for building proteins. Without proteins there is no life.

There is one more thing you need to know; namely, that proteins are made up of strands of amino acids. There are twenty types of amino acids in the human body (that can form proteins). Amino acids are small atom clusters that are always built according to a fixed plan. Amino acids are threaded like a pearl necklace to form a protein. This long strand of amino acids folds itself into a specific shape, such as a ball, a rod, or a hollow cylinder, forming a specific protein. This folding is possible because the atoms of which the strand is made are positively or negatively charged and can attract or repel one another.

The relationship between atoms, amino acids, and proteins can be pictured as follows. Just as there are various types of Lego blocks with different colors and sizes, there are also different atoms, for example hydrogen, oxygen, carbon, and so forth. Just as Lego blocks can build small basic structures, such as walls, windows, or roofs, atoms can build the twenty different amino acids. And just as these small basic Lego structures can build houses, amino acids can build proteins. A protein can consist of a few dozen of amino acids (a small house) or up to many thousands (a gigantic palace). Readers who want to learn more about proteins and amino acids can find more details at the end of the book, in the section "Additional Reading."

Proteins, and therefore amino acids, are found primarily in meat. Meat consists mainly of muscle cells, which are full of proteins. Fish, eggs, and cheese also contain a lot of proteins; and the proteins we eat do not only come from animals—plants contain proteins as well. Rich sources of vegetable proteins are nuts, legumes, tofu, and certain vegetables, such as broccoli. As we will discuss later, vegetable proteins are healthier than animal proteins.

SUMMARY

Proteins are the **building blocks** and **workhorses** of our cells. Proteins are found both within and outside of the cells; for example, in the bloodstream or surrounding the cells.

Animal sources of proteins are meat, fish, cheese, and eggs.
Vegetable sources of proteins are nuts, seeds, legumes (peas, beans, and lentils), quinoa (a pseudo-grain related to spinach), and tofu.

Vegetable sources of proteins are healthier than animal protein sources.

THE ROLE OF PROTEINS IN AGING

Why am I explaining all this? Because proteins play an important role in the aging process. A cell contains millions of proteins. These proteins are continuously built up and broken down by the cell. They are continuously recycled, but this recycling process does not always run smoothly. Every now and then, a protein escapes the process: It is not broken down but remains in the cell. At first there are only a few proteins, but as the decades pass, more and more proteins linger around in the cell. They also tend to cluster together, so that unbreakable protein clumps eventually fill up the cell. As time goes by, our cells become so filled with aggregated proteins that they no longer function well. That causes them to age: Heart cells no longer contract properly; nerve cells do not transmit signals efficiently; digestive cells do not absorb food as well as they used to. Finally, many cells simply die, strangled in a web of proteins. You can compare this to a deteriorating factory. A well-functioning factory (the cell) has the right number of personnel (proteins): not too many and not too few. But imagine that suddenly more and more personnel are added. Over time, the work areas, offices, and hallways are crowded with people, people who are not just hanging out but who also cluster in groups, becoming entangled in one another's arms and legs. Such a factory no longer functions properly, and as even more people are added, it can no longer produce goods. Ultimately, it bursts at the seams. This is what happens almost literally in our cells: As the decades pass, they become so stuffed with clumps of proteins that they can no longer function—they age and ultimately they die.

Take the heart, for instance. The heart is composed of heart muscle cells. Those cells slowly fill up with proteins. As a result they can no longer fully contract because all those proteins get in the way and the heart pumps less efficiently. As we get older, the heart's ability to pump blood through the body is compromised.

A similar process occurs in the brain. One of the most feared aging-related diseases is Alzheimer's disease. Alzheimer's is a form of dementia. There are several forms of dementia; the most common is Alzheimer's, which occurs in 65 percent of dementia cases. Alzheimer's disease is caused by proteins that accumulate both in and around brain cells. In the long term, the brain cells are literally smothered by this agglomeration of proteins and they die. Once about a quarter of the approximately 86 billion brain cells have disappeared that way, people develop the first signs of Alzheimer's: forgetfulness, difficulty finding words, and problems with orientation.

On average Alzheimer's lasts for eight to ten years from its first appearance until death. The cognitive capacities of the patients deteriorate to such an extent that they become bedridden and cannot do anything themselves. Even eating is difficult, and patients can, for example, die from pneumonia caused by food that has entered the airways. Or they may develop a blood clot in a leg due to lack of movement and that blood clot may then migrate to the lungs; or they die as a result of a bladder infection because they can no longer use the restroom by themselves.

We call Alzheimer's a disease but since this agglomeration of proteins is a typical phenomenon of aging, something similar also occurs in normally aging healthy people as well, but it happens more slowly. We can see that in the statistics: Starting at age 65, the risk of Alzheimer's disease doubles every five years, with the result that one in three people between the ages of 85 and 90 has Alzheimer's. In other words, if we grow old enough, everyone gets a degree of dementia because it is inherent in the aging process. We usually call it a disease when the process moves faster, about ten years from the first symptoms until death, or if it starts much earlier, such as at age 60. This is possible because some people have certain mutations in specific brain proteins. These brain proteins are built differently and agglomerate more rapidly.

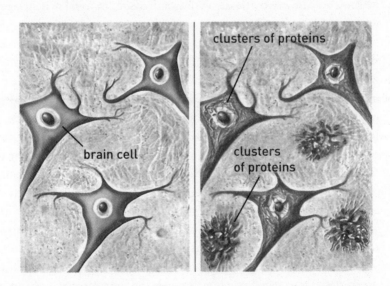

Healthy brain cells (left) and brain cells with Alzheimer's disease (right). Proteins form lumps and strands both inside and outside the cells. The brain cells are ultimately strangled by the excess proteins. (Source: the National Institute of Aging.)

Another brain disease caused by agglomeration of proteins is Parkinson's disease. In this disease it is mainly another protein, alpha-synuclein, which forms clumps, called Lewy bodies, primarily in areas of the brain that are responsible for the ability to make effortless and refined movements. As a result patients develop tremors in their extremities and their body movements become rigid. In addition, initiating movement becomes very difficult. Normally it is no problem to lift our feet to begin walking, but for someone with Parkinson's, this can be very difficult. When a line is drawn on the floor and a Parkinson's patient is asked to step over it, he cannot do it or only with great difficulty. This is because the areas of the brain involved in initiating movement do not function well anymore. Once he has taken the first step, he is able to go on. Since speaking also requires movement (it is muscles that make the vocal cords vibrate), speech also deteriorates. This can vary from stuttering to not being able to speak at all. In the final phases of the disease, cognitive problems and dementia may occur as well.

In short, agglomeration of proteins plays an important role in all kinds of aging-related diseases of the brain. Since all these brain diseases share the same underlying mechanism—clumping of proteins—it is sometimes difficult for physicians to distinguish one brain disease from another, especially because there are also brain diseases with simultaneous movement deficiencies resembling Parkinson's and dementia resembling Alzheimer's. Such diseases are referred to as "Parkinson's-plus syndromes." One disease begins with damage primarily in the movement areas of the brain, another begins with visual disturbances, and in another, memory or personality problems are first to appear. When I was a medical student, I remember one patient who suddenly became very religious. She had even sold her house and given all her money to religious charities. Eventually it became clear that she had frontotemporal dementia, a form of dementia that in its first stages affects in particular the personality of the patient, because inhibitions disappear. The frontal cortex of the brain (an area that mainly occupies the part of the brain behind the forehead) plays an important role in personality and moral behavior. This area puts the brake, as it were, on impulsive thoughts and plans, so that you can behave properly as a member of society. It prevents you from throwing a chair across the room when you are angry, from becoming belligerent at the supermarket checkout when you have to wait too long, or putting your fist through the wall in frustration. Patients with frontotemporal dementia often no longer have any social inhibitions, so they may urinate in public, become abusive or hypersexual, or start shoplifting.

Accumulation of proteins in the brain plays a large role in various diseases that can occur as we age. As we have already seen, however, proteins cluster everywhere in the body, including the heart. It is for this reason that researchers consider some forms of heart failure to be a form of Alzheimer's disease of the heart.[5] Proteins can cluster, not only in the heart and the brain but also in the blood vessel walls anywhere in the body.

After Alzheimer's disease, vascular dementia is the second most common form of dementia, responsible for 15 to 25 percent of dementia cases. Vascular dementia is caused when small blood vessels in the brain become obstructed or burst. When that happens, part of the brain does not get any blood and dies. These small, micro-infarcts can occur anywhere in the brain and eventually result in a diffuse cognitive decline, with forgetfulness, confusion, concentration problems, and difficulty with moving or urinating. One of the processes that contribute to these micro-infarcts is protein agglomeration in the blood vessel walls in the brain. These blood vessels then become brittle and can more easily break, resulting in bleeding in the brain. However, proteins also cluster, for example, in the walls of blood vessels in the intestine, so that the risk of an intestinal infarct (the tearing or obstruction of an intestinal blood vessel) increases. Part of the intestine dies, the content of the intestine then leaks into the abdomen, and eventually causes a massive infection that often quickly leads to death.

Proteins also cluster in the nerve cells in the spinal cord. This decreases the ability of the nerve cells to send out electrical signals, so that our reflexes deteriorate, also a typical symptom of aging. That is why a twenty-year-old can easily stand on one foot for a whole minute, whereas this may more difficult for a 50-year-old, and a 70-year-old should not try this without support. This deterioration of the nerve reflexes also causes older people to have difficulty regulating their body temperature, for the nerve cells are also involved in regulating body temperature: They make the muscles shiver or raise the hair on our arms when we are cold, or they make us sweat to cool us down on a hot summer's day. The older we get, however, the less we are able to regulate our body temperature, until the moment arrives that we want to go south for the winter.

Clusters of proteins can also be found in the lungs, making them lose their flexibility. Less flexible lungs cannot expand well when we breathe, allowing bacteria to more easily nestle in the lung and cause infections. Consequently, older people are more susceptible to pneumonia, one of the most common causes of death in the age group over 75 (of course, other aging processes also increase the risk of pneumonia, like a deteriorating immune system and cross-links, as we will see later).

Protein agglomeration can eventually cut down even the toughest people. These are the supercentenarians, people who reach age 110 or more (a regular centenarian is between 100 and 109 years old). Supercentenarians have such a strong body that they can last 110 years or more. It is not surprising, therefore, that they attract the attention of physicians and scientists who want to know how it is possible that they live so long, as well as what eventually kills them. Research has shown that these supercentenarians often die of a disease we call amyloidosis. Some researchers even believe that 70 percent of deaths of super-centenarians is due to amyloidosis.[6] This is actually a generalized agglomeration of proteins everywhere in the body. One type of protein in particular clusters in the body and causes extensive damage; namely, transthyretin.

Every one of us has transthyretin circulating in our bloodstream. It trans-ports substances in the blood; for example, thyroid hormones and vitamin A. The problem, however, is that transthyretin can easily agglomerate anywhere in the body. It does not form lumps, but strands that will begin to adhere everywhere, including in the walls of the blood vessels. This can cause the blood vessels to clog up or become brittle, causing a heart infarct, brain infarct, or bowel infarct, depending on the organ in which a large blood vessel fails. The transthyretin proteins also leak through the blood vessel walls and creep into the tissues, to form more clusters and strands there. If this happens in the lungs, it makes the lungs stiff, causing lung fibrosis, which is one of the reasons why supercentenarians become more susceptible to lung infections. The proteins can also cluster in the heart and cause heart failure; or around the nerve cells, causing nerve pain in the arms and legs. When such old people die, it is often said that they died of old age. But that is not true; people always die of something specific. In the case of supercentenarians, amyloidosis is a better explanation than old age. After more than a hundred years of protein agglomeration, their lungs, heart, or brain finally give up.

There is also a genetic disorder in which, due to a mutation in the trans-thyretin protein, the agglomeration is accelerated. This is Corino de Andrade disease, also called familial amyloid polyneuropathy (FAP). Symptoms appear at a young age, sometimes even in childhood—symptoms that we usually associate with aging: nerve pain, deterioration of reflexes, heart failure, high blood pressure, erectile problems, lung fibrosis, muscle weakness, and kidney problems. The disease is usually fatal about ten years after the first appearance of symptoms.

We have seen how protein agglomeration is one reason that we age. But what causes proteins to cluster to begin with? Has nature not found a way to prevent it? Well, nature did. One way to prevent that agglomeration is by making the proteins as perfect as possible. Imperfect proteins, with a slightly different shape, can clump together more easily. Some animal species are better able to build proteins with fewer imperfections, which increases their life span. One of these is our old friend the naked mole rat. These rodents live 30 years or more, whereas most rodents, such as mice or rats, have a lifespan of only a few years. Researchers have discovered that the naked mole rat's body makes more precise proteins with fewer imperfections so that they do not cluster as much.[7] That is one of the reasons why naked mole rats can live that long.

Another way to prevent protein agglomeration is via the incinerators in our cells. These incinerators, called lysosomes, are small sacs within in our cells. These sacs are full of digestive proteins called digestive enzymes. An enzyme is a protein that is able to break down substances, such as fats, sugars, and other proteins, into smaller pieces to digest them. Digestion is actually the breaking down of a substance into smaller pieces. It is the job of the lysosomal proteins to digest all the debris, such as damaged or clustered proteins, that enters the lysosomes.

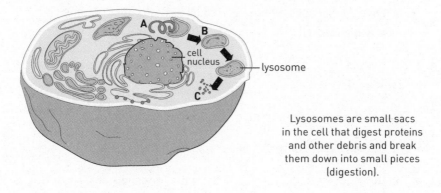

A

B

cell nucleus

lysosome

C

Lysosomes are small sacs in the cell that digest proteins and other debris and break them down into small pieces (digestion).

The older we get, the less efficient our lysosomes become, clogging up with proteins and other debris that they can no longer break down. When they can no longer do their job, the surrounding cell fills up with protein and other debris. You could compare an aging cell with a city where the trash incinerators (the lysosomes) are out of order. The garbage then piles up everywhere: in the buildings, the streets and the squares, blocking the roads and clogging the sewage system, so no one can go outside anymore and the city can no longer function.

There are other mini-incinerators in our body that also have the job of breaking down proteins; namely, the ubiquitin-proteasome system. But the older we get, the less efficient these garbage incinerators become in preventing the agglomeration of proteins. As a result, our cells are filled to the brim with proteins, which plays a role in Alzheimer's disease, heart failure, bowel infarcts, and nerve damage. Not only people with a normal life span but even the toughest supercentenarians (over the age of 110) are bound to be defeated by this agglomeration of proteins. Fortunately scientists all across the world are trying to find a solution. In addition, certain substances in our diet, and our diet itself, can slow down the agglomeration of proteins in our cells.

SUMMARY

Agglomeration of proteins in an around the cells plays an important role in aging and aging-related diseases. Proteins cluster, among others, in

- The **brain** (which plays a role in Alzheimer's, Huntington's, and Parkinson's diseases, characterized by forgetfulness, speech, or mobility disorders)

- The **nerves** (slowing down reflexes, impairing body temperature regulation)

- The **heart** (inefficient pumping of the heart, heart failure)

- The **blood vessels** (strokes, bowel infarctions)

- The **lungs** (decreasing the elasticity of the lungs, greater risk of pneumonia)

Generalized protein agglomeration is often the ultimate cause of death in **supercentenarians**.

Lysosomes are small bags in the cell that digest (break into small pieces) debris in the cell, such as proteins.

PROTEINS, NUTRITION, AND AGING

We have seen how protein agglomeration is one reason that we age. This is an important point because it can also tell us something about our diet. Our diet consists of proteins, in addition to carbohydrates (sugars) and fats. Proteins are found mainly in animal products, such as meat, fish, eggs, and cheese. In view of the role of proteins in aging, could eating lots of proteins accelerate aging? After all, if we eat more proteins, more proteins can agglomerate in our cells, thereby aging the body faster, and that is exactly what happens. Consuming too much protein can also indirectly make the body to age faster.

In the first place, a high intake of proteins serves as a signal to the body to grow. Proteins are the building blocks of our cells and if we take in more building blocks via our diet, more can be built and produced: more protein production, more hormone production, more building of other cell components. However, more growth also means that everything can pile up and clump together faster, resulting in an accelerated aging process. It is therefore not surprising that when we feed amino acids to worms and fruit flies, they age faster.[8] The same is true for rats and mice. Since the 1960s it has been known that the more proteins rodents eat, the shorter their life span. The reverse is true as well: The less protein they eat, the longer they live.[9–11] Even a diet from which a single essential amino acid is removed can extend the life span. Essential amino acids cannot be made by the body; they need to be taken in continually via food. A well-known essential amino acid is methionine. This amino acid is important because methionine is always the first amino acid with which an amino acid chain, which ultimately forms a protein, is built. Without methionine, protein building cannot get started. Various research studies have shown that methionine-restricted diets extend the life span of rodents.[12, 13] And here again, the reverse is true as well: When you feed rats a diet with a lot of methionine (2 percent of total calories), their blood vessels age much faster and they die earlier.[14] Another large study with hundreds of mice shows that it is not so much the number of calories but particularly the lower number of proteins that extends the life span of the mice.[15] Alzheimer's disease can be slowed down in mice via protein restriction cycles. Every other week, the mice were fed a diet that did not contain essential amino acids. The result was that the mice developed Alzheimer's at a slower rate and they scored higher on cognitive tests than did their fellow mice that were fed their regular diet, for there was less agglomeration of proteins in their brain that would cause the disease.[16] That said, I do not recommend that readers try eating fewer essential amino acids, because a lack of amino acids can also be bad for your health. It will take many more years of research to find out what the ideal dose and duration of such dietary patterns is for us humans.

Numerous studies show that an excess of proteins accelerates the aging process. Of course, one could point out that this pertains only to studies with animals and not with humans and that the results therefore do not necessarily apply to us. Another argument is that rats do not normally eat a lot of protein, so it is not surprising that when you feed them a high-protein diet, they die earlier. Nevertheless, these studies are meaningful, for their conclusions apply to all kinds of animals, from simple yeast cells and worms to mice and rats. There is a good chance, therefore, that they may also apply to humans. These dietary patterns influence aging mechanisms that have been preserved via evolution for hundreds of millions of years in many different animal species. Why would humans be any different? Some researchers suggest that, if a certain substance or intervention allows various kinds of experimental animals to live longer, affects known aging mechanisms, and decreases the risk of all kinds of aging-related diseases in humans (as we shall see later), we can be fairly certain that these substances or interventions can also slow down human aging and extend our life span.

Let's see what studies in humans tell us about this, starting with a quotation by researchers at the University of Cincinnati, who study obesity and aging-related diseases, including type 2 diabetes:

> There is increasing evidence that elevated dietary protein consumption also contributes to this syndrome [of metabolic abnormalities due to over-nutrition]. This observation is consistent with the approximate 33 percent rise in the consumption of processed meat over the last 50 years and with the association of high-protein diets with glucose intolerance, insulin resistance, and an increased incidence of type 2 diabetes.
>
> —"Nutrient overload, insulin resistance, and ribosomal protein S6 kinase 1, S6K1," *Cell Metabolism* (2006)

For most people in the West, the primary source of proteins is meat. How often have we not been told that we must eat meat to grow big and strong? Indeed, meat makes you big and strong, but there are also vegetarians who participate in triathlons and large, strong animals, such as elephants, that never eat meat. We see, however, that eating too much meat is not healthy. A study with 120,000 participants shows that their risk of a heart attack increased by 20 percent with each daily portion of meat they consumed. There was also a clear link between meat consumption and an increased risk of diabetes, cancer, and an overall increase in mortality.[17] Another study, which followed almost 450,000 Europeans over time, shows that participants who ate more than 160 grams of processed meat per day (about 5.5 ounces, the weight of one slice of bacon and two small sausages) had an 18 to 44 percent higher risk of dying during the study than those who ate little meat.[18]

Meat also increases the risk of all kinds of aging-related diseases, such as macular degeneration (AMD). This eye disease is caused by an accumulation of debris in the macular area of the retina, which leads to the death of cells in the retina, loss of central vision, and sometimes total blindness. People who eat red meat at least ten times per week have a 47 percent higher risk of developing macular degeneration than do those who eat red meat five times per week or less.[19] Other studies show a relationship between meat consumption and cancer. That is logical because cancer is the uncontrolled division of cells, and what do cancer cells need to divide and grow? Amino acids (and fast sugars, as we will discuss later). If you eat meat often, you activate all kinds of growth mechanisms in the cells so that regular cells can more quickly turn into cancer cells, while also fueling their growth. To study the effect of proteins on cancer growth, researchers have implanted tumor cells in mice. Then, one group of mice was put on a low-protein diet and another group of mice was put on a high-protein diet. The result was that in the mice that were on a high-protein diet, the tumors had grown several times faster and were larger than in the mice that were on a low-protein diet (see the figure on p. 44).[20]

And what about humans? A study done in 2006 shows that people who ate a lot of meat had a twice as high risk of non-Hodgkin's lymphoma, a cancer of the blood.[21] Women who ate meat every day had twice as high a risk of breast cancer compared to women who ate meat less than three times per week.[22] Too much meat, particularly red meat, also increases the risk of colon cancer. These are only a few examples of many studies that show that too much meat is unhealthy. That is why, in many countries, the dietary guidelines put out by government health organizations finally recommend eating less red meat.

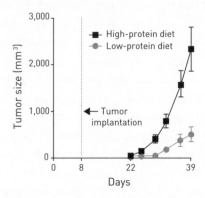

In mice on a high-protein diet, the cancer cells grow more rapidly.

However, not all types of meat are made equal. We just discussed red meat and processed meat. Many studies that investigate the relationship between meat and disease point especially to red meat as the culprit. Red meat comes from cows, sheep, and pigs. White meat comes from poultry (chicken and turkey). White meat is healthier than red meat. Each portion of red meat you replace with a portion of white meat reduces your risk of mortality by 14 percent.[17] Why is white meat healthier than red meat, even though both types of meat contain practically the same amount of protein? Contrary to white meat, red meat often contains a number of unhealthy substances, for example, certain fats that can stimulate inflammation, salt, preservatives, and coloring agents. Processed red meat, such as hot dogs, bacon, and salami, is the worst kind. If you really want to eat animal protein, it is best to replace red meat with white meat.

Some people are proponents of diets that are rich in meat, such as the classic paleo diet or the Atkins diet. Since more and more studies have been published showing that too much meat, particularly red meat, is not healthy, the proponents of these meat-rich diets argue that not all meat is bad. Meat from free-range animals or animals in the wild (as was the case in prehistoric times) is healthier than meat from animals that grow up in mega-barns and are fed grain products, such as corn.

Up to a point they are correct. Mega-barn cows are fattened up as fast as possible with grain-based feed, whereas free-range cows usually eat fresh grass. Research shows that, indeed, meat from grain-fed cows is less healthy; the ratio between unhealthy inflammation-stimulating omega-6 fatty acids and healthy omega-3 fatty acids is five times as high compared to grass-fed cows and contains far more unhealthy omega-6 fatty acids. The ratio of omega-3 fatty acids versus omega-6 fatty acids is twenty times better in eggs from grass-fed chickens compared to eggs from grain-fed chickens.[23, 24] I recommend buying eggs specifically from grass-fed chickens rather than free-range chickens, which often still get unhealthy feed. Research shows that there is even a difference in composition between meat from cows in pastures at different altitudes, such as in the Swiss Alps, where the grass contains more omega-3 fatty acids, and with different plant growth. One pasture is not the same as another.[25]

In the industrialized countries, we are feeding unhealthy food not only to ourselves but to our animals as well, making their meat, eggs, and milk less healthy. The proponents of the paleo diet, therefore, do have a point, in that meat from happy, stress-free, antibiotic-free animals that eat grass in a nice green pasture is healthier than meat from overstressed, overcrowded, antibiotic-stuffed, grain-fed animals in mega-barns. That does not alter the fact, however, that too much protein from any animal can accelerate aging. Meat is meat and contains animal protein, regardless whether it comes from a mega-barn cow or a grass-fed cow. It makes no difference whether it is red meat, white meat, eggs, or fish; it is still animal protein. Numerous studies point to a clear relationship between animal proteins (not only red meat) and a greater risk of all kinds of aging-related diseases.[26–29] One large study investigated more 6,000 people over an average period of eighteen years. The results show that people who ate a lot of animal protein had a four times higher risk of getting cancer, a five times higher risk of developing diabetes, and an almost twice as high a risk of dying, compared to people who ate few proteins.[20] In people over age 65, more protein appeared not to increase their risk of cancer, but their risk of developing diabetes remained high. So, it is not surprising that many researchers warn against high-protein diets, including the paleo diet.[28] (However, the paleo diet also has some good points, like shunning grains and milk, to which we will come back later.)

Some readers may point out that these studies show only associations and that an association is not necessarily a cause. For example, there is an association between the annual sale of ice cream and the number of people who are attacked by sharks. That does not mean that ice cream *causes* shark attacks.

There just happens to be an association because in the summer people flock to beaches and buy ice cream and when they take a dip in the sea, they may be attacked by sharks.

Still, an excess of proteins proves not to be merely an association but an actual cause of aging. That follows not only from our insights into the aging process (e.g., agglomeration of proteins) and from numerous animal experiments but also from experiments with humans. For example, when you increase the amino acid concentration in the blood (via protein-rich food or an infusion of amino acid), insulin sensitivity decreases immediately—the link could not be more causal.[30, 31] The less insulin sensitive your body is, the unhealthier you are, because your body is less able to process carbohydrates (sugars). When we age, insulin sensitivity decreases, which explains why many people after middle age develop an expanded waistline and are increasingly at risk of developing type 2 diabetes and all kinds of other aging-related diseases, like Alzheimer's or atherosclerosis (the clogging up of the arteries).

Too much animal protein can accelerate aging. But it turns out that this is not true for vegetable protein (from nuts, legumes, tofu, or mushrooms). Vegetable protein does not increase the risk of aging-related diseases. Why is that? Is a protein not always a protein, regardless of whether it comes from plants or animals? No, not really. Vegetable proteins generally have a different composition than animal proteins. They contain less sulfuric amino acids and less growth-stimulating methionine, and they do not stimulate aging pathways like mTOR or the release of age-accelerating growth hormones such as IGF, as much as animal proteins do.[32] Therefore, it is also not surprising that vegetarians often live longer. According to some studies, vegetarians live four to seven years longer than do people who eat meat and suffer from aging-related diseases less frequently.[33, 34] Eating less meat plays an important role in this.

Physicians have noticed for a long time that very old people often do not eat much meat. Furthermore, scientists have mapped various areas where people live longer (the so-called blue zones), which do not include any areas where people grow very old by eating lots of meat. There are zones in Italy that are home to many centenarians and where little meat was consumed, if only because before and after World War II meat was usually too expensive to buy in those regions.[35] In such areas you will find such people as Salvatore Caruso who, at 108 years of age, is the second-oldest Italian. He followed a plant-based diet all his life, just like most people in the small Italian village where he lives, which is one of the villages with the most centenarians per capita in the world.

Another, even more famous Italian who ate differently and became very old is Luigi Cornaro. He was a nobleman from Venice who lived in the sixteenth century. Cornaro was one of the first authors who wrote about nutrition, healthy aging, and a longer life. He became famous through his book *Discorsi della Vita Sobria* (Discourses on the sober life). In this book he describes how for many years, as a young nobleman, he had enjoyed rich banquets, with roast meat, sausages, pigs' heads on platters, and other delicacies. As a result, at around age 35, he began to suffer from all kinds of diseases and distress. Cornaro decided to switch to a completely different lifestyle. He began eating much less meat, eggs and other animal protein and also less starches and sugars. He died in 1566 at the age of 98 (although some sources claim he was only 85). His new lifestyle was drastically different from the banquets where an abundance of food—and meat in particular—was a sign of wealth (he still ate meat, eggs, bread, and other foods, but much less than before; in fact, far less than the average daily requirement for an adult, making his eating habits resemble caloric restriction—more on that later). Luigi Cornaro is sometimes called the Leonardo da Vinci of gerontology, because he was the first to provide clear guidelines for living as healthy as possible for as long as possible, and because he considered old age the best period of life, provided that one lives a healthy lifestyle.

Now that we better understand the role of proteins in aging, we may wonder why it is that animal-protein-rich diets are still so often highly recommended for losing weight (this includes whey protein, which is made from milk proteins). In supermarkets and drugstores you can find racks full of protein-rich foods for losing weight. There are several reasons for this. First and foremost, it is because people do indeed lose weight, sometimes a spectacular amount, by eating a lot of protein and few carbohydrates. Not only that, but the fats in their blood also decrease, their sugar levels improve, and they feel fitter and healthier, making them think that they are engaging in healthy living. However, these are all short-term effects. If we look at the long term, a diet rich in animal protein is not healthy—it accelerates aging and increases the risk of heart attack, type 2 diabetes, cancer, macular degeneration, and so forth.

We must therefore be critical of studies that show that eating more animal protein is healthy. Usually these studies last only a few weeks or months, or at most a few years. But what if you eat like that for many years or decades?

It also appears that the weight loss may only be temporary. Studies show that six years after following a high-protein diet 90 percent (!) of the trial subjects weigh just as much after the protein diet as before. In addition, an excess of proteins can overload the liver and kidneys, which have the task of breaking down all these proteins. The risk of autoimmune diseases may also increase because the gut immune system may recognize the poorly digested proteins as foreign substances and may become overactive, so that it starts attacking your own body.[36]

Another important reason high-protein diets are still so popular is that they are a money-making scheme. The extra proteins are sold in prepared protein drinks, protein bars, protein powders, and so on. In one specific protein diet, people must spend $600 or more on protein foods every month if they want to be faithful to their diet.

A final reason for the popularity of high-protein diets is that they are often actively promoted by the proponents of the paleo diet. This diet is based on prehistoric dietary patterns. It is assumed that prehistoric humans ate a lot of protein-rich food, such as meat. Followers of the paleo diet believe that it is the healthiest diet ever and that the body is made to eat that kind of food since our forefathers have eaten like that for hundreds of thousands of years. They claim that our body is best adapted to that type of food.

There are two important reservations that can be made about this. In the first place, we cannot be sure that prehistoric man ate a lot of meat. Some researchers believe that prehistoric humans ate mainly vegetables, fruit, seeds, nuts, insects, roots, mushrooms, alternated with wild meat or fish, and thus not mainly meat. Second, even if in prehistoric times people ate a lot of meat that does not automatically mean that it is healthy. Nature and humans have two different agendas. We want to live and stay healthy as long as possible but that is not what nature wants. Nature wants you to reproduce, preferably before you perish from external causes such as a predator, human enemy, or accident. It is possible, therefore, that a diet rich in meat enabled prehistoric humans to reproduce as much as possible. After all, all those animal proteins gave them a big, strong, muscular body and increased their production of growth hormones and sex hormones, such as testosterone, all of which improved their libido, strength, and stamina, so that they could impress the opposite sex, fight jealous rivals, and from time to time bring home a hunting trophy. However, all those animal proteins, male hormones, and growth factors may in the long term accelerate aging. Nature did not care that you might get a heart attack at age 65 because, in most cases, long before then you would be eaten, killed in an accident, murdered, or succumbed to an infectious disease. In short, the argument that a paleo diet is always the best diet because people have eaten this way for hundreds of thousands of years does not hold water, because nature and humans have different long-term goals.

Is the paleo diet unhealthy? Yes and no. The paleo diet does have some good points. After all it also promotes eating vegetables, fruit, mushrooms, and nuts, which are all healthy foods. Milk and grain products, such as bread, rice, and pasta, are discouraged, because these are all recent inventions resulting from the development of agriculture, some 10,000 years ago. If you eat fewer grain products and more vegetables, nuts, seeds, fruit, and fish, you will indeed start feeling healthier and often lose weight as well. Meat is still eaten, but processed red meat from grain-fed mega-barn animals is replaced by unprocessed meat from grass-fed or wild animals, which is somewhat healthier. In other words, a moderate paleo diet, which does not contain too many animal proteins, can indeed be healthy, but a paleo diet is not healthy if it contains large amounts of animal protein. Some proponents of paleo or prehistoric diets and followers of high-protein diets, eat a breakfast of four eggs and bacon, a lunch of salmon and vegetables, and a dinner consisting of a large chunk of beef with broccoli. That kind of paleo diet is not healthy because it contains too much animal protein and therefore accelerates aging.

So, should you eat fewer animal proteins? There are two things you can do. First, you can try to replace red and processed meat (bacon, hot dogs, hamburgers, sausages) more often with healthier animal sources of protein, such as white meat (chicken or turkey) and fatty fish. This will already decrease your risk of dying but you can do better. Even chicken and fish contain animal protein. Second, you could replace animal sources of protein (meat, fish, cheese, and eggs) more often with vegetable sources of protein (nuts, seeds, tofu, legumes, and protein-rich vegetables such as broccoli). You can even become a vegetarian and eat exclusively vegetable proteins. It is important that overall you take in enough proteins (animal or vegetable), because if you do not eat enough protein, you may start to feel weak or tired, or develop aching muscles. You should also take extra vitamin B_{12}, which is paramount (more on B vitamins later on).

This chapter is not meant to convert the reader to vegetarianism. First, it warns against eating too much red meat, and particularly processed meat, such as bacon, hamburgers, and sausages. For many ages, meat has been the symbol of wealth and prosperity, and it still has a prominent place on our plates. But less is more. For example, you could eat meat every other day or only twice a week. If you do eat red meat, have a smaller portion; for example, a piece the size of a deck of cards.

High-protein diets are also not recommended because they are not healthy. In the short term they may improve some health parameters, but in the long term they accelerate aging. Therefore, do not buy protein powders, bars, or drinks to lose weight and do not eat large amounts of meat, fish, and eggs just because proponents of high-protein diets or fitness fanatics say so. Maybe you will lose some weight in the beginning or become more muscular, but in the long term these diets accelerate aging. For older people, eating enough protein is important. Some researchers suggest that sufficient protein intake can decrease the risk of *sarcopenia*, weakening of the muscles. However, not enough studies have been done to conclude that a higher protein intake in the elderly reduces mortality.[37]

The food industry, of course, would like nothing better than to increase protein intake in older people, and in all people, for that matter, because it would like to sell that mountain of meat (285 million tons worldwide per year) and that ocean of milk (150 billion gallons per year) they produce. This is unsustainable. There will come a time when people will simply start eating less meat, not only for their own sake but for the sake of the environment as well. For every 2 pounds of beef that ends up on your plate, about 4,000 gallons of water are required to produce it, both to feed the animals and to grow the grain to feed them. By comparison, 2 pounds of tomatoes require only about 53 gallons of water. By eating once 1 pound less of meat, you save more water than by not showering for three months. All the livestock on earth together use one third of all available drinking water. In reality we do not live on a planet but on a gigantic farm; 40 percent of the total ice-free land surface is used to feed humanity, and 30 percent of this land is used to produce meat. For every American, an average of 270 pounds of meat is produced annually. For every resident of Bangladesh, it is only 4 pounds per year. If everyone would eat as much meat as is the norm in the West, we would need to produce so much meat that our earth could not support it, and the meat industry knows that. Eating less meat is healthier not only for yourself but also for our planet, and then we have not even mentioned the well-being of the animals that have to grow up in overcrowded mega-barns, only to be slaughtered in the end.

SUMMARY

Eating a lot of **animal protein** accelerates **aging** and increases the risk of cancer and aging-related diseases, including type 2 diabetes, heart disease, and macular degeneration.

Protein-rich diets cause

- In the **short term**, weight loss, and sometimes improved physical parameters, including lower blood pressure and better sugar levels

- In the **long term**, accelerated aging.

In order, the unhealthiest to the healthiest sources of protein:

- **Processed red meat** (cow, pig, and sheep): salami, bacon, ham, sausage, hot dogs, etc.

- **Red meat** from grain-fed mega barn animals

- **Red meat** from free-range, grass-fed animals

- **White meat** (chicken and turkey), preferably free-range and grass-fed

- **Fish**, particularly fatty fish that contain high levels of omega-3 fatty acids, such as salmon, herring, anchovies, and sardines

- **Vegetable proteins**, including nuts, legumes (peas, beans, and lentils), vegetables (broccoli, spinach, cabbage, brussels sprouts), tofu, mushrooms, and fungi-based meat substitutes

Replace **red meat** with **white meat (poultry)**, **fish**, **tofu**, or **fungi-based meat substitutes** more often.

Replace **animal protein** with **plant-based sources of protein** more often.

Carbohydrates

Like proteins, carbohydrates also play a role in the aging process. Carbohydrates have been both a blessing and a curse for our civilization and our health. Actually, the West currently follows a high-carbohydrate diet, and this contributes substantially to the massive epidemic of type 2 diabetes, obesity, and aging-related diseases. Let me first give you a short explanation of what carbohydrates are, because there is great confusion about that. This confusion also means we often eat much more carbohydrates than we think.

Carbohydrates are also called sugars. There are many different types of carbohydrates. There are *short (or simple)* carbohydrates, such as glucose, fructose, and sucrose (the white sugar we put in our tea), which form short chains, and there are *long (or complex)* carbohydrates, such as starch, which consists of long chains of glucose. Potatoes, bread, rice, and pasta are composed of starch; thus these products consist mainly of sugars, long chains of glucose that form starch. Many people are surprised to learn that their potatoes or their bread is made of sugars. We will come back to this important point later.

Actually this is pretty much all you need to know to understand the following discussion about carbohydrates and sugars. If you would like to know more, or see images of carbohydrates, you will find them in the sources listed in "Additional Reading" at the end of the book.

One more thing you do need to know is how the body digests and absorbs sugars. The gut can absorb only short sugars, such as glucose and fructose. Long sugar chains consisting of two or more sugars such as starch (which consists of thousands of glucose units) cannot be absorbed by the gut. That is why the gut cells produce enzymes (proteins), which they release into the gut. These digestive enzymes break down the longer sugar chains so that only separate pieces of glucose and fructose remain. These can then be absorbed by the gut so that these sugars can end up in the bloodstream. When your doctor measures your blood sugar, that means the glucose units in your blood.

This explains why there are *fast* carbohydrates and *slow* carbohydrates. The fast carbohydrates are short carbohydrates, such as glucose, which can enter the bloodstream quickly. A tablet of pure glucose consists of such loose glucose units. That is why glucose is an immediate pick-me-up for people with a low blood sugar level. The slow carbohydrates, such as starch, are composed of long glucose chains. It takes time to break those chains down until only the glucose remains, which can then be absorbed by the cells in the intestines. That is why long carbohydrates do not cause high sugar peaks in the blood as quickly as do the short carbohydrates. However, they often do still cause considerably high sugar peaks and long-term elevated blood sugar levels, which is not healthy.

There is one more type of carbohydrate we have not discussed yet: fiber. Fibers are long carbohydrate chains (composed of glucose or fructose) that cannot be broken down by the gut. Our body does not contain the digestive proteins (enzymes) necessary to break down these chains, and as a result we cannot absorb these fibers. They do not enter the gut cells and then the bloodstream. Some animals, such as horses and cows, do have the proteins to break down these fibers, so they can eat grass. Grass is full of tough sugar chains (fibers) that cannot be digested by humans. That is a pity because it would be practical if mowing your lawn would also provide your dinner. However, fibers are important for our health. They cannot feed us but they can feed the bacteria that dwell in our gut. These bacteria especially love water-soluble fibers, such as those in vegetables, fruit, and mushrooms. The more of these good fibers, the more happy bacteria, which produce all kinds of healthy substances, including vitamin K and short-chain fatty acids, and send them into the bloodstream.

SUMMARY

Carbohydrates are also called **sugars**.

Short, **fast**, or **simple**, carbohydrates are glucose, fructose, or sucrose. These are **quickly** absorbed by the gut cells and released into the bloodstream, where they cause **very high** sugar peaks.

Long, **slow**, or **complex**, carbohydrates are starch. Starch consists of thousands of glucose units that are linked together. Despite the term *slow*, these often still can cause **high** and **broad** sugar peaks: prolonged, elevated blood sugar levels.

Fibers are indigestible long carbohydrates. They are not absorbed and released into the bloodstream but serve as food for our good intestinal bacteria.

THE ROLE OF CARBOHYDRATES IN AGING

The impact of sugars in the body plays an important role in the aging process. In the first place, the intake of carbohydrates, and particularly of fast sugars, triggers the production of all kinds of hormones that accelerate aging.

This happens as follows. Imagine that you eat a piece of cake. The sugars in the cake, such as glucose, are absorbed by the gut cells and released into the bloodstream. These sugars are now circulating in the blood, but they cannot continue to circulate indefinitely and must eventually be absorbed by our cells, where they will provide energy. For the sugars to move out of the bloodstream and into the cells, they need an important hormone: insulin. Insulin is a small protein produced by the pancreas. When the pancreas becomes aware that the level of sugar in the blood rises, it releases insulin into the bloodstream. The insulin then moves through the entire body and encourages cells to open up their doors to allow the insulin to enter. It is particularly the cells that specialize in storing and processing sugar, such as the liver cells, fat cells, and muscle cells, that will allow the sugars in.

In addition to insulin, another important hormone will be released after a carbohydrate-rich meal. That hormone is insulin-like growth factor, or IGF, a very small protein that resembles insulin, hence its name. IGF affixes itself to cells via proteins designed specifically for that purpose, which protrude from the surface of the cell and are called IGF receptors. The IGF then orders the cells to grow or to speed up their activity. It is logical that IGF is released after a sugar-rich meal. A lot of sugar is then circulating in the bloodstream and provides enough energy for the cells to grow and rev up their activity. IGF spreads the message to the cells to work as hard as they can. However, the harder something works and grows, the faster it ages.

The sequence is as follows:

Glucose (from the cake) causes a glucose peak in the blood, which causes the release of **insulin** and **IGF**:

- **Insulin** ensures that cells can absorb glucose and boosts the activity of the cells.

- **IGF** urges the cells to grow and stimulates the activity of the cells.

Insulin and IGF together increase the metabolism of the cells but that also causes them to age faster. For example, the cells start to produce more proteins, and these proteins then clump together and ultimately cause aging-related diseases. The cells also fail to clean up, so that less debris is burned up in the incinerators of the cells. Why would they bother, if lots of energy and building blocks are available anyway? Fewer substances are produced that protect and maintain the cells. Growth and production are the only things that count. With a lot of insulin and IGF in the vicinity, the cells become intense production factories that want to produce more and more and faster and faster, and invest less in the maintenance of the factory and the machinery. This causes the factory to deteriorate more rapidly.

It is interesting to mention that in addition to sugar, amino acids also stimulate the production of IGF. What you eat, therefore, has a direct effect on the amount of hormonelike substances in your blood, such as insulin and IGF, that accelerate aging.

There is one other important growth-hormone-like substance we have not talked about yet, and that is the growth hormone (GH). We call insulin and IGF growth-hormone-like substances, but there is also the actual growth hormone, which induces production of IGF.

Scientists have succeeded in extending the life span of all kinds of organisms. How do they do that? By decreasing the amount of insulin, IGF, and growth hormone or by making the body less sensitive to these substances. Mice that produce less growth hormone and less IGF live up to 100 percent longer than regular mice.[38, 39] Not only do they live much longer but they are also less likely to suffer from cancer and all kinds of aging-related diseases, including cardiovascular disease, cataracts, arthritis, and diabetes. Scientists have succeeded in creating the oldest living mouse ever by allowing it to produce much less IGF. That mouse lived for almost five years, whereas regular mice usually live for only two years. Translated into human years, that is almost 180 years. Such mice live much longer, but they are smaller than their regular fellow mice because they were exposed less to growth-hormone-like stimuli.

Apparently, you do not have to be large, strong, and muscular to grow very old. This is seen in slim, 100-year-old Japanese ladies in Okinawa who consume a mainly plant-based diet and also in bodybuilders, who gobble up whey protein shakes and carb-rich foods and inject themselves with growth-hormone-like substances and have a heart attack at age 40. This does not mean that bodybuilders are doomed to die early or that slim women can grow very old. These two extremes merely give a hint that extra growth-hormone-like substances (and an abundance of fast sugars and amino acids) can accelerate aging.

The less IGF and growth hormone, the less you grow. It is not a coincidence, therefore, that smaller animals live longer than larger animals of the same species. Great Danes, for example, have an average life span of six to eight years, whereas Chihuahuas can live to be twenty years old. The smaller animals were exposed less to growth hormone and IGF when they were young, allowing them to grow less and be smaller, but reach longer life spans. However, this principle applies to members of the same species. If we look across different species, then the opposite is true. Elephants, which are much larger than dogs, can grow much older than dogs but, on average, a small elephant will grow older than a large elephant.

What about humans? Many studies show that small people on average live longer. A study with more than 600 people found that people who were taller than five foot three (1.61 meters) lived two years less on average than did those who were shorter.[40] The taller the people, the more pronounced these differences were. Another study of 8,000 people showed that people who are smaller than five foot two (1.58 meters) had a greater chance of becoming 95 years old. In addition, the smaller people also had less insulin in their bloodstream, which decreased their risk of cancer (insulin and IGF promote growth, which in turn encourages the growth of cancer cells).[41] A study to investigate the relationship between body size and cancer, performed with 1.2 million people, found that for every four inches (ten centimeters) a person is taller than five eleven (1.52 meters), the risk of cancer increases by 16 percent.[42] Should tall people worry about their size? Not necessarily. In the first place, these studies compared many thousands of people—only then does a relationship show up. For individual people it is virtually impossible to make predictions about their life span based only on their height, since so many other factors also play a role in how long they will live.

On average, however, smaller people live longer or have less risk of cancer and aging-related diseases. An extreme example of this is people who have a form of dwarfism called Laron syndrome. People with Laron syndrome are very small because they produce less IGF. The syndrome is seen, in particular, in certain remote villages in Ecuador. These villages are a known destination for medical researchers involved in the study of aging. Laron dwarfs live longer than average (taking into account their height) and in addition they are almost immune to aging-related diseases, such as cancer and diabetes.

Of the 100 Laron dwarfs who were followed for many years, none developed diabetes and there was only one case of a nonterminal cancer, whereas among family members with no Laron syndrome, 17 percent developed cancer and 5 percent, diabetes. Laron syndrome can provide interesting insights to combat cancer and diabetes. Researchers have discovered that dwarfs produce less IGF and also less insulin, which better protects their cells against damage and aging. For example, when their cells were placed in a petri dish and exposed to toxic materials, such as hydrogen peroxide, their DNA suffered less damage.[43] Laron dwarfs have already provided important insights to researchers about the aging process, which can be used to develop medications to combat aging-related diseases. Among other things, researchers want to give people substances that slow down the production of growth hormone and IGF, to see whether their risk of aging-related diseases then diminishes.

The opposite also exists: gigantism. Is it the case that, just as dwarfs stay small and live longer, giants grow tall and live shorter? Certain people have a condition called acromegaly that makes them grow too tall. Most often this excessive growth is caused by a tumor in the pituitary gland, located at the bottom of the brain, where growth hormone is produced. The tumor produces too much growth hormone and the body then also produces too much IGF. This disease can occur at any age, even in adulthood, when one is already fully grown. Acromegaly makes even adults continue to grow. The first signs of the disease may include having problems fitting into one's shoes, or a wedding ring that no longer fits. Speech changes as a result of a larger tongue. The forehead and chin become longer and more pronounced.

That is not all. Now that we know that excessive growth is also related to accelerated aging, it should not surprise us that people with acromegaly have a much greater risk of early death. They have at least three times as much risk of a heart attack, and have a higher risk of developing high blood pressure, diabetes, cancer, kidney problems, arthritis, and autoimmune diseases. Most of the many acromegaly patients who have appeared in the *Guinness World Records* books in the past several decades because of their large stature, died at a young age due to complications of their conditions. Leonid Stadnyk, who is said to have been eight foot three (2.52 meters), died at the age of 44 of a stroke. Robert Wadlow, the tallest man ever, was eight foot eleven (2.72 meters) and weighed 438 pounds. He died at the age of 22 from an infection in his ankle, further complicated by an autoimmune disease. Scientists are now investigating whether a medication that is prescribed for acromegaly can also help prevent aging-related diseases, including diabetes and cardiovascular disease.

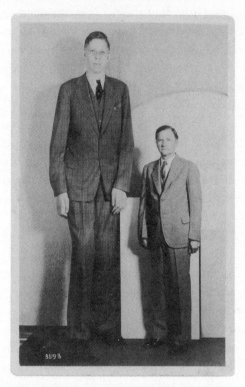

Robert Wadlow, the tallest man ever, was eight foot eleven (2.72 meters) and weighed 438 pounds. In this picture he is standing next to his father.

Too much growth is not healthy. Small animals, people, and dwarfs live longer; large animals, people, and giants on average live shorter. It is ironic, therefore, that growth hormone is recommended on numerous Internet sites and in all kinds of magazines as a miracle drug to slow down aging, whereas in reality it accelerates aging. Worn-out stockbrokers over age 50 or performance-oriented managers are prescribed growth hormone (and testosterone, which in too high doses also accelerates aging, as we have seen in the chapter about sex and lifespan). Often they do indeed feel better, not only from the placebo effect but also because they grow more muscle mass, while their fat mass shrinks. Some will even develop more stamina, but these are all short-term effects. In the long term an excess of growth hormone accelerates aging. There is a reason that the medical leaflets for growth hormone warn its use increases the risk of cancer and type 2 diabetes. Compare this to a Ferrari engine that is built into a small compact car. At first the car will go faster, but it will also wear down much faster.

Of course, people who have a real shortage of growth hormone (for example, because their pituitary gland has been damaged in a car accident or a fall from a horse) do benefit from taking growth hormone, to return the levels of the hormone to what is normal for their age.

Carbohydrates increase the production of insulin and IGF, growth-hormone-like substances that turn on all kinds of aging switches in our cells. But sugars can also *directly* play a role in aging. They do this by forming sugar cross-links. Cross-links are connections. Sugars can form connections between the proteins that build up our bodies. These sugar cross-links make the proteins stick together, much as sugary jam makes your fingers stick together.

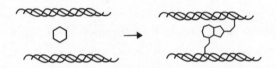

Sugar (glucose) forms a connection (cross-link) between two proteins. The cross-link makes the proteins stick together, so that the tissues that are made up of these proteins become less flexible, which causes wrinkles, cataracts, or high blood pressure. (Source: Johan Svantesson.)

When, for example, the collagen proteins that form our skin are glued together by cross-links, the skin becomes stiffer and less elastic and wrinkles appear. Compare this with toast. When you make toast in the morning, the heat in the toaster causes sugar cross-links to form between the proteins in the bread—this is what makes the toast crisp. Something similar happens in our skin. In that case is does not last four minutes, as in the toaster, but some 40 years before our skin also becomes crisp and wrinkly. This is also what causes fried or roasted meat to brown: Cross-links are formed between the proteins on the surface of the meat. Cross-links are found everywhere in nature. Bark on trees is so hard due to the many cross-links in the bark. In short, if you are ever asked what the relationship is between toast, wrinkles, and tree bark, you will know that the answer is cross-links.

Sugar cross-links are not only involved in forming wrinkles; they also play a role in all kinds of aging-related diseases. One example is cataracts. As we grow older, more and more sugar cross-links form between the transparent proteins that make up the lens of the eye. This makes these proteins stick together, which plays a role in the formation of a cataract, a typical disease of aging. Sugar cross-links between the proteins in the walls of our blood vessels, make the walls stiffer. This contributes to high blood pressure in old age. Particularly in the West, where we ingest a lot of fast sugars via soft drinks, breakfast grains, and white bread, high blood pressure is common. More than 60 percent of people over age 60 have high blood pressure. If we grow old enough, almost everyone will develop high blood pressure to a greater or lesser extent. Stiff blood vessels are also more brittle, making them more prone to breaking, just as a porcelain tube breaks more easily than a rubber tube. When this happens in the brain, it is called a brain hemorrhage or stroke.

Cross-links in the many small vessels in the kidneys that filter the blood, make kidney function deteriorate when we get older. From about age 30 on, kidney function decreases by 10 percent every ten years, and cross-links play a role in this. Cross-links form in the lungs as well, such as between elastin proteins and collagen proteins in the lung tissues, resulting in loss of elasticity. This makes the lungs more susceptible to infection, so that older people have a considerable risk of dying from pneumonia. Cross-links also form in and between the heart muscle cells, making the heart as a whole stiffer and less able to pump blood. This particularly plays a role in diastolic heart failure. This disease occurs when a stiff heart muscle cannot relax well enough to fill up with blood in between two heartbeats, so that each time too little blood is pumped around in the body. The formation of cross-links, or glycation, of cholesterol particles makes these stickier, so that they more easily stick to the blood vessel wall and make the vessel clog up. Cross-linking in the cartilage in our joints causes joint pain and stiffness. Cross-linking in the bladder makes it stiffer, less able to expand, so that older people's ability to retain urine in the bladder declines and they may have to get up several times during the night to urinate.

Cross-links and protein agglomeration are two reasons we age. However much a nuisance they may be individually, together they are even worse. These two mechanisms work together to accelerate aging. When proteins are cross-linked or glycated (glycated means that sugars attached themselves to the protein), they cannot easily be broken down by the cell and will more readily clump together in the cell. The proteins that form clumps and remain in the cell too long, run the risk of becoming cross-linked and glycated even more, which in turn makes the proteins clump together ever faster. Take, for example, the stiff blood vessels: They become stiffer not only because of cross-links, but also from protein agglomeration in the blood vessel wall.

Now we have an idea of the role of sugars, insulin, and IGF in the aging process. Let's see how we can use these insights with respect to nutrition.

CARBOHYDRATES, NUTRITION, AND AGING

Since an excess of sugars accelerates aging, it would be advisable to reduce our sugar intake. Reducing the amount of sugar we eat reduces the number of cross-links, so that our risk of wrinkles, cataracts, and heart disease declines. Eating less sugar also reduces the production of insulin and other growth-hormone-like substances that make our cells age faster.

Of course, when we think of reducing sugar-rich foods and drinks, we immediately think of the classics: soft drinks; candy; and baked goods, such as cakes, cookies, and pastries. These are indeed the products we all know to be unhealthy. A study with more than 2,500 people found that those who drank soft drinks daily had a 43 percent higher risk of a heart attack.[44] In another study with more than 40,000 participants, people who ate many sugar-rich products had a 275 percent higher risk of a heart attack.[45] These and many other studies prompted the mayor of New York to ban large soft drink cups and resulted in a guideline by the World Health Organization to get no more than 5 percent of daily calories from sugar. For an adult, this boils down to a maximum of six teaspoons of sugar (glucose, fructose, or sucrose) per day. One can of soft drink already contains about ten teaspoons.

These recommendations concern short-chain sugars (also called simple or fast sugars), including glucose, fructose, and sucrose, which are added to such products as soft drinks, cakes, cookies, and other baked goods. These sugars are also found in products that we would not immediately suspect contain it. Tomato ketchup, for example, contains 25 percent sugar. Some seemingly healthy products often contain a lot of sugar, such as salad dressings (particularly the so-called healthy, low-fat varieties), sauces (such as barbecue or pasta sauce), yogurts (which can contain lots of sugar), breakfast cereals, and store-bought fruit juices, which are all considered healthy. It would be better for your health to replace these products with low-sugar varieties, but it is particularly important to reduce the most serious culprits, such as soft drinks, baked goods, and candy (tasty alternatives will be presented later in the book). You can also directly replace sugars like sucrose (table sugar) with *natural sweeteners* like stevia or sugar-alcohols like erythritol, which do not cause sugar peaks in the blood. However, do not use even these natural sweeteners too much, because they will maintain your sweet tooth and make you crave and eat too many real sweets. Also, if you use stevia, be aware to use 100 percent stevia (like stevia droplets) and not stevia powder or "cubes" that often contain only 2 percent stevia and still 98 percent "dextrose" (which is just another name for glucose). Stay away from so-called healthy sugar substitutes, like coconut sugar, molasses, (organic) honey, and maple syrup; they are for the most part made of sucrose, glucose, or fructose.

But is it enough to simply consume fewer soft drinks, baked goods, and candy to reverse this epidemic of obesity and type 2 diabetes, let alone slow down the aging process? For most people this will not be enough. Sugars can assume all kinds of disguises. The sweet products mentioned here contain short-chain sugars ("simple sugars"), such as glucose, fructose, and sucrose, but we also need to cut down on products that contain long-chain sugars, such as starch. Starch is also sugar, even though we might not think so at first sight. Potatoes, bread, rice, and pasta are made of starch, which are long chains of glucose. Therefore these foods can also cause high sugar peaks. Boiled potatoes cause even higher sugar peaks in the blood than can regular white table sugar.[46] It is those sugar peaks that are not healthy: They cause the formation of sugar cross-links and increase the production of insulin and other aging hormones. That is why scientists at Harvard University—one of the most renowned universities in the world—have placed potatoes in the "use sparingly" section at the top of their Healthy Eating Pyramid, together with sweets and soft drinks. It gives food for thought that these Harvard scientists put potatoes in the same category as sweets and soft drinks. Or, to quote the professor Fredrik Nyström:

> If you eat potatoes you might as well eat candy. Potatoes contain glucose units in a chain, which is converted to sugar in the GI [gastrointestinal] tract. Such a diet causes blood sugar, and then the hormone insulin, to skyrocket.

Potatoes (boiled, mashed, french fries, or patties) cause high sugar peaks, similarly to other starchy products, such as white bread, white rice, and pasta made of white flour. Therefore, we should eat fewer of these products. It is often recommended to replace these items with their whole grain variants, such as whole grain bread, whole grain pasta, or brown rice. These are thought to be healthier because they cause lower sugar peaks. They also have more fiber, and fiber packages the sugar so that it is released into the bloodstream more slowly. However, even these whole grain products consist mainly of glucose in the form of starch, which all need to be processed by the body (these products have a high glycemic load: They supply a large load of sugars). A well-known example is whole grain pasta, which indeed causes lower sugar peaks than white pasta, but it does cause long-lasting elevated blood sugar levels and an overworked pancreas, which must produce a lot of insulin to process all that glucose. That is why so many people who eat a lot of "super healthy" whole grain foods cannot lose weight, because they are still consuming too many starchy carbohydrates.

Isn't that strange? Have we not always been told that whole grains are healthy? One study with more than 100,000 participants found that people who ate a lot of whole grains had a 9 percent lower risk of a heart attack.[47] Such studies are often extensively quoted in the media, and this plays nicely into the hands of the agricultural and food industries, which of course make a lot of money with the production and sale of whole grain products.

What we should not forget is that it can always be *more* healthy. Indeed, whole grain foods will always be healthy if you compare them with something *less* healthy. In many studies, people who eat whole grain products are compared with people who eat white bread, white rice, or white pasta. It is logical that whole grain foods come out looking better. However, this diet can be even better—a point that many health experts seem to be missing. If you would do a study to compare eating whole grain foods with eating vegetables, nuts, legumes, and mushrooms, you would find that the latter diet is considerably better. For example, a meta-analysis study found that a diet *without* starchy foods like bread, potatoes, pasta, and rice, could better treat metabolic syndrome (high blood pressure, elevated fats in the blood, increased waist circumference, elevated sugar levels) than the *official guidelines* of various countries (however, the diet still allowed too much intake of animal protein).[48] Furthermore, people who eat more whole grain foods may be healthier because they also eat more fruit and vegetables, smoke less, and exercise more. According to some scientists, whole grain products are more of a yardstick of whether you have a healthy lifestyle, than being a real important cause of good health.

In clinical practice you can see clearly that people can drastically improve their health by eating a diet with less starchy foods, including whole grain varieties. You cannot reverse type 2 diabetes by continuing a diet with lots of potatoes and whole grain bread (as is recommended in many official guidelines), but you can reverse it even within several weeks by refraining from eating bread, potatoes, pasta, and rice.[49] Many physicians and organizations in various countries reverse type 2 diabetes in patients by going further than the official guidelines and reducing the amount of starchy foods.[50] In the past people often said, "Once diabetes, always diabetes." In other words, once you are diabetic, things can only go downhill. First you get pills, and as the years go by, you have to take more and more pills, and ultimately you have to take insulin by injection. However, many diabetes patients have been able to stop their medications (pills, and insulin injections) by eating much less starch: Their blood sugar levels stabilize, not by medication but by healthy eating. (Warning: Diabetes patients who wish to decrease their medications by changing their diet should only do so under a doctor's supervision.) It is not a coincidence that many scientists recommend eating fewer carbohydrates as the most important first step in the treatment of diabetes patients.[51] With good reason they urge official institutions (diabetes federations) to finally adopt these new insights (we will discuss later why this is taking so long).

Weight loss is another example. People who want to lose weight often stop eating sugar-rich foods, such as soft drinks, baked goods, and candy. They also replace their white bread with whole grain bread. They even exercise regularly, but despite all these good intentions they lose very little weight. On the contrary, as the years go by, the pounds keep piling up, despite their much healthier lifestyle. To quote physician and researcher Peter Attia, who tried to lose weight by first adhering to the classical advice:

> Despite exercising 3 or 4 hours every single day and following the food pyramid to the letter, I gained a lot of weight and developed something called metabolic syndrome [which is characterized by hypertension, elevated fats and sugars in the blood, and increased abdominal fat]. I had become insulin resistant.

How is that possible? If people still eat a large amount of whole grain foods, they still get a large load of sugars (glucose, given that starch is entirely made up of glucose chains), which makes them fat and increases their risk of aging-related diseases. However, if these same people begin to eat fewer of these whole grain foods, they can lose a lot of weight. This change can sometimes be quite dramatic. I remember a professor, about 50 years old, who had tried all kinds of diets (more whole grains, a low-fat diet, etc.), but he could not lose weight until the day he decided to eliminate almost all starchy foods, such as potatoes, bread, and pasta. His weight loss was spectacular, so much even that he began to worry that he might have cancer. He has now been eating like this for many years and he feels great. This story illustrates what can happen if you also reduce your intake of starchy foods. In short, many people won't lose weight if they only cut out the sugary foods like soda and candy bars, but still eat five whole grain servings at breakfast, the same for lunch, and a plate of whole grain pasta for dinner. These starchy foods deliver too much glucose, hampering weight loss, reprogramming the body to pile on fat (as we will see later), and making you ask "Why do I hardly lose weight despite following my diet to the letter?"

Does this mean that whole grains are unhealthy? This question cannot be answered with a straight yes or no, as some nutrition gurus do (by saying yes) and some nutrition scientists do (by saying no). The answer is more complex than that. When you replace white bread with whole wheat bread, the latter is healthier (as some studies show), but it can be even healthier by replacing the whole grain bread with sourdough rye bread (the sourdough causes lower sugar peaks and rye is healthier than wheat). And it can be even healthier by replacing the sourdough rye bread with oatmeal (because of the water-soluble beta-glucan fibers and other good substances in oatmeal). You could make it even healthier by alternating the oatmeal with nuts, vegetables, or fruit (the sugar in fruit is packaged in fibers, so that it is released into the bloodstream more slowly, and in addition it contains thousands of substances that are good for the body, as we will discuss later).

In any case, in the West we eat too many starchy products, whether whole grain or not. Bread, rice, pasta, or potatoes three times per day requires the body to process large quantities of sugar on a continuous basis. The older you get, the less the body is able to do that, and that is certainly true if you already have diabetes or metabolic syndrome, which puts you at greater risk of cardiovascular disease or dementia. It is not surprising, therefore, that many studies show that a too high intake of carbohydrates is not healthy. A diet with a high glycemic index (food that causes high sugar peaks) and a high glycemic load (food that supplies many carbohydrates) increases the risk of all kinds of aging-related diseases. A study that followed 75,000 women over ten years, found that women who ate a lot of food with a high glycemic load, had a 98 percent higher risk of a heart attack.[52] Another study that followed 15,000 women over nine years, shows that women who often ate foods with a high glycemic load, had a 78 percent higher risk of a heart attack.[53] In a study of 44,000 Italians, researchers found that those participants who followed a diet with a high glycemic index had a twice higher risk of a stroke.[54] In short, diets that cause high sugar peaks (a high glycemic index or GI) and are high in simple sugars and starches overall (a high glycemic load or GL) are unhealthy, particularly in the long term.

One organ may be better able to process that continuous excess of carbohydrates than another. The brain, in particular, is very sensitive to too many sugars, since it is directly dependent on them. Brain cells operate mainly on sugars (and ketones, as we will discuss shortly); hence they cannot rely on fats for energy. Their dependence on sugars is also their weakness: The brain can quickly become sick from a bombardment of carbohydrates. A study shows that older people who eat a lot of carbohydrates have an almost twice as high risk of mild cognitive impairment, often a precursor of Alzheimer's disease. People with this condition have problems with memory, thinking, and reasoning. This study also shows that people who ate more healthy fats had a 44 percent lower risk of mild cognitive impairment.[55] Too many sugars can literally shrink the brain. People with somewhat higher—but still normal—blood sugar levels (what physicians call "high-normal") have up to 10 percent more shrinkage of certain areas of the brain.[56] The researchers concluded that even in the case of *normal blood sugar* levels and in the absence of diabetes, monitoring blood sugar levels can have an influence on the health of the brain.

A good way to estimate how much glycation (sugar sticking to proteins and other molecules) has taken place in your body is by measuring your HbA1c. HbA1c is a yardstick for the glycation of a specific protein in your blood, called hemoglobin. The higher your HbA1c, the more glycated your body is. If you eat a lot of sugar, your HbA1c will go up. People with a high HbA1c (5.9 to 9.0 percent) have twice as much loss of brain mass as do people with a low HbA1c (between 4.4 and 5.2 percent).[57] Some neurologists call a sugar-rich diet toxic for the brain, and by that they do not only mean soft drinks but also too much bread and potatoes.[58] Other researchers call Alzheimer's disease "type-3 diabetes" because Alzheimer's is like diabetes of the brain.

Of course, the agricultural and food industries do not like to hear about these studies. They minimize the impact of the glycemic index (the level of the sugar peaks) and they like to ignore the findings of studies that measure the glycemic load as well (a more accurate measurement than the glycemic index because it also takes the amount of carbohydrates into account). They emphasize the importance of healthy carbohydrates, such as whole grain bread or pasta, and brown rice. Those are supposedly essential for our body and our health. They often argue that without them we would not have enough energy to get through the day. This is just advertising-speak. Let's put carbohydrates and, more specifically grain products, in a broader perspective.

The human species (*Homo sapiens*) is roughly 200,000 years old. About 10,000 years ago, our ancestors switched from a hunter-gatherer to an agricultural subsistence. Thus, it is only for the past 10,000 years that we have practiced agriculture and begun to eat grain products, such as bread. Potatoes (cultivated for the first time about 8,000 years ago) and pasta (invented about 4,000 years ago in China in the form of noodles) were added later. Potatoes were not introduced in the West until the sixteenth century. In short, for more than 190,000 years, the human species did not eat bread, potatoes pasta, or rice. Now, these foods are suddenly essential for our body and our health? We could live without these products for 190,000 years, under much harder and more demanding conditions, but today a chair-bound office worker cannot get through the day without them?

The contrary appears to be true. We see that since the advent of agriculture with its grain products, humans have become *less* healthy. A subsistence based on agriculture made our diet less diverse at the expense of our health.[59] Hunter-gatherers ate a very diverse diet, including vegetables, fruit, nuts, seeds, fish, shellfish, mushrooms, and herbs. Farmers ate mostly grains. Researchers can tell that people's health deteriorated, among other things by comparing the skeletons of hunter-gatherers from tens of thousands of years ago (before the advent of agriculture) with the skeletons of farmers from several thousands of years ago. The skeletons of the farmers were much less healthy: Their body size is smaller and their skeletons and teeth are malformed and weak, which points to a significant lack of vitamins and minerals. It is estimated that hunter-gatherers before the agricultural revolution were on average about five foot eight inches (1.73 meters) tall. Since the advent of agriculture body size shrank by about six inches due to a serious lack of all kinds of healthy nutrients. Even in the eighteenth century a man on average was only five foot four (1.62 meters), and it was not until the mid-twentieth century that people were again as large as before the advent of agriculture.[60] A study that looked at 800 skeletons of primitive farmers and compared them to the skeletons of hunter-gatherers, found that these primitive farmers had a four times greater risk of anemia (which can cause a condition of the bone called porotic hyperostosis), a 50 percent greater risk of malnutrition (which affects the teeth enamel, for example), and three times as many abnormalities in the bones caused by infections (because the immune system is weakened by a lack of nutrients in the diet). The vertebrae were also more damaged, which may be due to the heavy work on the land because, compared to hunting and gathering nuts and berries, farming was a time-consuming and heavy job.[61]

Of course, agriculture also had great advantages. An ever more efficient agriculture made it possible to feed many more people. Thanks to agriculture, farmers could produce a food surplus, which meant that part of the population could do other things. Then, villages and cities could appear, where inventors, scientists, writers, craftsmen, and shopkeepers could feed themselves with the fruits of agriculture, and our civilization advanced with great strides. However, this took place at the expense of our health. We were inundated with an oversupply of starchy products that contained too little variety of healthy nutrients. To quote the late anthropologist George Armelagos: "Humanity paid a heavy biological cost for agriculture, especially when it came to the variety of nutrients. Even now, about 60 percent of our calories comes from corn, rice and wheat." In other words, in view of the past 200,000 years, the argument that lots of whole grain products are essential for good health comes across mainly as a cheap marketing ploy.

Another frequently heard argument is that carbohydrates are necessary to provide enough energy. Without carbohydrates, we are said to be unable to get through the day, become weak and sluggish, hardly able to withstand the busy daily life that demands so much of us. We know, however, that our ancestors in prehistoric times walked an average of ten miles per day to hunt or gather food. They did that without so-called energy sources, such as potatoes, bread, or pasta. Now we are suddenly asked to believe that we would not get through the day without these grain products, even though most of the time we sit behind a desk or in a car? This energy argument is also prominent in advertisements for sugar-rich breakfast cereals addressed to children, claiming that children need a lot of energy and that breakfast cereals are the ideal way to get it.

Finally, there is yet another often heard argument, namely, that starchy foods like potatoes, bread, pasta, and rice are excellent sources of vitamins, minerals, and fibers. "Potatoes contain vitamin C" has become the slogan of potato farmers everywhere. However, these vitamins, minerals, and fibers are also found, and in larger quantities, in foods that are a lot healthier, such as vegetables, fruit, nuts, legumes, and mushrooms. The contrary is true: Bread, potatoes, pasta, and rice are mainly empty calories that actually contain very few vitamins and minerals, compared to vegetables, fruit, and nuts, which contain not only far more vitamins and minerals but also thousands of very healthy substances, like flavonols, flavanones, flavonoids, catechins, proanthocyanidins, isoflavones, lignans, phenolic acids, stilbenes, and omega-3 fatty acids, to name a few.

But what about people in Asia, who eat "lots of rice" but are often healthy and live to a ripe old age? The Japanese have an average life expectancy of around 85 years, several years more than people in most Western countries, where the average life expectancy is about 81 years. However, compared to the West, people in Asia often consume fewer (fast) carbohydrates, so far at least. Asians consume less bread and fewer breakfast cereals, baked goods, and soft drinks. Asians do not fill their plate with mashed potatoes, french fries, or pasta. Whereas in Asia people eat a cup of rice with lots of vegetables, we in the West fill our plate with a hamburger (red meat and white bread) or pasta, followed by sweets or ice cream. The authentic Chinese or Japanese diet contains, besides rice, lots of vegetables, legumes, soy, healthier drinks, such as tea, and more foods that are rich in omega-3, such as fish—all foods that are not prominent in the Western diet. Furthermore, research shows that eating too much rice is unhealthy for Asians as well. A study that followed 64,000 Chinese people over many years, shows that the more foods with both a high glycemic index and glycemic load, particularly white rice, were consumed, the more the risk of type 2 diabetes increased.[62] As more people in Asia are beginning to eat like we do in the West, we also see a large increase in the occurrence of diabetes and obesity in such countries as China.

What about people in the Mediterranean? Is it not true that they have less cardiovascular disease or dementia, despite that baguette or plate of pasta that they eat regularly? We should not equate the "modern" Mediterranean diet, containing a lot of pasta and bread products (and red meat), with a more classic Mediterranean diet. Such a Mediterranean diet is healthier than the typical Western diet, because it already contains more vegetables, fruit, nuts, fish, and olive oil. It also contains less bread, pasta, and other carbohydrates. The typical Western diet contains on average 50 percent carbohydrates (sometimes even more than 60 percent), 35 percent fats, and 15 percent proteins. The Mediterranean diet contains only 38 percent carbohydrates, 46 percent fats, and 16 percent proteins.[63] Thus, it contains more fats and fewer carbohydrates. That is one reason it is healthier, but it could be even healthier if even less bread and pasta was consumed. This was also confirmed in some studies that show no health benefits in a Mediterranean diet, probably because this diet still contains too many carbohydrates, making it resemble a typical Western diet too much.[64, 65] Just to give you an idea of a real vintage, classical Mediterranean dish as prepared in the 1920s: Imagine a grandmother taking a big kettle, adding eggplants, zucchinis, paprika, tomatoes, lots of olive oil, garlic, lemon juice, and all kinds of herbs like oregano and sage, mixing it all together and letting it simmer for hours. Such a Mediterranean dish is something completely different from a big-crusted pizza topped with red meat and cheese.

That one's diet can always be healthier is exemplified by the food recommendations of scientists who study aging. These recommendations often go far beyond those issued by the government or official institutions. Not only do these scientists want to reduce weight gain but they also want to slow down the aging process and drastically reduce the risk of aging-related diseases. Often, these aging scientists suggest consuming much less carbohydrates, such as fast sugars, but also bread, potatoes, pasta, and rice. Professor Michael Rose, who became famous for his experiments in which he extended the life span of fruit flies, has the following to say about grain products: "Don't eat anything that comes from a grain or grass of any type—that includes rice and corn."

Cynthia Kenyon, a renowned researcher in the area of aging, says about her diet:

"There's a lot of these [healthy] diets . . . and what they all have in common is low carb—actually, low glycaemic index carbs. That's not eating the kind of carbohydrates where the sugar gets into your bloodstream very quickly [and stimulates production of insulin]." This means: No desserts. No sweets. No potatoes. No rice. No bread. No pasta. "When I say 'no,' I mean 'no, or not much.' Instead, eat green vegetables. I have a fabulous blood profile. My triglyceride level is only 30, and anything below 200 is good." Kenyon is shocked by the general lack of knowledge about nutrition. "It is a bit embarrassing to say that scientists actually don't know what to eat. . . . We can target particular oncogenes [genes that are involved in initiating cancer] but we don't know what we should eat. Crazy." Does her diet represent a return to scientists experimenting on themselves? "I don't think so—you have to eat something, and you just have to make your best judgment. And that's my best judgment. Plus, I feel better. Plus, I'm thin—I weigh what I weighed when I was in college. I feel great—you feel like you're a kid again. It's amazing."
                                        —"In Methuselah's mould," *PLoS Biology* (2004)

It is interesting that scientists who study aging, although working in a completely different field from nutrition science, still come to the same conclusions as recent research on nutrition: A diet with too many animal proteins and carbohydrates is not healthy. Does that mean that we should no longer eat any bread, pasta, rice, or potatoes, like Professor Kenyon? That may not be necessary, but we can certainly eat much less of these products. For breakfast, instead of bread or cereal, we can have healthier alternatives, such as nuts, seeds, fruit, soy yogurt, oatmeal, chia seed porridge, and dark chocolate. Instead of toast with jam, for example, we could fill a bowl with nuts, flaxseed, almond milk, pieces of pear and blueberries, and have a piece of dark chocolate for dessert. Or instead of eggs with bacon, you can prepare mushrooms, tofu, and spinach in a pan. For lunch or dinner, potatoes, pasta, and rice can be replaced by legumes (peas, beans, lentils), mushrooms, or an extra portion of vegetables (mashed broccoli or cauliflower instead of mashed potatoes, for instance). You can choose how far you want to go with that.

People with metabolic disorders, diabetes, or cardiovascular disease can take it quite far. Some diabetes patients can decide to eat no bread, potatoes, rice, and pasta, or very little; that is not a low-carbohydrate, ketogenic (ketone-inducing) diet (ketones are created by the body as fuel for the brain when there is not enough sugar) as it still contains carbohydrates from vegetables, mushrooms, legumes, and fruit. This is important, because often when people hear "no or much less bread, potatoes, pasta and rice," they automatically assume this diet involves a low-carb, but high (animal) protein diet, which is indeed not healthy in the long term. But the dietary pattern recommended here is not a low-carb diet, but a "low glycemic load, low glycemic index, healthy macronutrient diet," in which the macronutrient ratio (the proportion of carbs, fats, and proteins) leans more toward the classical Mediterranean diet, with a bit more emphasis on healthy fats and less on carbs, including starches. So instead of drastically reducing the carbs, fats, or proteins, like in many popular diets, I mainly focus on replacing the carbs with healthier alternatives (replacing bread, potatoes, rice, and pasta with more vegetables, legumes, and mushrooms), replacing the proteins more with healthier possibilities (processed red meat with poultry, fish, and vegetable protein) and replacing unhealthy fats with healthier ones, like fats from olives, olive oil, nuts, seeds or avocadoes—this is what the term "healthy macronutrient" entails. I discussed this diet in detail my previous book, called *The Food Hourglass*. It is the first diet that takes into account knowledge of the aging process and uses nutrition as a way to slow down the aging process and reduce the risk of aging-related diseases (more about that later).

Another misunderstanding lurks just around the corner, however: an undue fear of carbs. Some physicians and scientists were so shocked by the unhealthy effects of too many carbohydrates that they swung over to the complete opposite. They strictly prohibit not only bread, pasta, rice, and potatoes but also discourage eating fruit, legumes, and oatmeal, because these still contain too many carbohydrates. That is regrettable. First of all, the sugars in fruit, legumes, and oatmeal are packaged in fibers, so that the sugars are released into the bloodstream more slowly. Most types of fruit do not cause high sugar peaks. In addition, it is not only about sugar peaks: Fruit contains thousands of good substances that can help the body age more slowly. It would not only be a pity to stop eating delicious fruit but it would also be bad for your health. Another problem with the carbohydrate phobia is that the carbs that are cut from the diet are often replaced with . . . more proteins. As we have seen in the previous section, however, animal proteins (particularly processed red meat) actually accelerate aging.

In this section we have discussed the role of sugars in the aging process. We have seen that people in the West often eat lots of carbohydrates. But what about fats? What role do fats play in the aging process?

Oatmeal Versus Whole Wheat Bread

Despite that oats are a grain, they can be an interesting exception to the rule "less grain products." Oatmeal (the porridge made of oats) can be a convenient alternative for whole wheat bread, especially in the morning. There are several reasons for this. Oatmeal (not oats) has an average glycemic index (about 55) but a low glycemic load (a GL of 7 for an equally large (!) portion of bread). By comparison, the glycemic index of whole wheat bread is about 74 and the glycemic load is 30. Thus whole wheat bread delivers a lot more carbohydrates (GL), which then also cause higher sugar peaks than oatmeal (GI).

When looking up GL and GI, keep in mind that I refer to oatmeal and not oats. Oatmeal is porridge made with water or plant-based milk, and not just only the dry rolled oats (without the water or vegetable milk). The glycemic load of oatmeal is therefore much lower compared to dry rolled oats and whole wheat bread because, for the most part, the oatmeal consists of water or plant-based milk, which contains no or very few carbs. Also, when you compare the glycemic load of foods, make sure they have the same weight (for example, 100 g of bread with 100 g of oatmeal). Additionally, glycemic index and load tables can differ considerably from source to source, because many factors influence blood sugar levels and thus the measurements (one factor is the age of the participants—young people tend to have lower blood sugar levels than do older people).

Many types of whole wheat bread cause sugar peaks that are just as high as those caused by white bread. One reason is that whole wheat bread is made of genetically modified wheat. This wheat contains large amounts of amylopectin A, a kind of superstarch that causes high sugar peaks. This genetically modified wheat also contains more immunogenic (immune response–provoking) proteins, such as gluten or agglutinins, which can irritate the gut lining and the gut immune system (so it is not only about gluten). Whole wheat bread also contains few healthy, water-soluble fibers, such as beta-glucans. Oatmeal, on the other hand, contains large amounts of beta-glucans, hardly any gluten, and all kinds of substances that are healthy for the heart, such avenanthramides, which have anti-inflammatory properties. The beta-glucans in oatmeal are converted by bacteria in the intestine to short-chain fatty acids that have a positive effect on metabolism. This is one of the reasons why oatmeal has received an official health claim authorized by the European Union, in contrast to whole wheat products, such as bread or pasta, which did not get such a claim. Oatmeal can be prepared with plant-based milk, such as soy or almond milk. Add walnuts, flaxseeds, blueberries, cinnamon, ginger, nutmeg, dark chocolate or cacao to it to make it even tastier and healthier. Cooking oatmeal does not increase the glycemic index because the water-soluble fibers form a thick jelly in the intestine, which is slow to release sugars. However, use regular oats and not instant oats. Instant oats cause higher sugar peaks because they are more processed (pressed, rolled, cut), so that they release their sugars faster. Regular oats have longer cooking times than instant oats (around twenty minutes versus two minutes). Also, instant oatmeal often contains extra added sugar.

What About Fruit Juices?

Now this is an interesting topic. Fruit juices have received some bad press in recent years because they "contain lots of sugar." However, some researchers make a distinction between commercial, store-bought fruit juices with hardly any fiber, and fresh, homemade fruit juices with lots of fiber. The fiber is important, because it slows down the absorption of the sugars. Also, commercial fruit juices often contain a lot of extra sugars (usually in the form of "fruit concentrates"). These fruit juices, therefore, cause high sugar peaks. You can, however, make fruit juices (smoothies) yourself in a blender. In a blender you can mix, for example, an apple, a pear, and some blueberries. Although you are getting lots of sugars, you are also drinking fibers, so that the sugar peaks are not quite as high as when you drink commercial fruit juice. Additionally, compared to store-bought fruit juices, the healthy nutrients in homemade fruit juice are very fresh. You can also specifically choose low sugar fruits like blueberries, and you can be sure that you didn't add extra amounts of sugar or sugar-rich fruit concentrates (like fruit juice manufacturers often do). One study found that homemade fruit juice is healthier than commercial fruit juice and also reduces your risk of type 2 diabetes or metabolic syndrome.[66] The great advantage of smoothies is that to get more fruit into your daily diet, you simply can drink your fruit. It is even better to make your smoothies with vegetables, because vegetables contain less sugar than fruit and also contain all kinds of other healthy substances that you do not find in fruit. Try making a smoothie with vegetables or with vegetables, fruit, and nuts. Nuts give a more creamy texture to your smoothies. This way you are starting the day with a lot of healthy nutrients.

Several studies even suggest that despite the sugars in fruit juices, they can confer health benefits. One study with close to 2,000 participants showed that people who regularly drank fruit and vegetable juices had a lower risk of Alzheimer's disease.[67] Another study showed that in people who regularly drank pomegranate juice, the blood vessels do not clog up as fast.[68] Older people who consumed blueberry juice for three months had improved memory and cognitive skills and lower glucose levels.[69] Other studies show that drinking blueberry juice can protect against DNA damage[70] and even improve insulin resistance in obese people.[71] Could it be that specific fruit juices contain such healthy compounds that even despite the sugar, they can have beneficial effects?

In summary, one glass of fiber-rich smoothie a day, especially made of low sugar fruit like blueberries, raspberries or strawberries, together with very low sugar vegetables, can be a healthy habit.

SUMMARY

Carbohydrates (sugars and starches)

- Increase **insulin, IGF,** and other **growth-hormone-like substances** that accelerate aging

- Form **sugar cross-links** that make the proteins in our tissues stick together and give us, among other things
  - Wrinkles
  - Stiffer blood vessels
  - Cataracts
  - Deteriorating kidney function
  - A stiffer bladder
  - A stiffer heart.

Laron dwarfs have less IGF and insulin circulating in their blood and are almost immune to cancer and diabetes.

Larger people and animals have a greater risk of cancer and of dying early.

A diet with a **low glycemic index** (fewer high sugar peaks) and a **low glycemic load** (fewer carbohydrates) reduces the risk of all kinds of aging-related diseases, including type 2 diabetes, heart attacks, and strokes.

Whole grain products are healthier than other grain products, such as white bread or white pasta, but still contain **many carbohydrates**. This also applies to spelt bread.

In order, these are the unhealthiest to the healthiest carbohydrate-rich foods:

- White bread, white pasta, white rice, potatoes

- Whole grain bread or pasta, brown rice

- Oatmeal, vegetables, legumes, mushrooms, quinoa, fruit

Fruit contains sugars but also fibers (so that the sugars in the fruit are more slowly released) and thousands of other healthy substances that are not found in bread, pasta, or rice.

Consume far fewer **short**, **simple**, or **fast sugars** (glucose, fructose, and sucrose), including soft drinks, commercial fruit juices, baked goods, and candy.

Also consume fewer **long**, **complex** or **slow sugars**, including bread, potatoes, rice, pasta, and breakfast cereals.

For **breakfast**, replace bread or breakfast cereals with

- Oatmeal, chia seed pudding, nuts, seeds, fruit, dark chocolate, (sautéed) vegetables such as spinach and tomato with tofu, legumes, fungi-based meat substitutes, and/or eggs (a few eggs per week are permitted)

For **lunch** or **dinner**, replace potatoes, pasta, or rice with

- Legumes (peas, beans, lentils, soybeans)

- Mushrooms (oyster mushrooms, button mushrooms, shiitake, enokitake, etc.)

- An extra portion of vegetables (such as mashed cauliflower instead of mashed potatoes). Vegetables should be the basis of your diet, not potatoes and grains (in the US potatoes are considered a vegetable, while in many European countries potatoes are not regarded as a vegetable, but rather as a staple food, like corn or wheat).

Fats

For decades, fats have had an undeserved bad reputation. Several generations of people have been scared away from fats, although the story is much more complex and interesting. But first, let's consider what fats really are.

To put it simply, fats resemble a kind of molecular squid. They consist of a head (consisting of several dozens of atoms) and two or three arms, which are called fatty acids.

```
        H H H H H H H H H H H H H H H H O   H
        | | | | | | | | | | | | | | | | ||  |
    H-C-C-C-C-C-C-C-C-C-C-C-C-C-C-C-C-C-O-C-H
        | | | | | | | | | | | | | | | |        |
        H H H H H H H H H H H H H H H H         |
                                                |
        H H H H H H H H H H H H H H H H O       |
        | | | | | | | | | | | | | | | | ||      |
    H-C-C-C-C-C-C-C-C-C-C-C-C-C-C-C-C-C-O-C-H
        | | | | | | | | | | | | | | | |        |
        H H H H H H H H H H H H H H H H         |
                                                |
        H H H H H H H H H H H H H H H H O       |
        | | | | | | | | | | | | | | | | ||      |
    H-C-C-C-C-C-C-C-C-C-C-C-C-C-C-C-C-C-O-C-H
        | | | | | | | | | | | | | | | |        |
        H H H H H H H H H H H H H H H H         H
```

This is what a fat looks like. The three long arms on the left are the tails, or fatty acids. The tails are attached to the head, which consists of three carbon (C) atoms, to which several oxygen (O) and hydrogen (H) atoms are attached.

Thousands of billions of these squids together form a drop of fat. When we eat fats, such as a piece of cheese or a walnut, the fats enter our digestive system, where the digestive enzymes (a certain type of proteins) separate the arms from the head—the squids are amputated, as it were. That is necessary because the intestinal cells cannot absorb the squids whole. The arms (fatty acids) are absorbed by the intestinal cells and end up in the bloodstream. Fat cells absorb the fatty acids and attach them to a new head to create a new squid again. Fat cells, therefore, are filled with squids (fats) but it is mainly the arms (fatty acids) that circulate in the bloodstream. Often the terms *fats* and *fatty acids* are used interchangeably, which is OK in most cases.

There are several types of fatty acids (or fats). On the one hand, there are saturated fatty acids. This means that the fatty acid is saturated with hydrogen atoms. You can compare this with a Christmas tree branch hung with ornaments: The branch is saturated (filled) with ornaments (hydrogen atoms). Since these ornaments are so close together, they push against one another and they actually keep the branch straight: Therefore, saturated fatty acids are straight. In unsaturated fatty acids, on the other hand, two hydrogen atoms (ornaments) are missing in specific places, so that the fatty acid is bent at the place where normally the hydrogens atoms should be: Unsaturated fatty acids have a kink.

In saturated fatty acids (right), the tail is completely saturated with hydrogen (H) atoms, resulting in a straight tail. In unsaturated fatty acids (left) the tail is not saturated with hydrogen atoms: Two are missing and the tail is bent.

Saturated (straight) fatty acids are often found in animal products, such as meat, cheese, butter, and milk. Vegetable sources of saturated fatty acids are palm oil, coconut oil, and the cocoa butter in chocolate. Unsaturated (bent) fatty acids are omega-3 fatty acids, which are found in fatty fish or walnuts. Other unsaturated fatty acids are the omega-6 fatty acids, such as those in meat, sunflower oil, or corn oil.

The last type of fat is trans fats. Trans fats are strange fats. They are straight fats, although they are missing several hydrogen atoms. So they share some characteristics with both the saturated fats—being straight—and with the unsaturated fats—missing a few hydrogen atoms.

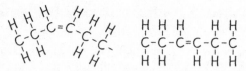

The tail of trans fats (right) is straight, although the tail is unsaturated (it is missing two hydrogen atoms). Compare this to the bent tail of unsaturated fats (left): The tail of the trans fatty acid is straight because the hydrogen atoms are located on opposite sides of the bend.

These unusual fats are found in industrially prepared foods, including baked goods, snack bars, fats for deep frying, fast food, and some margarines. Research has shown that trans fats are very unhealthy and increase the risk of cardiovascular disease. The effects of saturated and unsaturated fats are not as clear-cut, as we shall see.

SUMMARY

Saturated (straight) fats are found in

- Animal sources: meat (imagine the fatty edges and veins in the meat), cheese, butter, and milk

- Vegetable sources: palm oil, coconut oil, and cocoa butter (in chocolate).

Unsaturated (bent) fats are found in

- Omega-3 fatty acids: fatty fish, walnuts, flaxseeds

- Omega-6 fatty acids: meat, sunflower oil, corn oil

- Other unsaturated fatty acids: olive oil.

Trans fats (straight fats) are found in

- Industrially prepared foods, baked goods, snack bars, fried foods, fast food, and some margarines.

THE ROLE OF FATS IN AGING

In the course of our life, fat makes a strange journey through our body. When we are young, most fat is located under the skin. As we grow older, more and more fat will settle in the abdomen, between the organs. Many people will notice that in the form of a potbelly. If you eat an unhealthy diet and drink a lot of soft drinks and alcohol, you will develop that potbelly sooner. When we are past 70, more and more fat will accumulate in the strangest places in the body, such as in the bone marrow, our organs, and our blood vessels, all places where it does not belong. It is as if the more we age, the more the fat starts encroaching into areas where it shouldn't be. The location of the fat tells us a lot about our health. Under the skin is a good place for fat; this is actually healthy fat. In women, it is found mostly around the buttocks, which gives women the typical *pear* shape, and it is also a symbol of beauty and fertility.

Fat that accumulates in the abdomen, however, is not healthy. People with a lot of abdominal fat often have an *apple* shape. That abdominal fat produces all kinds of inflammatory substances that are released into the bloodstream. These substances make the blood vessels clog up faster, putting you at greater risk of a heart attack and dementia. People with abdominal fat have three times a greater risk of dementia.[72] A study found that people with a waist circumference that is 80 percent of their height die on average twenty years earlier.[73] Normally the waist is the smallest area between the hips and the lower ribs, somewhat above or below the navel. Ideally your waist should be half the size of your height. For example, someone who is five foot two (62 inches) should have a waist of 31 inches. However, even in people with a normal waistline, there may still be a lot of fat in the abdomen, in between the organs. These people are sometimes referred to as TOFI (thin on the outside, fat on the inside). Although they are slim and do not have a potbelly, TOFIs still have a higher risk of cardiovascular disease because they have too much unhealthy internal fat in between the organs.

Why is it that in the course of our life, fat moves out from under the skin and ultimately all through our body? That is because, as we age, fat cells fail to do the job they are made for: storing fat. A lifelong bombardment of insulin, IGF, amino acids and other substances, makes the fat cells age. When they fail to properly store fat, it migrates to other places and accumulates in places where it does not belong, including the abdomen, the liver (fatty liver disease), or in the blood vessel walls, which plays a role in atherosclerosis. Since people tend to gain weight as they grow older, it is often assumed that their fat cells function too well because they store too much fat. The opposite seems to be true, however: Fat begins to migrate and accumulate in the wrong places because fat cells are not doing their job. We are in good health when our fat cells are functioning well.

FATS, NUTRITION, AND AGING

Fats have had a bad reputation for decades, and they still do. Fats have been blamed for causing clogged blood vessels, heart attacks, and weight gain. For decades, government organizations have urged people to eat less fat, which they did. However, even though we eat less fat, we see an increasing incidence of cardiovascular disease, type 2 diabetes, and obesity. To combat this epidemic of obesity, millions of people were put on low-fat diets, but the results were dismal, as we will discuss later. A low-fat diet seems to be a logical choice to lose weight because fats contain lots of calories and are said to be "bad for the heart." But it is not that simple.

This fat phobia is regrettable and largely unwarranted. Fats are very important to our body. If you look at the human body, it naturally contains much fat compared to other animals. Humans are particularly fatty. On average, men consist of 15 percent fat and women even of 25 percent; that's one quarter of the body! Our closest relatives, the apes, have much less fat in their body. The body of a young ape consists of 3 percent fat, whereas the body of a human child contains at least five times as much fat. An adult chimpanzee contains about 6 percent fat; a human adult, between 15 and 25 percent. In short, the fact that a healthy human body contains that much fat indicates that fat fulfills an important function in our body, something that did not go unnoticed among scientists.

For many years, scientists have asked themselves why humans contain so much fat. Some scientists suggested that it is because our ancestors often lived near the water. Other mammals that contain a lot of fat are whales. These animals need fat to stay warm in cold waters. Since our ancestors often lived near water to gather fish and shellfish, maybe they, too, developed a protective layer of fat under the skin to keep warm. At first sight this may seem a far-fetched explanation, but we should not forget that the process of evolution can be very powerful. Whales are descendants of wolflike animals that began to live close to water more than 60 million years ago and ultimately moved into the water. Whales, therefore, descended from land-dwelling animals. However, the idea of the human as a water-primate has proven to be wrong. One reason would be that in many places in the world they would have to share the water with big, not very friendly animals, such as crocodiles and hippos. There are many better explanations of why humans contain so much fat.

One reason our body contains so much fat is that we have such a large brain. We are so fatty because we are so smart. The fat in our body is what builds our brain and keeps it functioning. The brain consists largely of fat: About 60 percent of the dry weight (with all the water removed) of the brain is fat. That is also the reason that the body of human children contain so much fat (compared to other primates, such as chimpanzees): Those fats are necessary for the building and further growth of their brain in their first years of life.

We also need a good supply of fat to keep our brain running on a continuous basis. Our brain uses a lot of energy: Twenty percent of our energy goes to that 2.6 pounds of thinking jelly in our skull. That energy provides us with self-consciousness, emotions, and a whole lot of worries. The problem is that this energy needs to be available at all times; you cannot turn the brain off. Fat is the ideal source of continuous energy supply: 100 grams (3.5 ounces) of fat contain 900 calories of energy. Fat can serve as a large reserve of energy to bridge periods of scarcity. One problem, however, is that the brain cannot use fats as a source of energy directly because the brain actually runs primarily on sugar. Fortunately the body has found a solution for that: Fats can be converted into ketones. Ketones are substances that can be used as energy by the brain. In prehistoric times this was important in periods of scarcity, which occurred quite often. If our ancestors were unable to find any food for a few days, the fat stored in their body ensured that their energy-guzzling brain could still be kept running.

An energy reserve rich in fat was necessary not only to build a large brain and keep it running but also to ensure long-lasting endurance. Endurance was extremely important for our ancestors, since they were actually very incompetent hunters. Compared to other animals, humans are excruciatingly slow because they have only two legs instead of four. A cheetah can run about 75 miles per hour, a goat can run twice as fast as the fastest human, and even a squirrel, which is so much smaller than a human, is faster than we are—just try to catch one. Strength is not our best feature either: An average chimpanzee, which weighs about 40 pounds less than a human, is twice as strong as the strongest human athletes. That is why chimpanzees are so dangerous. From time to time, we hear that a zookeeper was dragged away by a chimpanzee and later found dead or savagely wounded. In a confrontation with most animals, we, with our weak and slow bodies, are the losers. In terms of our body, humans are nature's lemons.

It was not easy for our ancestors to catch animals that were almost always stronger and faster. Nevertheless, they succeeded. How? One way was to use a special technique called *persistence hunting*. This involved following a prey for hours, sometimes days, by just walking behind it, until the animal succumbed to stress and exhaustion. The structure of the human body shows that we are particularly adapted to this form of hunting. The large amount of fat in our body enables us to follow prey for days without eating but with no real lack of energy—in contrast to the zebra or gazelle, which quickly become completely exhausted.

In addition to a large fat reserve, our body has other characteristics that are adapted to persistence hunting. Two of these are typical for a human being: our hairless skin and our ability to sweat profusely. Most other mammals have a coat of hair and few sweat glands. Most have no *eccrine* sweat glands (sweat glands that are spread out over the body), whereas humans have millions of them (The other type of sweat glands are *apocrine* sweat glands, which are concentrated in certain regions, such as the armpits and near the reproductive organs, and they produce a different scent). Since mammals can hardly sweat, they must cool themselves in other ways; for example, dogs do it by panting; kangaroos and lions by lying in the shade in the hot afternoon; and pigs, by rolling in mud. Humans, by contrast, are able to sweat profusely —as much as one gallon per hour—and that, in combination with a hairless skin, enables them to cool themselves quickly. This was useful during the hot afternoons on the African savanna, whereas other mammals, such as zebras and gazelles, sweat very little and can easily become overheated. In addition they have a coat, which also makes cooling off more difficult. In other words, the reason we humans are naked, and why we have clothing stores and deodorant factories, is that in prehistoric times these qualities helped us to hunt better. Thanks also to a large fat reserve, we were feared hunters who did not rely on speed and strength but on patience and persistence. That also allowed us to roam around for days in search of fruits, nuts, seeds, and plants and to explore new territory.

Fat is also very important for reproduction. Our large fat reserve enabled us to reproduce faster. It gave women the necessary energy to allow the fetus to grow (particularly its brain), to breastfeed, and to raise children, which in periods of scarcity may mean eating less to give the children more. A woman with a lot of body fat could reproduce faster; she could breastfeed one child, give her own food to an older child (she has enough energy in the form of fat), and become pregnant again all at the same time. Women can have three times as many children as chimpanzees.[60, 74] For that reason, women on average have more fat than men (25 percent instead of 15 percent). The fact that humans could reproduce faster was a contributing factor to the speed with which our species was able to spread across the world.

Omega-3 Fatty Acids

When we look at the evolutionary history of the human species, we can see that fats helped us think better, hunt better, and have more children. The importance of fat also becomes clear when we look at the structure of our body, which contains a lot of fat compared to that of other mammals. It is not surprising, therefore, that fats are important for our health. People who eat foods that contain more healthy fats are less at risk of all kinds of diseases in old age. A great example is omega-3 fatty acids. They can be found in fish (particularly fatty fish, including salmon, herring, mackerel, and anchovies), nuts (such as walnuts), and flaxseeds. Eating more of such fatty foods can slow down the aging process and decrease the risk of aging-related diseases.

An example of such a disease is macular degeneration. In this disease, cells in the retina of the eye die because all kinds of protein and other debris have collected there. This leads to blindness in the central field of vision, which can spread outward until complete blindness follows. Macular degeneration is a typical aging-related disease in the West: Twenty percent of people over the age of 65 has it. However, keep in mind that with many aging-related diseases, if you get old enough, everyone will experience such diseases to a greater or lesser degree. Various studies show that even by eating fish once a week, you can better protect yourself against macular degeneration. In a study in which people ate ample omega-3 fatty acids, they had 45 percent less risk of developing macular degeneration than did those who ate few omega-3 fatty acids.[75–78]

Rheumatoid arthritis is another disease we often associate with aging. This disease causes inflammation of the joints. For example, a study of more than 32,000 women shows that women who ate one portion of fatty fish per week (which provides at least 210 mg of omega-3 fatty acids) had a 35 percent lower risk of arthritis.[79] Other studies show that people who eat fish regularly have less degeneration of the brain.[80, 81] Besides fish, walnuts also contain many healthy fats, including omega-3 fats. When mice and rats are fed walnuts, they have less cognitive decline or are less likely to develop Alzheimer's disease.[82] In an experiment, mice with a mutation that caused them to develop Alzheimer's were divided into three groups: One group was given food consisting of 6 percent walnuts, one group received food with 9 percent walnuts, and the third group did not eat walnuts. The brain of the mice that were fed 9 percent walnuts degenerated less from Alzheimer's disease and made 45 percent fewer errors in a test measuring memory compared to the mice that did not eat walnuts.[83] The researchers concluded that "walnuts can have a positive effect on decreasing Alzheimer's disease, as well as slowing down or preventing it." People who eat a lot of walnuts have a faster and healthier brain.[84, 85] In addition, walnuts are good for the heart and the blood vessels. According to a study with 120,000 participants, people who ate a handful of walnuts daily had a 45 percent lower risk of heart attack.[86]

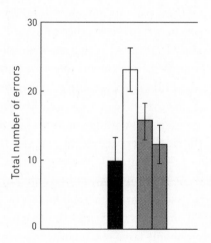

Mice with Alzheimer's disease that were fed walnuts (gray bars) make fewer errors compared to the mice with Alzheimer's that did not get walnuts (white bar). The black bar shows the group control mice that have no Alzheimer's mutation and cannot develop the disease. (Source: "Dietary supplementation of walnuts improves memory deficits and learning skills in transgenic mouse model of Alzheimer's disease," *Journal of Alzheimer's Disease* [2014].)

A greater intake of healthy fats from fish, nuts, and seeds can reduce the risk of all kinds of aging-related diseases. The problem is that we in the West eat too few healthy fats, such as omega-3 fatty acids. Since not everyone can or wants to eat fish or nuts, people sometimes take omega-3 supplements. There are numerous studies showing that omega-3 supplements can decrease the risk of various diseases, such as heart-rhythm abnormalities,[87-89] heart attacks,[90, 91] and even psychoses.[92] On the other hand, there are also some studies showing that omega-3 supplements are not very effective, or that they do not improve overall mortality. According to a study with more than 68,000 patients, there was only a 9 percent decrease in the risk of dying from a heart attack by taking omega-3 supplements, and that 9 percent was considered "statistically insignificant."[93]

In such cases, the media or certain experts are quick to announce that omega-3 fatty acids do not work. But it is not that simple. In such studies, the participants are often heart patients who take all kinds of other drugs, such as aspirin, blood pressure–lowering drugs, and statins, as well as follow a healthier diet, so that their risk of a heart attack has already decreased substantially. A potential additional effect of omega-3 can then be negligible, or in any case considerably less than if these patients took only omega-3 fatty acids. Indeed, studies show that, when no or very few other drugs are taken, the effect of omega-3 is much greater.[94] In the studies that show no effect, researchers may use different types of omega-3 supplements, or some supplements may be of inferior quality. The fatty acids may, for example, be contaminated or oxidized, which makes them less effective and can even cause liver function problems in some patients. There are a number of different forms of omega-3 fatty acids in supplements, such as the ethyl ester, triglyceride, or phospholipid form, which may have different effects. The source of the omega-3 fatty acids may also play a role: fatty fish, algae, or krill (tiny shrimplike animals). Manufacturers of triglyceride omega-3 fatty acids claim that their form is the best, whereas those who make phospholipid omega-3 fatty acids insist that they sell the best form. Finally, these studies often only last a few months or a year, which is too short to test the effect of a substance on the progression of an aging-related disease that needs decades to manifest itself. You could compare this to a house that has been wasting away for 30 years and is about to collapse. Will replacing the gutters at the last minute be able to save the house? In some cases maybe, but most likely not because you have not taken care of the flooded basement, or the cracks in the wall, or the leaking roof. But that does not mean that replacing the gutters has no effect. It is important to maintain the gutters, provided that you combine that with other maintenance (like other nutrients). That is why I specifically advocate eating foods rich in omega-3 rather than relying only on supplements. Fatty fish, nuts, and flaxseeds contain not only omega-3 fatty acids but all kinds of other healthy substances, such as furan fatty acids, iodine, various forms of vitamin E, fiber, and hundreds of other, as yet undiscovered, substances that have healthy effects on the body and that you will not find in an omega-3 supplement.

We can see that in research as well. Take Alzheimer's disease, for example. Some studies show that omega-3 fatty acids help slow down the progression of this disease, whereas other studies show no effect. This is not surprising because Alzheimer's is a serious disease that occurs after a person has been exposed for decades to a variety of factors, such as bad nutrition, toxins, stress, lack of exercise, lack of sleep, depression, and so forth. To repair the gutters at the last moment (give the person omega-3 fatty acids, usually for a short period) will often not have a significant effect on preventing the house from collapse. But what if you do not wait to take omega-3 fatty acids until you have Alzheimer's, but do it years earlier by eating a healthy diet that includes omega-3 fatty acids? According to one study, people who eat fish once a week or more have a 60 percent lower risk of developing Alzheimer's disease than do people who eat fish rarely or never.[95, 96] A study that followed more than 8,000 people over the age of 65 over many years, found that those who ate fish less than once a week had a 47 percent greater risk of dementia. People who ate fish daily, however, had a 44 percent lower risk. Older people who regularly ate oils rich in omega-3, such as walnut or flaxseed oil, had a 60 percent lower risk of dementia.[97]

Of course, people who eat more fish or walnuts are often more educated, eat other healthy foods, exercise more, and smoke less. Researchers try as much as possible to take these factors into account when they estimate the importance of healthy fats. Be that what it may, the conclusion remains the same: A healthy lifestyle and a diet with more healthy fats can lower your risk of aging-related diseases, such as Alzheimer's, macular degeneration, and cardiovascular disease. That is also the reason why the American Heart Association and the European Cardiologic Society recommend a higher intake of omega-3 fatty acids, by eating fish at least twice a week, as well as nuts, flaxseed, olives, avocados, and other healthy food rich in fats.

Cholesterol

One of the reasons why fats have been considered to be unhealthy for so long has to do with cholesterol, because this substance is often considered to be a fat as well. Cholesterol has a different structure than a typical fat, but since cholesterol is also difficult to dissolve in water, it is often called a fat. We are always told that a high cholesterol level is unhealthy. But it is not that simple.

Various large studies show that there is *no* relationship between an elevated cholesterol level and the risk of a heart attack.[98, 99] Yes, you are reading it correctly: High cholesterol does not increase the risk of a heart attack. That is not really surprising, since 75 percent of the people who arrive in the emergency room with a heart attack actually have normal cholesterol.[100] There are, of course, rare genetic diseases that cause some people to have an exceptionally high cholesterol level and may increase their risk of a heart attack, but these are exceptions. In this condition, the cholesterol levels are called supraphysiological, which means that they are so extremely high that interpretations that apply to healthy people are of little use. Remarkably, of people with this genetic condition—called familial hypercholesterolemia—40 percent have a normal life span.[101]

An elevated cholesterol, therefore, is not necessarily unhealthy. Professor George Mann, one of the investigators in the well-known Framingham Heart Study, says the following about this:

> The diet heart hypothesis that suggest that a high intake of fat or cholesterol causes heart disease has been repeatedly shown to be wrong, and yet, for complicated reasons or pride, profit and prejudice, the hypothesis continues to be exploited by scientists, fund-raising enterprise, food companies, and even governmental agencies. The public is being deceived by the greatest health scam of the century.

The food and pharmaceutical industries like the idea that high cholesterol is bad for you, because the food industry can then promote cholesterol-lowering margarine and the pharmaceutical industry can sell billions of dollars of cholesterol-lowering drugs. Despite all the scientific research that shows otherwise, we can still see television commercials promoting the use heart-healthy margarine, which supposedly lowers cholesterol (and is full of inflammation-increasing omega-6 fatty acids).

Due to all that fear of high cholesterol, we might almost forget that cholesterol is an important substance in the body. Similar to omega-3 fatty acids, cholesterol is part of the cell walls (cell membranes). The more cholesterol our cell walls contain, the more liquid and flexible they are. This allows the cells to better communicate with one another. That is particularly good for our brain cells, which like nothing better than to communicate and thereby generate our consciousness. Our brain cells are chock-full of cholesterol. Although the weight of our brain is only 2 percent of our body weight, it contains 25 percent of all cholesterol in our body. Your brain needs cholesterol to function. That helps to explain why people with a so-called healthy lower cholesterol level in the blood (less than 200 mg/dl or 5.17 mmol/l), are more forgetful and perform less well on cognitive tests than people with a moderately high cholesterol (between 200 and 239 mg/dl or between 5.17 and 6.18 mmol/l).[102] This is even more pronounced in older people.

Yet even more interesting is that people with high cholesterol often live longer than do those with low cholesterol. In a study published in the well-known medical journal the *Lancet*, very old people were followed over a period of ten years (the average age of the participants was 98 years). Not only does this study show that there was no relationship between high cholesterol and the risk of a heart attack but it also shows that the people with the highest cholesterol were the ones who lived longest! People with high cholesterol also had a lower risk of cancer and infections (probably due to the fact that cholesterol allows the immune system to be more effective).[103, 104] Women with high cholesterol have a lower risk of Parkinson's disease: The more cholesterol in the blood, the less the risk of Parkinson's.[105] Patients with amyotrophic lateral sclerosis (ALS, or Lou Gehrig's disease) live longer on average if they have high cholesterol levels.[106] In short, having too much cholesterol is not always bad for your health; people with high cholesterol levels in the blood even seem to live longer.

That there is no relationship between high cholesterol and, for example, the risk of a heart attack eventually became clear to even the most fervent believers in the "cholesterol is bad" myth. Therefore, they put forth a second, more refined, hypothesis. According to this hypothesis, there are two types of cholesterol: bad cholesterol (LDL cholesterol) and good cholesterol (HDL cholesterol). The more LDL cholesterol, the more your blood vessels clog up; the more HDL cholesterol, the healthier your blood vessels. However, even this approach is too simple. It happens all too often that even people with normal HDL and LDL cholesterol values still are at higher risk of a heart attack and die early. Other studies show, for instance, that people with low LDL cholesterol in their blood still have a several times' higher risk of

Parkinson's disease.[107] Increasing the good HDL cholesterol with medications also does not help lower the risk of a heart attack, and genetic variations in people that makes them produce more, or less, good cholesterol does not predict their risk of a heart attack.[108]

We need to look further than the amount and type of cholesterol. Cholesterol is not really harmful in itself. But it becomes very harmful when it is glycated, oxidized, and small. If the LDL cholesterol particles in the blood have become glycated from too much sugar in our diet, or oxidized because we eat too little fruit and vegetables, the cholesterol particles become sticky. Then, they stick to the blood vessel wall more easily and trigger inflammation, causing the blood vessel to clog up. Another thing that makes cholesterol dangerous is its size. Small cholesterol particles are particularly dangerous because due to their small size they can more easily creep into the blood vessel wall and pile up there. We see that people who have a mutation that makes them produce large cholesterol particles have a greater chance of reaching the age of 100.[109] Also, a diet high in carbohydrates makes the cholesterol particles smaller and therefore more harmful.

All this does not mean to say that more refined LDL and HDL cholesterol measurements are useless: They can tell you something about your risk profile, taking the overall picture into account. Nor does it mean that statins (cholesterol-lowering drugs) are not useful: Statins can reduce the risk of a heart attack. However, it becomes more and more apparent that statins can also do this by other mechanisms than by lowering cholesterol: Statins reduce inflammation in the body, improve the functioning of the cells in the blood vessel walls, and affect the stickiness of proteins. These are all different working mechanisms from "just lowering cholesterol." Each patient has his or her own unique risk profile, so when in doubt about your medication or your diet, it is best to discuss this with your physician.

Saturated Fats

So, after all, cholesterol is not as bad as we thought. Then, there is another type of fat that have all been lumped together and labeled as bad: saturated fats. Saturated fats can be found in animal products such as meat, butter, eggs, and cheese but also in plant-based foods like chocolate and coconut oil. For decades, nutritionists have discouraged people from eating saturated fats because these fats were thought to clog your blood vessels and increase your risk of a heart attack. But is it really that simple, namely, that *all* saturated fats are *always* unhealthy?

It seems to be more complex than that. For example, various large studies have showed that saturated fats do *not* increase your risk of a heart attack.[110, 111] On the contrary: The more carbohydrates you replace with saturated fats, the less risk of a heart attack. For every 5 percent of carbohydrates that are replaced with saturated fats, the risk of a heart attack decreases by 7 percent.[112–114] Such studies seem to suggest that too many carbohydrates in particular, rather than too many fats, are bad for your heart. The fewer carbohydrates and the more fats you eat, the healthier you are. That is not surprising in the light of what we know about aging. We have seen that too many carbohydrates accelerate the aging process.

Another problem is that all saturated fats are thrown together and described as "unhealthy." But not all saturated fats are the same. The short-chain saturated fatty acid butyrate has various health effects.[115, 116] Butyrate is even one of the reasons why you should eat food with lots of water-soluble fiber: these fibers are converted by the bacteria in your gut into butyrate, which has various beneficial effects on your gut health, immune system, metabolism and even your brain. Of course, this does not mean that all saturated fats are healthy and that you should gobble down loads of butter. There are unhealthy saturated fats and neutral saturated fats. But also healthy saturated fats. In many foods, their effects cancel each other out, and this is one of the reasons why many large studies have not found a relationship between saturated fats and the risk of a heart attack.

But why then, despite all these studies, do we still often hear from many governments that all saturated fats are unhealthy? There are several reasons for this.

One reason is the studies done by well-known nutrition expert Ancel Keys. Keys became famous for his Seven Countries Study, published in 1970. This study looked into the fat consumption in seven different countries. Keys discovered that in countries where people eat a lot of saturated fats, the risk of a heart attack was higher. Keys, who did not scorn publicity and was also very good at eloquently explaining his findings, went on a crusade against saturated fats, which he labeled as the main cause of cardiovascular disease. He also was a member of important advisory committees and managed to convince the American government that saturated fats were unhealthy, not an excess of carbohydrates. After all, in those days, there were also scientists who were convinced that not so much fats but particularly too many carbohydrates (soft drinks, bread, and baked goods) were unhealthy. After fierce debates, however, and by referring to his Seven Countries Study, Keys succeeded in convincing the authorities since his study shows clearly that in countries where the diet included many saturated fats, the risk of heart attack was higher. The authorities adopted his point of view, and since authorities tend to simplify matters to make them more understandable for the general public, the recommendation was to drastically reduce the consumption of all fats, not only saturated fats.

Therefore, for decades the message was spread that fats, and particularly saturated fats, were unhealthy. That was not good advice. For one thing, it became clear that Keys had not looked at the overall picture in his Seven Countries Study: He had studied quite a few more than seven countries. In fact, he had studied 21, but had chosen to highlight only the seven countries that corresponded with his point of view. Those were the countries where a relationship existed between the intake of saturated fats and the risk of a heart attack. However, he ignored the countries and populations where there was no relationship at all. There are numerous examples of this. The Inuit in Alaska, the Maasai tribes in Kenya, and the Samburu people in Uganda have diets that consist of 70 to 80 percent fats, including lots of saturated fats but nevertheless they have very little obesity or clogged blood vessels.[65] In his study Keys even ignored countries, such as France, Germany, and Switzerland, where the relationship between saturated fats and heart attacks was unclear. In Greece he studied only nine people, and not only that: Of the 12,770 people who participated in the Seven Countries Study, the eating patterns of only 3.9 percent were studied.

As if all this were not bad enough, Keys even drew a wrong conclusion from the seven countries that best fitted his views. A re-analysis of the Seven Countries Study done in 1999 shows a more significant relationship between heart attacks and the consumption of sugar, bread, and baked goods, than with eating animal products (which contain saturated fats).[117] How painful is that? Numerous government organizations have based their health recommendations on Keys' views for decades and many still do so today. Keys' view was also good news for many food manufacturers. With that information they can sell to the public cheap, *low-fat* but high-carbohydrate foods (bread, pasta, doughnuts, breakfast cereals, pizzas, etc.), and even proclaim that their products are healthy because they contain little fat or cholesterol.

Of course, we cannot blame it all on Dr. Keys. There are many other reasons that we believed for so long that fats are unhealthy. One is common sense. Studies shows that people with high levels of fats in their blood have a higher risk of a heart attack. Common sense would tell you that fats clog the blood vessels, and therefore you would be wise to reduce your fat intake. But what if the high levels of fats in your blood did not come from eating too much fat but from something else—carbohydrates, for instance?

Westerners have a completely different diet from that of people living hundreds of thousands of years ago. We eat large amounts of carbohydrates daily: for breakfast, a large bowl of sugary cereal or toast with jam; for lunch, a sandwich of white bread or a hamburger; and for dinner, rice, pasta, or potatoes, followed by a sweet dessert. Our liver has the task of processing this deluge of carbohydrates. That liver is the product of millions of years of evolution and for millions of years never had anything to do with toast with jam, french fries, or pies. Our poor liver cannot burn up or store all these carbohydrates, and the only way out is to convert the excess sugars into fats. This explains why people who eat many carbohydrates also often get a fatty liver and pile up fat everywhere in the abdomen (creating the typical potbelly), and have high levels of fat in their blood. Intuitively and at first sight, it would make sense to eat less fat in order to reduce the fats in in your blood. However, in medicine many things are not as simple as that. Ironically, the best way to reduce the fats in your blood is by eating fewer carbohydrates, not fewer fats.[118]

Yet another reason fats have had a bad name for so long is that there are indeed fats that are unhealthy. These mean cousins of most other fats have given fats in general a bad name. Now we are talking about the trans fats. These unhealthy fats are found in industrially prepared foods, such as baked goods, fried foods, fast food, and some margarines. They do indeed increase the risk of a heart attack. Furthermore, there are the omega-6 fatty acids: The counterparts of the omega-3 fatty acids, these are found in meat and oils, such as corn oil or sunflower oil. In large quantities, most omega-6 fatty acids can stimulate inflammation in the body. That is a problem in many industrialized countries: We eat too many omega-6 fatty acids and too few omega-3 fatty acids. Some margarines may contain hardly any trans fats, but they are still chock-full of omega-6 fatty acids, which is not recommended.

We have now seen that most fats are not unhealthy. Where do we go from here? Not long ago the front cover of *Time* magazine pictured a butter curl with the message, "Eat butter," and underneath it said, "Scientists labeled fat the enemy. Why they were wrong."

Does that mean that we can now eat entire gobs of butter? No, not really. Butter may not be as bad as was first thought, but that does not mean that we can eat big gobs of it with impunity. The fear of many products that contain saturated fats, such as butter, is indeed exaggerated. You can use butter or other products that contain saturated fats, such as coconut oil, sparingly, for example to cook with. As David Ludwig from Harvard University puts it, the next time you eat buttered toast, think of butter as actually the more health-ful component." This quote summarizes the shift in thinking that is going on in nutrition science: Instead of putting all the blame on fats, we finally see that too much carbohydrates plays an important role in disease and acceler-ated aging. And "too much carbohydrates" not only refers to fast sugars but also to the sacred starches, which have stayed out of range for too long.

Of course, we should not forget the really healthy fats, like omega-3 fatty acids from fish and nuts and the fats in olive oil, avocados, and dark chocolate (indeed, despite the fact that dark chocolate also contains lots of saturated fats it has various health effects, as we will see later). I particu-larly recommend these types of healthy fats. For example, a study shows that a Mediterranean diet with more fats obtained from olive oil and nuts was related to a 30 percent lower risk of strokes and heart attacks.[119] It is for good reason that scientists at Harvard University put fats from nuts, seeds, olives, avocados, and oils, such as olive oil and walnut oil, at the base of their food pyramid. A diet rich in omega-6 fats, such as margarines and corn oil, should be avoided as much as possible.

In short, more healthy fats, fewer fast carbohydrates, and not too many animal proteins would be the ideal recommendation for a long and healthy life.

SUMMARY

Saturated fats and **cholesterol** are not as unhealthy as previously thought.

A diet with **healthy fats** reduces the risk of aging-related diseases, including Alzheimer's disease, heart attacks, macular degeneration, and strokes.

Eat more healthy fats:

Via food: nuts, seeds, olives, avocados, fatty fish (salmon, mackerel, herring, anchovies, etc.)

Via oils: extra virgin olive oil (mechanically pressed without heat or added chemicals), walnut oil, flax oil. Many oils can be used in cold foods but not for cooking. Good oils **for cooking** are

- Olive oil

- Avocado oil

- Coconut oil

- Butter.

Eat fewer unhealthy fats:

- **Trans fats** (clog the blood vessels): particularly in industrially prepared foods, including baked goods, snack bars, fats for deep frying, fast food, and some margarines

- **Omega-6 fatty acids** (increase inflammation): corn oil, sunflower oil, sesame seed oil, and most margarines

Our Energy Generators and Their Role in Life, Death, and Aging

We have now discussed at length the effect of proteins, carbohydrates and fats in aging. However, there are other reasons why we age, besides protein clumps or sugar cross-links. For example, mitochondria also play an important role in the slow but definite progression into frailty and infirmity that we call aging.

Mitochondria are fascinating things. They are small structures in our cells, without which we would not be able to walk, think, feel, or talk. They literally form the life energy and life breath that keep us ticking. They are life itself because they produce the energy to make our cells function. Mitochondria are why you breathe 20,000 times per day and eat every day. Oxygen and food (particularly carbohydrates and fats) are the fuel for our mitochondria to produce energy. Mitochondria are why restaurants, supermarkets, snack dispensers, and agriculture exist. They made it possible for warm-blooded mammals to emerge and for life on this planet to become more complex than simple single-celled bacteria. And, before I forget, they also play a role in aging.

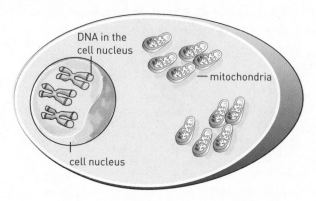

Mitochondria are small structures within the cell that provide energy for the cell. They resemble bacteria because they descended from them.

A body cell contains on average several hundreds to many thousands of mitochondria. Particularly those cells that have to continuously work hard, and therefore use a lot of energy, contain many mitochondria, such as brain cells, eye cells, and kidney cells (red blood cells are the only cells that do not contain mitochondria, but then again, they don't have to work hard). Knowing that the body contains about 40,000 billion cells, and cells on average contain several hundreds to many thousands of mitochondria, you can understand that your body must harbor an unfathomable amount of mitochondria. A rough estimate is that there about ten million billion mitochondria in your body. The reason there are so many is that they are so important.

What are mitochondria? Actually they are small cells in and of themselves. The walls of the mitochondria consist of fats, just like the walls of our cells. Furthermore, mitochondria also contain DNA, just like our cells (the *regular DNA* of our cells is found inside the cell nucleus. That DNA contains the building instructions for the proteins in the cell. The *mitochondrial DNA* is found inside the mitochondria and contains the instructions for building mitochondria—specifically, mitochondrial proteins).

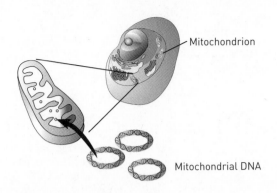

Mitochondrion

Mitochondrial DNA

Mitochondria contain their own DNA that forms little circles. This mitochondrial DNA contains the instructions for building mitochondrial proteins. The "regular" DNA is located in the cell nucleus. That nuclear DNA contains the instructions for building proteins for the cell. (Image: National Institutes of Health—National Human Genome Research Institute.)

There is an important reason that mitochondria are *cells within our cells* and have their own DNA. Billions of years ago the mitochondria were free-living bacteria. Life on earth originated about 3.8 billion years ago, at first only in the form of bacteria. They were simple, primitive cells, more or less small water-filled sacs with DNA and proteins, but without mitochondria. About two billion years ago, one of the most important events in the evolution of life on earth took place: A large bacteria had swallowed a small bacteria. However, instead of being digested, the small bacteria continued to exist inside the large bacteria. It did even more: It began producing energy for the large bacteria. Thus, the small bacteria became the first mitochondrion and the large bacteria became a real cell.

Mitochondria, therefore, are small ancient bacteria that produce energy for a larger bacteria, or cell. All cells in our body are descendants of this large bacterial cell containing small bacteria or mitochondria that produce that energy. Our mitochondria, therefore, are small ancient bacteria that produce our energy, so that we can talk, breathe, and walk. Since our cells contain hundreds or thousands of mitochondria, each human is literally a walking, talking colony of bacteria. Just as a car is propelled by its engine, our body is propelled by bacteria in the form of mitochondria.

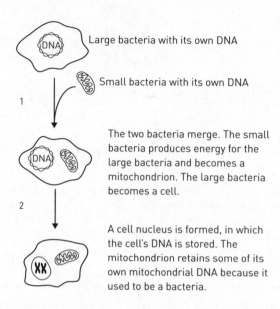

Large bacteria with its own DNA

Small bacteria with its own DNA

1

The two bacteria merge. The small bacteria produces energy for the large bacteria and becomes a mitochondrion. The large bacteria becomes a cell.

2

A cell nucleus is formed, in which the cell's DNA is stored. The mitochondrion retains some of its own mitochondrial DNA because it used to be a bacteria.

The growth of complex cells: A small bacteria merges with a large bacteria. The small bacteria produces energy for the large bacteria and thus becomes a mitochondrion. The large bacteria becomes a cell. Since there is now a source of energy available, the large bacteria can develop a cell nucleus to store its DNA (the mitochondria also have their own DNA). Cells with mitochondria and a cell nucleus are complex cells from which all complex life, such as jellyfish and humans, is formed.

The fact that mitochondria still have the characteristics of a bacteria can be seen from their behavior. For example, mitochondria can divide inside our cells and duplicate themselves, just as bacteria do. When a cell needs more mitochondria (such as when we exercise and need to produce more energy), the mitochondria divide into two, in the same way bacteria do. In addition, just like bacteria, mitochondria are sensitive to antibiotics. Therefore, some antibiotics are harmful for mitochondria since they are actually ancient bacteria. That explains why some antibiotics are very toxic for our body and thus are not used.

As we have seen, the most important task of mitochondria is to produce energy for our cells. But what is the energy that the mitochondria produce? Energy is often understood as something abstract, such as a flash of lightning or a spark of electricity. However, in our body, energy is an actual molecule, called adenosine triphosphate (ATP). ATP is sometimes considered the most important substance in the body after DNA.

ATP, the engine of all life, is a small molecule, built up of oxygen
atoms (O), phosphorous atoms (P), hydrogen atoms (H), and carbon atoms (C)
(not always shown; they are located on the corners). ATP tends to bind
to proteins, changes their structure, and thus allows them to function.

ATP is a small molecule that is produced continuously in gigantic quantities via the oxygen (that we breathe) and sugar and fats (that we eat) in the mitochondria. Why is ATP energy? Because it is a very reactive substance: It tends to bind to all kinds of proteins in our cells. This binding changes the structure of the proteins. ATP, therefore, creates a kind of domino effect in the proteins in our cells. When ATP binds to a protein, the protein then slightly changes in structure, which allows it to *function*. When ATP binds, for example, to a *channel protein* that is attached perpendicularly in the cell wall, the protein opens, so that certain substances can flow into the cell. When an ATP molecule binds to a *muscle protein*, the muscle protein slightly changes shape, making it shorter. If this happens simultaneously in hundreds of thousands of proteins in a muscle cell, and in the millions of muscle cells in our arms or legs, these muscles will contract and allow us to get up from a chair, or go for a walk, or turn this page.

In short, thanks to ATP we can move, breathe, and live. It is the substance that gives life to things, or more specifically, it makes them work. ATP changes the structure of tiny proteins, so that muscles can contract, stomach cells can produce stomach acid, channel proteins can open or close, and a whole body can be made to move and function. ATP is what distinguishes a living being from a stone or other lifeless object. Every day, thousands of billions of mitochondria in our body produce about 155 pounds of ATP! Of course, this ATP is also continuously broken down (by interaction with proteins) and

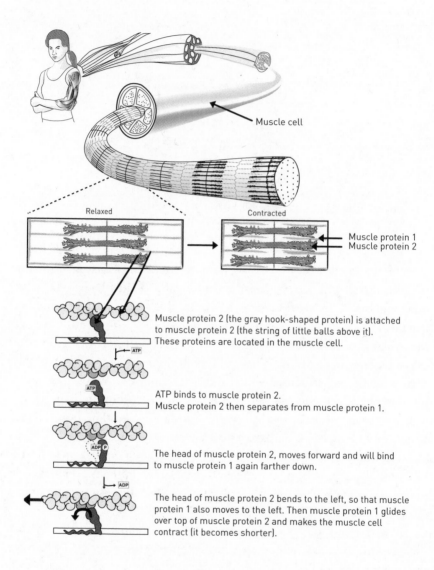

Muscle cell

Relaxed

Contracted

Muscle protein 1
Muscle protein 2

Muscle protein 2 (the gray hook-shaped protein) is attached to muscle protein 2 (the string of little balls above it). These proteins are located in the muscle cell.

ATP binds to muscle protein 2.
Muscle protein 2 then separates from muscle protein 1.

The head of muscle protein 2, moves forward and will bind to muscle protein 1 again farther down.

The head of muscle protein 2 bends to the left, so that muscle protein 1 also moves to the left. Then muscle protein 1 glides over top of muscle protein 2 and makes the muscle cell contract (it becomes shorter).

Muscle cells contain parallel strings of proteins (consisting of muscle protein 1 and muscle protein 2). These proteins hook into each other. When ATP binds to a muscle protein 1, muscle protein 2 will make muscle protein 1 move. When millions of proteins do this in millions of muscle cells, the whole muscle will contract, so that we can walk, breathe, and laugh.

built anew in the mitochondria. So, every day this quantity of ATP is being recycled in our body.

ATP is the life energy that directs almost all processes in our cells. This explains, for example, why cyanide is very toxic. Cyanide is a molecule that binds with an important mitochondrial protein, so that the mitochondrion is unable to function. A few hundred milligrams of cyanide is sufficient to shut down our mitochondria and cause death within minutes. Without ATP our cells no longer function and we die. The brain cells stop functioning, so that we become unconscious, the heart muscle cells stop contracting, and breathing comes to a halt.

ATP, therefore, explains why we can die. Dying almost always boils down to the same thing: a lack of oxygen, which makes it impossible for the mitochondria to produce ATP (unless you are crushed to death or evaporated by heat, for example). Whether you drown, have a heart attack, or bleed out after a car accident: Supply of oxygen via the blood stops. The mitochondria are no longer able to produce ATP, so that the cells stop functioning and you die. One could say that ATP is the *soul*, namely, the invisible, intangible substance that makes the body function. In a living person, there is a continuous production of millions of billions of ATP molecules per second that change the structure of vast numbers of proteins. In a dead person, the production of ATP has stopped and everything has shut down.

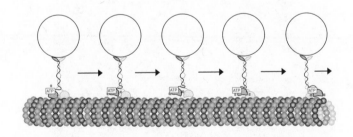

ATP ensures that transport proteins can transport sacs containing certain substances via the highways of the cell. These highways are long tubelike structures in the cell, each also composed of proteins. The transport protein has two feet, which can literally step over the highway. Each time an ATP molecule binds to one of the feet, the foot-shaped protein's structure changes, so that the foot takes a step forward and the protein can drag the sac along the tube. This is how all kinds of substances are transported in our cells.

Mitochondria are not only necessary to keep life going. They also gave a particular direction to life: They played an important role in the evolution of life on earth. Thanks to mitochondria, it was possible for intelligent life to emerge. Without mitochondria, there would be no animals, people, cities, or iPads, and the earth would be populated only by bacteria indifferently floating around in a pool of water.

Bacteria are small sacs of water in which the DNA floats around. In contrast to our cells, bacteria do not contain mitochondria and no cell nucleus where DNA is neatly stored. About two billion years ago, however, a large bacterium swallowed a small bacterium and thus mitochondria were formed, small bacteria that produced energy for their hosts. This provided the large bacteria (cells) with much more energy (ATP), allowing them to evolve further and become much more complex. Thanks to this additional energy, a cell nucleus could develop. The cell nucleus is the ball-shaped structure in the cell in which the DNA of the cell is stored neatly (as opposed to bacteria, in which the DNA simply floats around).

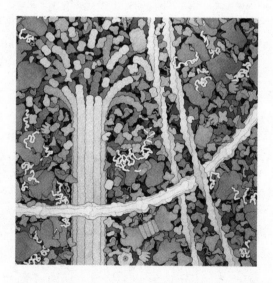

The inside of a cell. All the long proteins form the cell skeleton
that can make the cell move and give it a specific shape.
(Source: David S. Goodsell, the Scripps Research Institute.)

With the energy produced by the mitochondria, the large bacteria could also grow much larger: A bacterium is thousands of times smaller than a regular body cell, of which people (and all plants, animals, and fungi) are built. The mitochondria allowed large one-celled bacteria to now also build a cell skeleton: a complex framework consisting of many tens of thousands of hinged proteins that can make the cell move. White blood cells, for example, can grasp bacteria or viruses with their tentacles and devour them. With their cell skeleton, intestinal cells can form long protrusions, allowing them to absorb more nutrients from the intestine. It costs a lot of energy to move a cell skeleton (ATP needs to bind to the cell skeleton proteins everywhere to change the structure of the skeleton), and mitochondria provide this energy.

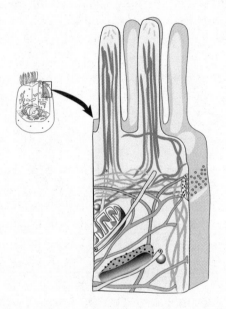

The protrusions at the top of this cell are long rods composed of many thousands of proteins. Such rods, threads, and tubes in the cell form the cell skeleton.

Thanks to mitochondria, cells could become much larger and more complex. Without mitochondria, life on earth would never have become more complex than bacteria. Some scientists argue that the emergence of mitochondria is a much more important and rarer event than the origin of life itself. After all, it looks like we live in a fairly biophilic universe. What this means is that it may not be that difficult for life to emerge from lifeless elements. Throw together some methane gas, phosphorous minerals, and carbon dioxide gases, and after about a week, amino acids, the building blocks of proteins and of life, will spontaneously appear. Even on meteorites, the building blocks of DNA have been found. Furthermore, recent research shows that life could fairly easily develop in the pores of hydrothermal vents at the bottom of the ocean.

Therefore, the emergence of life may not be such a remarkable event, but the emergence of *complex* life is probably a different story. This required a coincidental collaboration between two bacteria that worked out. That is how mitochondria could form and life could ultimately become much more complex. This successful bacterial merger may be a much rarer occurrence in the history of life than the origin of life itself. This can also explain why the evolution of life on this planet has been so slow. Life itself began very early on (barely several hundreds of millions years after the earth had cooled down sufficiently, about 3.8 billion years ago). But then it took almost two billion years before mitochondria developed from bacteria. For almost two billion years the most complex life-form on this planet was no more than bacteria. That is a long time. Perhaps our universe comprises numerous planets where simple life-forms such as bacteria abound but that have never developed mitochondria, so that they were never able to evolve into more complex life, such as jellyfish and people.

Mitochondria have been of enormous importance in the history of life. Furthermore, they are also responsible for making life finite, because they play an important role in aging. That is because mitochondria have a weakness: the DNA they store inside. That mitochondrial DNA contains the building and maintenance instructions for the mitochondria. It is very susceptible to damage, however, because it is inside the mitochondria, but that happens to be one of the worst places in a cell to store DNA.

The mitochondria are the energy generators of our cells; hence, continuous, intense chemical activity is taking place inside them, including the production of toxic, harmful, waste particles, or free radicals. Just as toxic smoke leaves a coal plant, the mitochondria release free radicals. These free radicals are small particles (atoms or molecules) that are very reactive; they attach themselves to all kinds of structures in our cells and damage them. Free radicals also react with the mitochondrial DNA, which is very close to the location where the free radicals are produced. That is a problem because the mitochondria need that DNA to build themselves, to reproduce (make copies of themselves), and to maintain and repair themselves. It is therefore not a good thing that vulnerable mitochondrial DNA is located inside the mitochondria. It would be similar to keeping the paper instructions for building your oven next to the hot oven itself, which continuously throws off hot sparks.

Mother Nature noticed that, too. That is why, during the past two billion years, she has tried to move as many pieces of mitochondrial DNA (genes) as possible out of the mitochondria and into the safety of the cell nucleus. It is much farther away from the free radical–producing mitochondria. More than a thousand mitochondrial genes (pieces of DNA that make up the code for proteins in the mitochondria) have already been moved to the cell nucleus—with the exception of 37 genes that code for about thirteen mitochondrial proteins. These genes are still located in the mitochondria, where they form the mitochondrial DNA that is susceptible to damage.

Babies have fresh, pristine mitochondria. Children have mitochondria that perform beautifully. Children can run around in the house and on the playground for hours without getting tired, with abundant energy. When you are 50, it is a different story. You tire more easily and it takes longer to recover from a long walk, or a game of tennis, or dancing the night away. As the decades pass, more and more mitochondrial DNA is damaged and your mitochondria do not function so well anymore. This is one of the causes of aging. The energy generators of our cells no longer function well, and we get all kinds of typical symptoms, problems, and diseases that come with aging. We tire more easily because our damaged mitochondria cannot produce enough energy (ATP). Old mitochondria in the brain provides less energy to the brain cells and cause a decline in functioning of the cells; as a result, your ability to learn new things declines, you have more difficulty retrieving words, and your thinking speed slows down. Old mitochondria in the heart provide less energy to the heart muscles, so that the heart pumps less well. Old mitochondria in the muscle cells weaken our muscle strength. Going upstairs becomes more difficult, one day you have a chairlift installed, and finally you are in a wheelchair. In short, the worse our mitochondria get, the less energy we have to move, to think, and ultimately to live.

Some people are born with a rare mitochondrial disease, whereby these typical symptoms of aging begin at a young age. Such diseases are caused because certain proteins in the mitochondria are not functioning well or not produced in sufficient quantities. It is not surprising that these diseases particularly affect tissues that use a lot of energy, like the brain, retina, heart, or muscles.

One example of such a mitochondrial diseases is MELAS (short for mitochondrial encephalopathy, lactate acidosis, and stroke-like episodes). This disease can occur in children of only a few years old. They suffer from muscle weakness and muscle aches because the mitochondria in the muscles do not produce sufficient energy. Sight and hearing decline because the eye cells and hearing cells produce insufficient energy and die because of that. These children can also have fierce headaches and epileptic episodes because the brain cells lack energy. Their heart and kidney function decreases, and they get diabetes. Finally they develop dementia, blindness, and deafness. It seems as if these children are affected decades too soon by all kinds of aging-related diseases that healthy people develop only at a much later age.

Another mitochondrial disease is the Kearns-Sayre syndrome (also called oculocraniosomatic neuromuscular disorder with unraveled red fibers in doctor's parlance). This disease usually begins with weakness of the eye muscles. These muscles need much energy to allow us to look around all day. When less of this energy is available due to a mitochondrial defect, the muscles around the eye are often the first to decline. The eyelid starts to droop because the small muscles that hold it up weaken (we see this in older people as well, and some opt for plastic surgery to correct it). People with this disease tend to move their head back to be able to see under the drooped eyelid. Next comes weakening of the muscles that move the eyeball, which you need to look around, the muscles in the arms and legs, and the muscles that enable you to swallow. Patients with this disease can also suffer vision loss, hearing loss, heart-rhythm disorders, movement disorders, and diabetes.

There are numerous other mitochondrial diseases. What they all have in common is that they cause all kinds of symptoms that we normally see in old age, such as muscle weakness, loss of vision and hearing, diabetes, or dementia. These are afflictions that most healthy people will develop with age when their mitochondrial functioning declines. Researchers have been able to induce all kinds of aging-related diseases in mice by giving them a toxic substance that interferes with the functioning of the mitochondria. In people, as well, functioning of the mitochondria can be disturbed by certain substances, the long-term effect of which is that they develop all kinds of conditions that mimic aging-related diseases. That substance can be a medication, for example a drug that is used to slow down HIV. One of the side effects of some HIV drugs is that they damage the mitochondria (fortunately, this does not apply to all HIV medications). HIV drugs aim to prevent the virus from replicating inside white blood cells (immune cells), which would otherwise lead to a severely incapacitated immune system. Without a proper immune system,

HIV patients would die from bacterial infections, viruses, and fungi—this stage of the disease we call AIDS. Like so many drugs, certain HIV medications can have side effects. These HIV drugs interfere with the functioning of a protein in the mitochondria. The mitochondria can then no longer properly multiply and mitochondrial function declines. The visible and tangible consequences manifest themselves only after patients have used this medication for many years. They develop nerve pain, often beginning in the feet because the nerves have been damaged by the poorly functioning mitochondria. They also develop all kinds of accelerated aging-related symptoms: Their blood vessels clog up faster, which increases their risk of a heart attack. They can also develop diabetes, as well as a syndrome called lipodystrophy. In this syndrome, fat disappears. That might seem like a good thing but the problem is that the fat moves from the right areas to the wrong ones. Fat under the skin, for example, moves from the face and the arms and legs to the abdomen. This causes thin arms and legs and a potbelly, which increases the risk of a heart attack, diabetes, and dementia. Such a belly is a typical phenomenon of aging. Since the fat disappears from under the skin, such as in the face, one gets sunken cheeks and looks older. The increased risk of heart attacks, diabetes, and lipodystrophy is the result of poorly functioning mitochondria, which can no longer properly burn and process fats and sugars.

Fortunately, not every patient who takes these particular HIV drugs develops these problems. The severity of problems also varies greatly from person to person and depends on whether the person exercises regularly and eats a healthy diet, which also has an effect on the health of the mitochondria. Furthermore, this medication is life-saving, for many people would prefer to live 25 years longer with this medication and then die of a side effect, such as a heart attack, than live without this medication and die within a few years of the adverse consequences of AIDS. As is often the case in medicine, one thing must be weighed against another.

Mitochondria also help explain why some population groups are more susceptible to certain aging-related diseases. People of African origin or from the Middle East are often more susceptible to various aging-related and affluence-related diseases resulting from an unhealthy lifestyle. It may be no coincidence that these are people who live in, or originate from, countries with a hot climate. In addition to energy (ATP), mitochondria also produce heat. The fact that warm-blooded mammals exist is due to mitochondria. Our constant body temperature of roughly 98°F is generated mainly by our mitochondria, which, as a by-product of their chemical activity, also produce heat. It was thanks to warm blood that mammals could emerge and subsequently colonize colder regions such as Europe, North America, and even the polar regions. This in contrast to cold-blooded animals, such as crocodiles, turtles, and lizards, which are found mainly in the warm tropics (their cells contain fewer mitochondria, so that they generate less heat and are therefore cold-blooded). The disadvantage of warm-bloodedness is that it costs a lot of energy: You need to eat much more, so that your mitochondria can continuously produce ATP and heat. That is why we eat at least three times per day—we need to feed our mitochondria. A cold-blooded snake can eat a goat and then go without food for two years, whereas people need to eat every few hours or they will get hungry again.

What does this have to do with a greater susceptibility to some aging-related diseases? Those whose ancestors have always lived in warm climates have differently functioning mitochondria. They produce less heat (because it is already warm enough), so that the production lines in the mitochondria move more slowly. They do not need to work as hard to create heat and keep the body temperature constant, but this also happens to increase the production of free radicals. Compare this with a production line in a coal plant. If it runs smoothly, fewer coals will drop off, but if the line moves more slowly and with stops and starts, more coals (free radicals) will drop down. That can be one reason why people whose ancestors lived in warm countries are more susceptible to all kinds of aging-related diseases: Their mitochondria get damaged faster. This can explain why, for example, people of African descent are more likely to develop cardiovascular disease and high blood pressure compared to those with European ancestors, who lived in colder regions for thousands of years. Even when African Americans live in the far north of the United States, they have inherited their mitochondria from their ancestors who lived in a warm country for thousands of years.[120]

In addition to people of African origin, a number of indigenous peoples are also more susceptible to affluence-related diseases. An example are the Pima people, who live on the border between Mexico and the United States. Almost 60 percent of adults there have type 2 diabetes. This enormous increase in diabetes began when they changed to a Western diet, with lots of white flour and processed red meat. These people have a greater risk of diabetes than Westerners (only about 10 percent of the European population has diabetes). So one population group may be much more sensitive than another to an unhealthy Western diet and aging-related diseases. Genetic differences play a role in this, including functioning of the mitochondria.

In the previous several pages we have discussed the role of mitochondria in the aging process. As times goes by, the functioning of the mitochondria declines as a result of their own ceaseless activity. Their strength is also their weakness: The mitochondria supply our life energy, literally and figuratively speaking. However, in the process of producing this energy, they slowly but definitely damage themselves. This mitochondrial decline plays a role in all kinds of problems that come with age: muscle weakness, fatigue, a heart that pumps less powerfully, forgetfulness, a potbelly, and diabetes. Some substances and certain drugs can also damage the mitochondria, so that the symptoms of aging occur faster. In the next chapters of the book we will discuss ways in which nutrition and future medical interventions can slow down the decline of our mitochondria and even make them young and healthy again.

SUMMARY

Mitochondria are the **power plants** of our cells. The ancestors of mitochondria were **small bacteria** that produced energy inside larger bacteria.

Mitochondria produce **ATP**: This is a small molecule that binds to proteins and activates or deactivates them (by changing the shape of the proteins).

ATP is the **life energy** that powers our body.

The mitochondria and the mitochondrial DNA they contain are damaged as we get older. As a result **less energy (ATP)** is produced, contributing to reduced functioning and the demise of

• Body cells: We tire faster and need more rest.

• Brain cells: Concentration, memory and thinking speed decline.

- Muscle cells: We experience loss of muscle mass, strength, and stamina.

- Heart cells: The heart cannot contract as well and weakens.

- Nerve cells: Reflexes become slower.

- Eye and ear cells: Sight and hearing diminish.

- Insulin and fat cells: We have an increased risk of type 2 diabetes.

Shoelaces and Strings

If we would believe the average health magazine or the numerous websites about health, it is clear why we age: DNA damage. That is one of the most frequently heard explanations of aging. Dietary supplements, expensive beauty creams, even more expensive facial serums, and all kinds of other antiaging treatments need to protect us from DNA damage as we get older.

But it is a bit more complicated than that. DNA is found in the innermost part of our cells, in the cell nucleus. It is actually a long string of atoms that contains the instructions for building proteins and to build our entire body, since almost all functions in the body are performed by proteins.

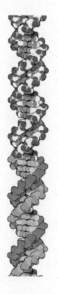

DNA is a long string of atoms shaped like a spiral staircase (each little ball is an atom). Each tread of the spiral staircase consists of certain molecules that contain the instructions for building proteins. These proteins perform almost all functions in the cell.

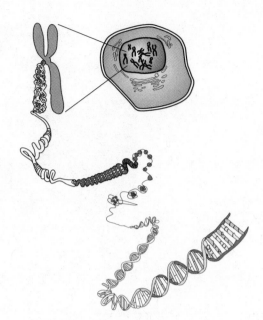

DNA is found in the cell nucleus. To fit itself into the cell nucleus it has to coil itself up tightly and thus forms the structures we call chromosomes.

The most popular explanation for aging is that DNA is damaged by free radicals. The more the DNA is damaged, the less clear the building instructions for making proteins. This decreases the functioning of our cells, hence they age. However, this DNA damage theory is not the whole story. First of all, most free radicals cannot reach our DNA, since it is stored safely in the cell nucleus. Nor is there a clear relationship between the speed at which the DNA of an animal species is damaged and its life span. Some animals suffer ongoing DNA damage but may still become very old.

Yet many people are convinced that it is mainly DNA damage that makes us age. They often refer to so-called accelerated aging diseases, diseases that makes people age at a faster rate. Most of these diseases are indeed caused by DNA damage. For that reason, many people think that DNA damage is the one and only contributor to aging. It is not that simple, however.

Consider the best-known accelerated aging disease, progeria, also called Hutchinson-Gilford's disease. Progeria patients age seven times faster than healthy people and on average live no more than about thirteen years. At that age they look as if they were 80: They are bald; have a thin, wrinkled, blue-veined skin; a pointed, hook-shaped nose; and thin arms and legs with very little muscle mass.

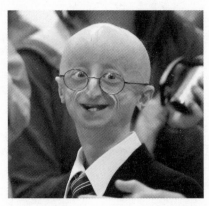

Young progeria patients look much older than they really are.
This is a photo of Sam Berns at age sixteen. His parents requested
that his lecture "My Philosophy for a Happy Life" be mentioned in
this book; it can be viewed on YouTube.
(Photo: Scott and Leslie Berns, The Progeria Foundation.)

Children with progeria also develop stiff joints (osteoarthritis) and vascular problems. They often die of a heart attack. Their intelligence remains normal and they are well aware of their accelerated aging process. How to deal with a body that ages rapidly and a short life is put into words by Sam Berns, a seventeen-year-old progeria patient, who gave a very inspiring lecture about his disease. It has been viewed millions of times on the Internet. Not long after giving this lecture, he died of the effects of progeria.

Progeria stems from heavy DNA damage. The DNA in the cell nucleus is damaged because the cell nucleus collapses, as it were. Normally, the cell nucleus is a robust, hollow ball with a wall built of proteins and fats, with DNA floating inside. In progeria, by contrast, a certain protein that builds up the wall of the cell nucleus has the wrong shape. Normally this protein functions as a kind of beam that supports the cell nucleus and gives it its round shape. Thousands of these proteins together shape the cell nucleus into a nice round ball. When these proteins have the wrong shape, however, the cell nucleus becomes unstable and becomes a weak structure with dents, much like a soccer ball that deflates. That is what causes the damage to the DNA. It makes progeria patients develop all kinds of problems, and they grow old faster. Because progeria patients age so quickly, and because the disease is caused by damaged DNA, many researchers thought that mainly DNA damage is responsible for normal aging. However, when we look at progeria in detail, we see that this disease is not really an imitation of the normal aging process. Progeria patients do experience certain typical aging symptoms, such as balding, cardiovascular disease, and arthritis, but they are exempt from others, such as Alzheimer's and Parkinson's disease, hearing and vision loss, weakening of the immune system, increased fats in the blood, and cataracts. In short, the symptoms of progeria do resemble those of aging to a certain extent, but many typical symptoms and diseases associated with aging do not occur.

DNA damage is not just the only reason we grow older. There are other processes involved, including sugar cross-linking, protein agglomeration, and defective mitochondria. These processes take decades to develop. Since progeria patients live only until their early teens, they do not have time to build up sufficient sugar cross-links, for example, to develop cataracts, or sufficient protein agglomeration in the brain that plays a role in Alzheimer's disease. Nevertheless, progeria patients do look like old people because in both progeria and normal aging, the end result is about the same: Cells die en masse. However, the cause is different: In progeria the cells die because their nuclei collapse, whereas in normal aging cells die of such factors as protein agglomeration, defective mitochondria, and cross-linking.

Such diseases as progeria show that DNA damage is not the whole story. Far from that even, because what happens *around* the DNA is also very important. This determines which parts of the DNA are active and therefore able to pass on instructions for building certain proteins. Let me explain this further. The DNA is rolled up tightly inside the cell nucleus. This happens by wrapping the DNA around spools (which in turn are proteins). These spools determine which pieces of DNA are rolled up tighter or looser. The more the DNA is unrolled, the more active and better able it is to pass on the building instructions for proteins. As we age, this process does not always run smoothly. Some pieces of DNA are unrolled too much; other pieces are rolled up too tightly. As a result, the cell no longer functions as well as it should. The science that studies this rolling and unrolling of DNA is called epigenetics, and it is a very interesting emerging field. (There are also other epigenetic mechanisms, but these are beyond the scope of this book.) It explains why DNA damage is only a part of the story. What happens around the DNA is probably more important.

In addition, another DNA-related process plays a role in aging, namely, shortening of the telomeres. Telomeres are pieces of DNA but not just any DNA; they are the end pieces of the DNA strings. The telomeres prevent unraveling of the DNA strings. You can compare the DNA in our cell nucleus with a collection of bundles of string. In each of our cell nuclei are 46 bundles of string; that is, 46 strings of DNA. One bundle of DNA strings is called a chromosome. If you would take one bundle of DNA string and unroll it to get one long string, the end pieces of this string are the telomeres. These telomeres themselves are also DNA, but they do not contain any instructions for building proteins.

What is the function of telomeres? Telomeres prevent the DNA string from unraveling at the ends. You can compare them to the small plastic sheaths or aglets on the ends of shoelaces, which prevent the shoelaces from unraveling. Nature invented such aglets in the form of telomeres at the ends of our DNA. What role do they play in in aging?

Each time our cells divide, the telomeres become a little bit shorter. That happens because the cellular machinery must unwind all those bundles of string to be able to duplicate them, and in the process always forgets a small piece at the end. After a certain number of cell divisions, usually about 60, the telomeres have become so short that they can no longer provide sufficient protection: The DNA starts to unravel and becomes unstable, similar to a fraying shoelace when its aglet is gone. With this unraveling, unstable DNA in the cell can no longer properly function, since it is the cell's DNA that contains the building instructions of all the proteins that maintain the cell and keep it alive.

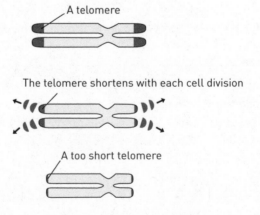

A telomere

The telomere shortens with each cell division

A too short telomere

The telomeres are the end pieces of the DNA string, or chromosome (bundle of string). The more often the cells divide, the more the telomeres shorten.

Telomeres can be considered a ticking clock that slowly counts down. With each tick—a cell division—the cell comes a little closer to its end because the telomeres shorten. Why would nature have created such a system? Would it not be better if our telomeres would always stay the same, so that our cells could stay young and healthy?

The main reason that they exist is that telomeres protect us against cancer. Telomeres function as a defense mechanism. Suppose that cells change into cancer cells and begin to divide uncontrollably. This will shorten the telomeres very rapidly (since they shorten with each cell division), causing the affected cells' DNA to unravel and the cancer cells to self-destruct. This protection mechanism, therefore, continuously protects us against new cancer cells in the body. Every day, thousands of cancer cells form in our body that are destroyed by this protection mechanism. This mechanism is not perfect, however. Every once in a while a mutation (a new characteristic) allows the cancer cell to avoid destruction and produce a protein that automatically lengthens the telomeres. This protein, *telomerase*, prevents the telomeres from shortening after each cell division and ensures that cancer cells can freely continue to divide and become immortal.

Some polyps and worms can also produce their own telomerase, which prevents them from aging, making them immortal. People produce telomerase only in the reproductive cells, which allows them to stay young (occasionally telomerase is also produced in white blood cells for a short time when they are forced to divide more often). As we have seen earlier, it is important for the reproductive cells to stay young, because babies need to be born fresh and young and not with Alzheimer's disease or heart failure.

There are a few congenital conditions whereby people are born with very short telomeres. That is unfair, because you are forced to start your life with a clock that has already counted halfway down. Think of a kitchen timer: For one person, it is set at 60 minutes; for another, at 40 minutes or ten minutes. In the mild form of this telomere-shortening disease, patients have moderately short telomeres. They often develop a disease called pulmonary fibrosis. Their lungs become filled with connective tissue, which causes shortness of breath and cough. As the disease progresses, they always feel out of breath and as if they may suffocate. They also become unable to do much because they run out of breath quickly. The fast-dividing cells that make the lung tissues flexible die too quickly due to shortening of the telomeres, and this makes the lungs stiff and breathing difficult. Pulmonary fibrosis usually begins when people are only 40 or 50 years old, which is much too young for the lungs to degenerate. It must be pointed out that only about 10 percent of cases of pulmonary fibrosis is caused by shortening of the telomeres; other forms of the disease are caused, for example, by autoimmune disease or silica dust.

Pulmonary fibrosis occurs when you have *moderately* short telomeres. When someone is born with *very* short telomeres, additional symptoms may appear at a younger age, often in childhood. One such disease is dyskeratosis congenita. Children with this disease get gray hair and become bald at a very young age. Their skin ages more rapidly, as well as the connective tissues in their lungs and liver. They have malformed nails that tend to fall off (nails are formed by rapidly dividing cells). Their immune system, too, declines rapidly—immune cells divide frequently (every hour billions of immune cells are produced in the body), which quickly shortens their telomeres. Immune cells are white blood cells that circulate in the bloodstream to track down such germs as bacteria, viruses, and parasites. With each division, the telomeres in the white blood cells become shorter, and in people born with already shorter telomeres, the time comes sooner when they can no longer make enough white blood cells. Patients often have a poorly functioning immune system at age ten, which makes them much more susceptible to infections and cancer (the immune system also cleans up cancer cells). In people with normal telomeres, this usually does not happen until they are 70 or older.

As is often the case in medicine, things can be even worse. People with Hoyeraal-Hreidarsson disease are born with even shorter telomeres than in dyskeratosis congenita. In this disease, the same kinds of symptoms occur at an even younger age: Often children in the first year of life have too much connective tissue in their organs, hair loss, continuous infections due to a failing immune system, and problems with nails and skin. The brain and the eyes are also affected. Usually these children live no more than a few years.

When telomeres are too short, they can cause all kinds of symptoms that we also see in normal aging, such as gray hair or deterioration of the immune system. However, some scientists are not convinced that telomeres play an important role in the aging process. There are, for example, also cells that divide very little, such as muscle cells and nerve cells, so their telomeres do not shorten much. Still, these cell age. There are also animals, such as mice, that have a short life span but have longer telomeres than humans. You would expect that the cells of mice with their longer telomeres could have many more divisions and thus a longer life span. Nevertheless, mice live to only two years old; and people for about 80 years.

Maybe it is not so much the length of the telomeres that plays a role (unless they are very short as in some diseases) but the *capacity* to lengthen or repair telomeres. All our cells have the capacity to produce a protein that can make short telomeres long again, namely, telomerase. This protein is active mainly in cells that need to divide frequently, such as sex cells or immune cells. Sometimes, however, telomerase can be active in other cells to make them younger. When mice are given telomerase, they live longer,[121] and when they are given a substance that inhibits telomerase, they die prematurely of all kinds of aging diseases. Researchers have discovered that Ashkenazi Jews, who tend to live to be very old, sometimes possess a particularly active form of telomerase, which ensures that their telomeres remain longer than usual.[122] Some worms, as well, can become immortal by activating telomerase in their body cells. They do this when they turn to sexless division. When the worms reproduce sexually (via egg cells and sperm cells), their body becomes mortal again because the capacity for immortality has then moved from the body cells to only the reproductive cells.

In short, the discussion about the role of telomeres in aging is ongoing. In any case, you, yourself, can ensure that your telomeres stay in good condition. People who follow a healthy Mediterranean diet generally have longer telomeres.[123] More exercise and less sitting (at our desks, in trains, and on sofas) can also help the telomeres to stay healthier.[124] Another study shows that a healthy life style can influence the activity of the telomerase protein and reduce the risk of prostate cancer.[125] Unhealthy foods, such as soft drinks, by contrast, lead to shorter telomeres.[126]

SUMMARY

DNA is a very long molecule that contains **building instructions** for our proteins, which are the building blocks and workhorses of our cells.

Telomeres are the **ends** of a DNA string (telomeres themselves also consist of DNA). They are the caps that ensure that the DNA string **does not unravel**.

Telomeres play a role in **aging**:

- With each cell division the telomeres shorten. When they become too short, the DNA is no longer protected (the caps are gone) and cell functioning declines. This particularly affects the stem cells because they must divide frequently.

- In cells that divide infrequently (muscle or nerve cells), the telomeres can still become damaged over time and send out signals that impair proper cellular functioning.

Cancer cells, reproductive cells, and some worms can become **immortal** by producing **telomerase**, a protein that lengthens the shortened telomeres.

Good nutrition and sufficient **exercise** can counteract the shortening of telomeres.

Progeria is often called an aging disease, but although it does imitate some symptoms of aging, it is not really an aging disease.

Other Causes and Conclusion

Aging is a complex process. We have discussed four important reasons why we age: protein agglomeration; an excess of carbohydrates, which produce IGF and sugar cross-links; defective mitochondria; and changes related to DNA, such as the telomeres and epigenetics. However, there are other reasons that we age, and it is very likely that in the future other aging mechanisms will be discovered. The four reasons we have discussed are the most important causes we know about today. They are the four horsemen of death and together they represent a formidable enemy that undermines our health as the decades pass. It starts with a lack of energy when you have to run to catch the train or bus, and the first gray hairs and crow's feet, and will gradually develop into a wide specter of aging diseases, such as cardiovascular disease or dementia.

These four forces make our cells age, not only our regular body cells but also our *stem cells*. These cells are spread throughout our body and create billions of new cells daily. Stem cells in the gut continuously produce new gut cells, since gut cells live only about five days. Stem cells in the bone marrow create two million red blood cells per second. Stem cells in the skin renew our entire skin every month. Stem cells in our bones rebuild our skeleton every ten years. It is our stem cells that make us on a regular basis. When they are damaged, however, by aging processes, such as protein agglomeration, cross-links, DNA damage, or short telomeres, they also age and ultimately stop working or die. As time goes by, hardly any functional stem cells remain, so that we cannot renew and replenish our precious tissues—we literally wither away. Our muscles are no longer maintained and restored, so that our arms and legs become thinner (sarcopenia). We have trouble going upstairs and we fall more easily, whether or not we break our already fragile bones. The fat cells under the skin of our face slowly disappear, giving us a bony, wrinkly face. Our skin is no longer renewed and becomes thinner and more fragile. Our hair turns gray, because the stem cells around the root of the hair die and produce fewer melanocytes. Melanocytes are cells that produce dark pig-ments, so that hair can be brown, black, or blond, depending on the amount of pigment (melanin) the hair contains. Interestingly, aging stem cells do not always have to wither away and die. Some aged stem cells just go into "off" mode. They become *senescent stem cells*, meaning that they stop divid-ing, so that the tissues cannot be replenished. Normal body cells (non–stem cells, like skin cells or liver cells) can also become *senescent cells*, as a defense mechanism against cancer. When a normal body cell becomes too damaged (mutated), it gets brakes put on, so that the cell cannot divide anymore. Such a damaged cell that cannot divide anymore is a senescent cell. That way, the senescent cell cannot further transform (mutate) into cancer cells that divide uncontrollably. Sounds good, but there is a drawback. Senescent stem cells also produce all kinds of toxic substances that damage the cellular environ-ment, impairing the proper functioning of the tissues, and making them age. For example, lots of senescent stem cells and senescent skin cells in our skin contribute to wrinkles, sagging skin and other undeniable signs of aging.

Some people who become very old have strong and long-lasting stem cells. An example is Hendrikje van Andel-Schipper, a Dutch woman who died at age 115. Researchers discovered that at the end of her life, this woman still produced mil-lions of blood cells, thanks to a few very strong and tenacious stem cells. A young person has about 1,300 active blood stem cells, which make billions of blood cells every day (red blood cells and white blood cells, which form the immune system). The older we get, the more of these blood stem cells are destroyed or switched off by aging. Mrs. Van Andel-Schipper had only a few functioning stem cells left (or to be more specific, only a few stem cell clones, which are groups of similar stem cells), which were responsible for producing her blood cells.[127]

Now that we have a better understanding of why we age, we can see what the future may bring. As scientists further investigate the aging process, they may be able to develop better ways to slow it down and ultimately potentially turn it back. That is what the next chapter is about.

3

The Longevity Staircase

What can we do to slow down the aging process? Scientists have learned a lot more about aging in the last decade than in the thousands of years before. New discoveries follow each other with unprecedented speed. To better organize these new insights and knowledge, and to make maximum use of their potential, I have designed a plan for living a longer and healthier life. It can be represented in the form of a staircase, which currently has four steps. Each step contains a method to slow down the aging process and stay young longer. At the bottom of the staircase, on step 1, you will find the simplest method but this may also be the least effective one. This method consists of consuming essential nutrients that the body needs to function properly, such as certain vitamins, minerals, and fats. The second step describes hormesis, a process that allows organisms to live longer. Step 3 tells you how growth stimulation can be reduced via your diet. The higher up we go, the more effective and promising the methods become. The top step consists of methods that are not yet available today or are used only to treat certain rare diseases but, as we shall see, in the future these methods may become accessible to everyone to slow down or even reverse aging. Since currently so much knowledge is circulating about aging, this staircase is a work in progress and new steps may be added as new discoveries are made.

The Longevity Staircase

Step 4: Reverse aging
Via new therapies, such as vaccines against protein agglomeration, lysosomal protein therapy, sugar cross-link breakers, mitochondrial repair, rejuvenating substances in the blood, stem cell therapy, or CRISPR proteins.*

Step 3: Reduce growth stimulation
Via foods that supply slower carbohydrates and animal proteins. Via calorie restriction or fasting.

Step 2: Stimulate hormesis
Via mildly toxic substances in foods (such as flavonoids) or exercise (such as high-intensity interval training [HIIT]).

Step 1: Avoid deficiencies
Via sufficient intake of relevant micronutrients from healthy foods and natural dietary supplements as needed.

* clustered regularly interspaced short palindromic repeats (genome editing technology)

Step 1: Avoid Deficiencies

It is remarkable that in the West millions of people are overweight but still suffer from malnutrition. They are overweight because they consume too many *macronutrients*, and they are malnourished due to a lack of *micronutrients*. Macronutrients are carbohydrates (sugars), fats, and proteins. These foods supply energy. Micronutrients are healthy substances, such as vitamins, flavonoids, stilbenes, phenolic acids, lignans, and omega-3 fatty acids. Micronutrients are needed for the proper functioning of the body. Much of the food we eat today consists mainly of macronutrients with very few micronutrients. Such foods are sometimes referred to as empty calories: soft drinks, fast food, bread, pasta, potatoes, rice, chips, and baked goods. These foods supply many calories but few micronutrients.

An important reason for this is the industrialization of our food. Thanks to recently invented industrial processes, enormous amounts of macronutrients can be produced very cheaply. Via these processes, beets, corn, sunflower seeds, cows, and chickens are turned into mountains of refined sugar, extracted oil, and packaged protein. These are then combined into new foods that never existed before, such as cakes and cookies, made of sugar, starch, and trans fats; hamburgers made from cheap red meat rich in omega-6 fatty acids from grain-fed, mega-barn cows, with the addition of salt and flavor enhancers to make them tasty; and soft drinks full of glucose and fructose, which can be made cheaply from corn and diluted with artificial flavorings and phosphates. All of these foods accelerate aging. Some physicians speak of "Frankenstein food" because these foods resemble a collection of dissected parts of nature concocted in a laboratory, not wholesome foods, such as nuts, vegetables, fruit, and fish that still look the way they are found in nature.

The result of this industrialization is that we fill ourselves up with food and drink that make us fat and supply few micronutrients. A deficiency of certain micronutrients can undermine our health in the short term as well as in the long term. In the short term, a deficiency can manifest itself in the form of all kinds of vague health problems, such as fatigue, poor concentration or brain fog, irritability, or muscle aches. After a while, many people consider these problems normal or an inevitable sign of aging. Sometimes these problems become so worrisome that people go to the doctor. He or she then orders various tests to see if the patients might have cancer, diabetes, or a serious neurological disorder. In most cases nothing is found, while the patients suffer from a deficiency of all kinds of micronutrients, such as omega-3 fatty acids, certain B vitamins, or magnesium, which standard blood tests cannot easily detect.

In the long term as well, a deficiency of micronutrients can harm our health. A chronic shortage of, say, magnesium, B vitamins, vitamin K, selenium, or potassium can increase the risk of all kinds of diseases related to aging. Many proteins in our body need these nutrients to function properly. You could view these proteins as small machines that can work only if there is a particular cogwheel, such as selenium or magnesium. These proteins are involved in energy metabolism, clotting of blood, detoxification, or removal of free radicals. A chronic deficiency of all kinds of micronutrients can undermine our long-term health.

Around this concept an entire industry has been established: the dietary supplement industry. It urges us to continuously use supplements to keep us healthy and protect us against all kinds of diseases. However, many large studies have shown that dietary supplements of minerals and vitamins do not decrease mortality (risk of dying). Whether you take vitamin and mineral supplements or not, you do not live longer according to these studies.[128–130] Does that mean that supplements are useless? No, it only means that studies show that many vitamin and mineral supplements do not really work—and that should not surprise us. But that doesn't mean that supplements are useless. Let me first explain why so many studies show no real effect of supplements on our health or life span.

First, the supplements usually contain doses that are much too small to have any effect. An average multivitamin supplement, for example, contains only 80 mg of magnesium and 50 mg of potassium. An adult ideally needs 300 to 600 mg of magnesium and about 5,400 mg of potassium per day. In prehistoric times, the average potassium intake was even 11,000 mg. It is no wonder that many studies of dietary supplements do not show a clear effect, since the doses they contain are too low.

Furthermore, supplements often come in a form that is poorly absorbed by the body. Take copper, for instance. Many supplements contain copper in the form of copper oxide, most of which is not absorbed by the gut.[131] The same is true for magnesium. Supplements often contain magnesium oxide, which is not nearly absorbed as well as, say, magnesium malate. Magnesium oxide is even so badly absorbed that it is also used as a laxative, because most of it stays in the gut, creating a purgative effect.

Furthermore, the substances in supplements, including those used in scientific studies, are often not combined in the right way. For example, there was a long-term study that found no effect of a supplement containing various vitamins and minerals, including zinc, but the supplement did not contain copper. If you give zinc to a person for a long time, you also need to add copper, because when you take zinc, you absorb less copper. Thus, if you take a supplement with a relatively high dose of zinc (20 mg)—as was done in this study—in the long term you could develop a copper deficiency. Both a deficiency and an excess of copper can increase the risk of cardiovascular disease, so the dose needs to be exactly right.

Even if the supplement contains the right dose of a substance, in an easily absorbed form, and in the right combination with other vitamins and minerals, problems can still occur. Many supplements contain only one form of a substance. Take, for example, vitamin E. There are eight different forms of this vitamin, but most supplements contain only alpha-tocopherol. If you take only one form, you absorb less of other forms of vitamin E, such as beta-tocopherol, gamma-tocopherol, and alpha-tocotrienol. The proteins in the gut wall that absorb vitamin E are then saturated with that one form of vitamin E, so that you absorb less of the other forms of the vitamin. This also applies to beta-carotene. Supplements that contain a high dose of beta-carotene prevent the absorption of other carotenes, so that your risk of cancer may increase.[132]

Not only the absorption but also the effectiveness of a substance may depend on the form. Take selenium, for instance. There are numerous different forms of selenium: selenium methionine, triphenyl phosphine selenide, isoselenocyanate, phosphine selenide, and so forth. One form of selenium can be a thousand times more active than another. One study shows that selenium methionine does not decrease the risk of cancer,[133] whereas another study found that people who take selenium yeast had half the risk of cancer.[134] Some researchers believe that this difference can be explained by the fact that selenium yeast contains other forms of selenium that have a stronger effect on the body than selenium methionine alone.

Finally, yet another reason dietary supplements used in studies often show no effect, is that the synergetic effect is ignored. Many substances work together, so if you do not include all of them in a supplement, there will be no, or only a minimal, effect. For example, vitamin A, vitamin D, and omega-3 fatty acids all attach to one particular protein, which then acts as a switch to activate the cells. If you take only vitamins A and D and too little omega-3 fatty acids, the protein will not function well. Compare it with a car that needs four wheels; if it has only three, it cannot run properly. A study in which only vitamin A is given, has no effect unless it is combined with vitamin D, omega-3 fatty acids, or other additions at the same time.

All in all, it is not surprising that many studies of dietary supplements do not show any effect. Then, people split into two camps. Some immediately conclude that all supplements are useless, but that is a superficial and hasty conclusion. On the other hand, there are those who continue to believe in supplements as a remedy for all kinds of ailments, but that is too optimistic. It is difficult to make physical ailments disappear with a few supplements. The body is very complex and it needs many substances to work properly, you cannot add them all into one supplement. Nevertheless, studies show that *some* supplements can be useful, for example because so many people have a deficiency of it despite having a varied diet or because those substances in high enough doses can have a positive influence on certain mechanisms in the body.

Take the B vitamins, for instance. They form a family: vitamins B_1, B_2, B_3, B_5, B_6, B_7, B_9 (folic acid, also called vitamin B_{11}), and vitamin B_{12}. Many proteins in our body need B vitamins to be able to function, certainly proteins involved in the metabolism. The B vitamins bind with these proteins, enabling them to work. The organ with the highest metabolism is the brain, so it is not surprising that it needs lots of B vitamins to keep functioning properly. Various studies show that older people who have few B vitamins in their blood have a greater risk of shrinking of the brain. This is a phenomenon that often occurs with aging. The brain can even shrink so much that the blood vessels between the brain and the skull come under pressure and break easily, so that, for example, a minor fall on the head can cause a substantial brain bleeding.

One study found that in people with little vitamin B_{12} in their blood, there can be six times greater shrinkage of the brain than in people with sufficient vitamin B_{12}.[135] Researchers who gave high doses of vitamins B_6, folic acid (B_9), and vitamin B_{12} to a group of elderly people, observed in brain scans that there was seven times less brain shrinkage in this group than in a group that did not take supplements.[136] The researchers concluded that "the disease process responsible for cognitive decline can be slowed down significantly and maybe even halted." A more recent study, however, in which participants were given high doses of only two types of B vitamins (B_9 and B_{12}) did not show an effect on cognition.[137] Does that mean that high doses of vitamin B are useless? Not according to scientists like Sudha Seshadri, a professor and Alzheimer's researcher, who stated, "The second study did not last long enough and the methods used to measure cognition were too crude." This method was the Mini-Mental State Examination. This test is very crude and only people with advanced dementia will score low on it (the test asks things like spelling "world" backwards or remembering a series of words; if you had a bad night of sleep you will score differently from when you are well-rested and after a nice cup of coffee). Furthermore, cognition does not decline all at once; rather, it is a very slow, creeping process that may take tens of years to develop. It may be asking too much to slow down this process with supplements to such an extent that it would be possible to detect obvious changes on a very insensitive test after a few months or even two years of supplementation. Besides, other studies show that high doses of B vitamins can indeed improve cognition in older people.[138, 139] Finally, in many vitamin B studies, only one or two B vitamins are used (usually vitamins B9 and B12), whereas other B vitamins are also important and work together; for example, vitamin B6, which plays an important role in various metabolic processes such as sugar and fat metabolism, works with vitamin B12 and B9 in various ways.

In short, B vitamins can be useful, but combined and often in higher doses than those found in most supplements. B vitamins can be taken in large doses, with the exception of vitamin B6 (the dose of this vitamin should be no more than 20 to 50 mg per day because an excess of it over long periods can cause nerve pain—the exact maximum amount varies from expert to expert and institute to institute). You can take B-vitamin supplements with several times the recommended dose of B vitamins. The B-vitamin doses in the aforementioned studies are often even higher. The best thing to do is to take a B-vitamin complex (vitamins B1 through B12), since they all work together to achieve optimum functioning of the body. It is regrettable that most people in the West do not get sufficient B vitamins from their diet, including many people who believe they are eating variedly and healthy.[140, 141]

Magnesium is another example of a micronutrient that is lacking in many people. Magnesium binds to all kinds of proteins to make them function better. Like the B vitamins, this mineral is important for our metabolism, including sugar metabolism. Magnesium improves the ability to process sugars.[142–144] That is important because the older we get, the less the body is able to process sugars, which increases our risk of various aging-related diseases, including type 2 diabetes, cardiovascular disease, and dementia. Magnesium can also lower blood pressure, which is good for the blood vessels.[145] It can also reduce the risk of heart-rhythm abnormalities, which are an important cause of death in older people.[146, 147] Heart-rhythm abnormalities can occur spontaneously because the heart has aged, but also after a heart attack. The heart attack damages the heart, making it more susceptible to rhythm abnormalities.

Many people do not get enough magnesium via their diet, even if they already eat quite healthy, so they can opt for supplements. Be sure to take a good form of magnesium. As we have seen, magnesium oxide is hardly absorbed in the gut. One of the best forms of magnesium is magnesium malate. It is much better absorbed and malate has also interesting health effects. Make sure the dose is high enough, such as 300 to 600 mg of magnesium per day.

But the best thing is to get as much as possible via your diet. Food contains forms of magnesium that can be more easily absorbed and are more active than that in supplements. That is because the magnesium in food is packaged together with all kinds of cofactors, substances that improve its activity and absorption, in contrast to the magnesium in supplements, which does not include these extra cofactors. A study with 60,000 participants shows that people who ate many foods rich in magnesium had a 50 percent lower risk of a heart attack.[148] These foods include green leafy vegetables, such as cabbage, lettuce, and spinach, as well as legumes (peas, beans, and lentils), nuts, and seeds.

Another example of a nutrient that is often deficient in the Western diet is selenium. Many people's own antioxidant proteins, which are thousand times better at counteracting free radicals than any antioxidant supplement, as well as many immune system proteins, need selenium for proper functioning. Selenium can also decrease the risk of cancer. Most Europeans get too little selenium because the soil in Europe contains very little of it. You could take a supplement, such as selenium yeast (instead of selenium methionine, as we have seen earlier). But be careful: Selenium is a powerful substance and you can easily take too much. A supplement containing no more than 100 mcg (micrograms, not milligrams) is best, since you will also get some selenium from your diet.

The best thing is to get selenium from your diet as much as possible, because food contains various forms of it as well as cofactors that allow it to be more easily absorbed and do its work. Seafood, such as oysters and fish, contains a lot of selenium. Seeds and nuts also contain selenium. One of the richest sources of selenium is Brazil nuts. One Brazil nut contains 60 to 90 mcg of selenium, which is a lot. Some people eat a Brazil nut from time to time instead of taking a supplement, but be careful: Too much selenium, including from Brazil nuts, is not healthy. Eat, for example, only a few Brazil nuts per week.

Many people also have a deficiency of vitamin D. Vitamin D is necessary for the immune system, metabolism, healthy bones, the brain, and many other body processes. A lack of vitamin D is related to a higher risk of a heart attack, cancer, and such diseases as multiple sclerosis and diabetes.[149, 150] Various large studies (meta-analyses) show that vitamin D supplements can reduce the risk of heart disease or death.[151–153] Some other studies do not show a significant effect of vitamin D on health.[154] The problem, however, is that often the amounts of vitamin D used were too low—400 to 800 units per day, whereas most researchers recommend at least 2,000 units—and that these studies did not last long enough. To see significant effect on mortality, you need to take the vitamin for several years, at least. A large study shows that a significant effect is obtained only when vitamin D is taken for longer than three years.[153] Another problem with many studies is that the wrong form of vitamin D is used, namely, ergocalciferol (vitamin D2), which does not work as well as cholecalciferol (vitamin D3). Studies show that vitamin D2 can even increase mortality, whereas vitamin D3 decreases it.[152] Currently better-designed studies are being conducted in which participants receive 2,000 units of vitamin D3 per day for five years. The first results will be available in the coming years.

Should you, or should you not, take vitamin D supplements? Many government authorities recommend them, particularly for older people or people wearing head scarves and therefore who get less sun exposure. Often, the recommended dose is 400 to 800 units of vitamin D per day (do not confuse units with micrograms). Some scientists believe this is too low, and that it should be more in the range of 2,000 units per day. It is best to have vitamin D level in your blood tested. If it is too low, you can take vitamin D supplements in the form of vitamin D3, or cholecalciferol. Ideally, you should have a minimum of 30 ng/ml (or 75 nmol/l) in your blood. On the other hand, you need to be careful not to take too much, such as more than 8,000 units per day for many months, because vitamin D is fat-soluble, which means that an excess cannot easily be removed via the urine. If 8,000 units sounds like a lot, take a look at one study[155] wherein older people were given a one-time injection of 500,000 units of vitamin D! (No wonder there was a higher risk of hip fractures instead of the lower risk that was expected. Too much of a good thing can be bad for you.)

In addition to taking supplements, there are other ways to increase your vitamin D level. Your body can make vitamin D via exposure to sunlight, which converts substances in your skin into vitamin D. The problem is that sunlight also ages the skin. Furthermore, many Western countries are far north of the equator, so that sunlight comes in at an angle so it is less effective and even exposing oneself to sunlight may not produce sufficient vitamin D. In addition to sunlight, you can also raise your vitamin D level via your food. Mushrooms and salmon, for example, contain vitamin D. A study found that people who ingested a lot of vitamin D via their diet had a lower risk of Alzheimer's disease.[156] This lower risk is not only due to vitamin D, of course, because food rich in vitamin D often also contains many other substances that are good for the brain, such as omega-3 fatty acids in salmon and certain polysaccharides in mushrooms. Anyhow, most foods contain little or no vitamin D, so that it is almost impossible to get sufficient vitamin D from our food, especially if you consume a Western diet. In this case, supplements can be a good solution.

In almost all studies in which vitamin D is given, this is done without adding another vitamin; namely, vitamin K. This vitamin works in combination with vitamin D. Vitamin K is sometimes called a forgotten vitamin because it is not well known. That is regrettable because we need it for strong bones and healthy blood vessels, two things that noticeably deteriorate when we get older. Our bones become weaker as we age, causing osteoporosis (also called brittle bones), and our blood vessels calcify, which increases the risk of heart attack and stroke. Brittle bones and calcified blood vessels are related: Physicians often see patients who present both problems at the same time. It seems as if the calcium leaves the bones and settles in the blood vessel walls. A lack of vitamin K may play a role in that process because it ensures that calcium in our body goes to the right place: to the bones and not the blood vessel walls. That is why vitamin K can at the same time decrease the risk of brittle bones and calcification of the blood vessels.

Osteoporosis is a common problem as we age, particularly for women. Osteoporosis can cause older people to fracture their hip in a fall, or even break their wrist by lifting a cup of coffee, simply because their bones are so fragile. A broken hip can be the beginning of the end for an older person; it is often followed by a serious hip operation and months-long revalidation and immobility. This then makes the person much more susceptible to cardiovascular disease, thrombosis, and a general accelerated decline. Vitamin K decreases the risk of osteoporosis, according to many studies. For example, one study found that women who took vitamin K supplements had an 81 percent lower risk of bone fractures.[157]

While the bones become more fragile as we age, the blood vessels harden and calcify. This accumulation of calcium in the blood vessels increases the risk of a heart attack. The more calcification, the greater the risk of a heart attack. Vitamin K can slow down this calcification as well. Rats that were given vitamin K had less calcification of the blood vessels;[158] people whose diet contains ample vitamin K have less blood vessel calcification.[159] On the other hand, people who take blood thinners, such as warfarin, which counteracts vitamin K, have a greater risk of calcification of the blood vessels and heart valves,[160] an effect that can be corrected by taking more vitamin K (however, people who take warfarin need to be careful with vitamin K—see box).[161] Vitamin K could even explain why people with severe osteoporosis have more wrinkles. How is that possible? A chronic lack of vitamin K prevents calcium from getting into the bones, causing osteoporosis. The free-floating calcium then binds with the elastin and collagen proteins in the skin, making the skin more rigid and wrinkly (other aging processes, like sugar cross-links, also play a role in wrinkles).

Our skin, blood vessels, and bones are all connected; hence, wrinkles, cardiovascular disease, and osteoporosis can be viewed as related symptoms. Of course, it is not only vitamin K that plays a role in all this. It also does not mean that everyone with lots of wrinkles has osteoporosis. But can vitamin K help prevent wrinkles? More research is needed to see if that is possible. We do know that there are people with rare diseases whose vitamin K metabolism is not working properly. These people have more wrinkles, skin folds, and flaccid skin.[162]

In addition, vitamin K also makes the mitochondria function better. That is a good thing because the longer our mitochondria remain healthy, the slower we age.[163] That is also one reason that sufficient intake of vitamin K decreases the risk of typical aging-related diseases, such as Alzheimer's disease, diabetes, and cardiovascular disease.[164–166]

So vitamin K is an important vitamin. How can we get more of it? There are two forms of it: vitamin K1, which is found in plants (green leafy vegetables, such as cabbage and spinach) and vitamin K2, found mainly in animal products, such as cheese. Vitamin K2 is the strongest form. Bacteria in our intestines convert vitamin K1 from plants to vitamin K2. Products like fermented soybeans (natto, miso, and tempeh) also contain a lot of vitamin K2 because bacteria in the soybeans produce this vitamin during the fermentation process. There are numerous variants of both vitamins K1 and K2, such as vitamin K2-7, K2-8, and so on. Most supplements contain only one form; namely, vitamin K2-7. However, there are many more forms of vitamin K than a supplement can contain. It is best, therefore, to get as much vitamin K as possible from food by eating more fermented foods (natto, miso, tempeh, and cheese), green leafy vegetables (like spinach, cabbage, and brussels sprouts), and herbs (such as parsley).

People whose diet contains ample vitamin K have an almost 60 percent lower risk to die of a heart attack.[167] The well-known Nurses' Health Study found that women who got a lot of vitamin K from their diet, on average had a 30 percent lower risk of breaking a hip.[168] According to a Japanese study, women who frequently ate natto had a lower risk of bone decalcification; according to the researchers, this was due to the high vitamin K content of natto.[169] Natto is one of the richest sources of vitamin K2. Despite its bad taste, in Japan natto is often eaten for breakfast. A little soy sauce and mustard may improve the taste somewhat, enabling you to get a good dose of vitamin K.

Vitamin K and Blood Thinners

Some patients who use "vitamin K antagonists" like warfarin must be careful. These drugs thin the blood by interfering with vitamin K metabolism. Warfarin reduces the effectiveness of vitamin K, and vitamin K in turn reduces the effectiveness of warfarin. As we have seen, vitamin K can reduce the risk of calcification of the blood vessels. In short, a physician must weigh which is more important: keeping the blood thin with warfarin (which is most important in many serious and potentially dangerous conditions, like atrial fibrillation, whereby the heart contracts irregularly and can then produce blood clots that could travel to the brain and cause a stroke) or a potentially higher risk of calcification of the blood vessels in the long term.[160, 170] Fortunately, other blood thinners have now been developed that do not have the side effects of warfarin.

As we have seen, dietary supplements often do not work because they are taken in too low doses. One example is the mineral potassium. Most supplements contain only about 50 mg of potassium. However, potassium is an important substance in the body. This mineral binds to proteins (and to the walls of our cells) and affects how well they function. Potassium in the body is the counterpart of sodium, which is found in the salt we use in our food (salt is also called sodium chloride). In the West, we eat too much sodium and too little potassium, which is found mainly in fruit, vegetables, and nuts. In prehistoric times, before the emergence of the agricultural industry, our ancestors consumed an average of 11 g of potassium per day and only 0.7 g of sodium. Today, the situation is reversed: We eat about 4 g of sodium per day and only 2.5 g of potassium. That is bad for our body, particularly in the long term and mainly for our heart and blood vessels. When the relationship between sodium and potassium is out of balance, it results in a higher risk of various aging-related diseases, such as high blood pressure, which in turn can dramatically increase the risk of heart attack or stroke. In many primitive tribes across the world high blood pressure is very rare, even in the elderly. One reason is the high intake of potassium via their diet.

For many years, we have been told that eating too much salt is unhealthy, but that is only half of the story: A lack of potassium also plays a role. That also explains why reducing salt intake has only a disappointing effect on reducing blood pressure. When people eat less salt but still too little potassium, the relationship is still unbalanced.[171] This illustrates how often in scientific studies things are viewed too narrowly: One substance is increased or decreased, in the hope there will be some change. When nothing happens, this is usually interpreted to mean that the substance does not work. However, as said earlier, a car needs all four of its wheels to be able to go.

Potassium can lower blood pressure.[172] That is particularly important to reduce the risk of a stroke. A too-high blood pressure damages the thousands of miles of hair-thin blood vessels in our brain, an organ that needs a continuously high supply of oxygen and nutrients and therefore has a very extensive network of blood vessels. For each gram of potassium we eat daily, the risk of a stroke decreases by 11 percent.[173] That is why it is important to take in more potassium. But supplements alone are not enough, because these contain very little or no potassium. The best way to get more potassium in your diet is by eating more vegetables, fruit, legumes, and nuts.

If you can find it, you could also use potassium salt instead of regular salt. Potassium salt is potassium chloride, whereas regular salt is sodium chloride. In some supermarkets you can find much healthier salt, for example a mixture of 70 percent potassium salt and 30 percent sodium salt. Regular salt is always about 100 percent sodium chloride. Do not be fooled by the so-called Himalayan salt or sea salt. These supposedly healthier salts still contain more than 99 percent sodium chloride (regular salt) and only a minuscule amount of other minerals. You can also use salt that contains more than 90 percent potassium salt but it is quite bitter. Some researchers believe that replacing regular salt with potassium salt was an important intervention in a famous study done in Finland. In this study, thousands of Fins were urged to eat a healthier diet, and they reduced their risk of heart attack by an average of 60 percent.[174] One way this result was achieved was by adding potassium salt. By using potassium salt, it is possible to get much higher daily doses of potassium than via the average supplement.

One final word about another nutrient many people are deficient of: iodine. This mineral is very important for our metabolism, energy levels, immune system and thyroid function. A deficiency can cause fatigue, muscle pains, concentration problems and all other kinds of subtle but bothersome issues. In most Western countries, there is a rampant deficiency in iodine, even despite some countries mandating to add iodine to bread. How is this possible? One reason is that the soil in many countries is too depleted in iodine. Another is that many people eat too little seafood. Fish, shellfish and seaweed contain lots of iodine (seaweed even contains huge amounts of iodine, so limit its consumption to one time per week). In prehistoric times, people often lived near coastlines, rivers, or lakes, so they got plenty of iodine from seafood. And prehistoric hunter-gatherers who lived inland could get iodine from eggs or from the thyroid glands they ate from hunted animals. But the average Westerner, who hardly eats any fish, let alone regularly a fresh thyroid gland, is often deficient in this nutrient. So a daily iodine supplement can be very useful for many people. The advised daily dose is 150 to maximum 200 microgram (not milligram) of iodine.

The first step of the longevity staircase involves having a diet with sufficient micronutrients. Lack of many micronutrients can accelerate the aging process and undermine health in the long term. Today's industrialized food provides too many empty calories, food that consists mainly of carbohydrates, fats, and proteins and contains very few micronutrients. Many thousands of micronutrients are important for our health, too many to get them all into one supplement. Dietary supplements are therefore not the solution, because people who have a lack of one nutrient, usually also have a lack of hundreds of other nutrients. These are nutrients like flavonoids, stilbenes, coumarins, isothiocyanates, indoles, omega-3 fatty acids, carotenes, lutein, and prebiotic fiber. These substances interact with important proteins, the genome, epigenome, microbiome, cell receptors, the cell membrane, and innumerable other mechanisms. Only a healthy, varied diet can provide all these substances. This is the first and most important step. But that does not mean that supplements are useless. Studies show that various specific supplements, if they contain the right substances in a high enough dose and in the correct form, can be useful for improving health or slowing down the aging process. These substances include magnesium (in the form of magnesium malate), selenium (from selenium yeast), potassium (in high enough amounts), vitamin D, vitamin K (in the right form), and iodine.

SUMMARY

Step 1: Ensuring a **sufficient intake of important micronutrients** can slow down the aging process and reduce the risk of aging-related diseases.

The **industrialization** of our food provides too many **empty calories** with many **macronutrients** (carbohydrates, fats, and proteins) and few **micronutrients** (such as vitamins and minerals).

Examples of important **micronutrients** are

B vitamins: reduce age-related shrinking of the brain and play an important role in energy metabolism, among other things.

Food rich in B vitamins:

- Seafood: salmon, mussels, shrimp

- Oatmeal

- Vegetables

- Nuts and seeds

- Chicken and eggs

Supplement: Best is a supplement that contains various B vitamins in sufficiently high doses.

Magnesium: good for the heart and blood vessels, plays an important role in the sugar and energy metabolism.

Food rich in magnesium:

- Green leafy vegetables: kale, brussels sprouts, spinach

- Nuts and seeds

- Legumes

Supplement: Best is a supplement in the form of magnesium malate providing 300 to 600 milligrams of magnesium per day.

Selenium: component of proteins that neutralizes free radicals or is involved in the immune system.

Food rich in selenium:

- Nuts: Brazil nuts—no more than a few per week

- Seeds and pits

- Seafood: salmon, sardines, tuna, crab, oysters, mussels, squid

- Mushrooms: portobello, shiitake, cremini

Supplement: selenium yeast, 100 micrograms per day.

Vitamin D: important for the immune system, metabolism, cardiovascular health, reduces the risk of osteoporosis.

Sunlight: produces vitamin D but ages the skin

Supplement: cholecalciferol (vitamin D_3), 1,000 to 2,000 units per day (monitoring via blood tests).

Vitamin K: counteracts hardening of the blood vessels, reduces the risk of osteoporosis, works in combination with vitamin D.

Food rich in vitamin K:

- Green leafy vegetables

- Fermented foods: natto, miso, tempeh, cheese

- Herbs: parsley, (dried) basil

Supplement: for example, vitamin K_{2-7}, 45 micrograms per day or a supplement that contains both vitamins K and D.

Potassium: can reduce the risk of high blood pressure and stroke.

Food rich in potassium:

- Green leafy vegetables: spinach, cabbage, brussels sprouts

- Legumes: beans, peas

- Fruit: apricots, peaches, plums, raisins, avocado, figs

Use potassium salt (potassium chloride) instead of standard sodium salt (sodium chloride).

Iodine: regulates the thyroid gland and metabolism.

Food rich in iodine:

- Mainly seafood: fish, shellfish, seaweed

Supplement: maximum 200 micrograms per day.

Supplements contain only a few micronutrients. A **varied, healthy diet** in the form of vegetables, fruit, nuts, seeds, legumes, fish, poultry, dark chocolate, green tea, coffee, herbs, mushrooms, and many other foods provides **thousands of other micronutrients** that interact with important proteins, the genome, epigenome, microbiome, cell receptors, the cell membrane, and many other structures.

Step 2: Stimulate Hormesis

Once upon a time, a Dutch journal for professional sheep farmers published an article titled "Thirty Sheep Killed by Poisonous Weed." The unfortunate sheep had eaten a poisonous plant that was growing at the edge of their pasture, *Galega officinalis*, also known as goat's rue. It is a beautiful plant with mauve or white flowers, and it is also used in the garden. Although the goat's rue killed 30 sheep within a day and a half, this plant has saved millions of lives. A substance from goat's rue is the basis for the most prescribed medication for one of the most widespread diseases in the West: metformin.

Metformin is the drug most frequently used for treating type 2 diabetes. As far back as the Middle Ages, goat's rue was used to alleviate the symptoms of diabetes, but it was not until the twentieth century that researchers were able to extract the active substance from the plant to produce metformin. Thus, this toxic plant formed the basis for one of the most successful pharmaceutical products in the world.

Metformin is special because it is one of the few medications that can extend the life span and slow down the aging process in various species of animals. Mice treated with metformin live longer and have a reduced risk of getting cancer and aging-related diseases. In humans, it can not only prevent or slow down the progression of type 2 diabetes but also decrease the risk of other aging-related diseases, such heart attack and Parkinson's disease.[175, 176] One study found that diabetes patients who took metformin lived 15 percent longer than healthy people.[177] This is all the more remarkable because diabetes is actually a disease that would otherwise shorten the life span by several years.

Metformin acts by making the body more sensitive to insulin, so that less insulin is needed and sugars in the body are processed more quickly. The health and life-extending effects in lab animals and people have even prompted some healthy people to take metformin to slow down aging. However, metformin is a drug, which means that there are always potential side effects. With metformin these are usually mild: The feared lactate acidosis or acidification of the blood, which was associated with high doses of metformin, has been proven to be exaggerated.[178, 179]

Goat's rue illustrates an important principle in medicine: Harmful things in small doses can be healthy. That principle is called hormesis. Those harmful things can be actual substances, such as toxins, but also heat, cold, radioactive radiation, and exercise. Metformin, as it happens, is mildly toxic to the mitochondria, the energy generators that activate the cells in our body. This causes the mitochondria to better fortify and repair themselves, making them less prone to aging. This, in turn, causes the body to improve its capacity to process insulin and sugars.

Exercise is also a form of hormesis. The most important reason why exercising is healthy is because it damages the body. An hour of cycling or swimming makes our cells work much harder than they usually do. They become overtaxed and slightly damaged, which you can feel the next day when you wake up with sore muscles. However, this damage shakes our cells awake and prompts them to repair and better protect themselves for the next time you go for a bike ride or dive into the pool. As the cells keep arming themselves against that kind of damage, they are then also better protected against other kinds of damage, such as that caused by aging processes. This is one important reason why exercising can decrease the risk of all kinds of aging-related diseases, such as heart disease and dementia.

Some exercise methods aim to cause as much damage as possible in a short time. An example is high-intensity interval training (HIIT). This method consists of, for example, putting out as much effort as you can by pedaling or running really fast for one minute, then resting for one minute, then putting out as much effort as you can for another minute, and slowing down for one minute by pedaling or walking at a slower pace. By performing this sequence ten times or more you force your mitochondria, and your cells, to work very hard each time, which causes damage and is healthy. In one study, sedentary people aged 45 on average, who had not exercised for at least one year, were put on an HIIT regime. They had to participate in HIIT for twenty minutes, three times per week, not counting a few minutes of warmup. After two weeks their metabolism had substantially improved and the insulin sensitivity of their body had increased by 35 percent.[180] The higher the insulin sensitivity, the better the body can process sugars and the less risk you have of diabetes, heart disease, and dementia. HIIT also stimulates the mitochondrial biogenesis, which means that the number of mitochondria in your cells increases.[181] This is very healthy because the more mitochondria, the more they can share the work between them, and the more slowly they age. HIIT may also be interesting to people who have little time, because even five times 30 seconds of maximum effort with 30 seconds recovery each time can already yield considerable health effects, even though the total duration of this exercise is only five minutes.

Exercising or movement does not always have to be as intense as HIIT, however; even regular walking is enough to put lazy cells to work and damage them slightly, certainly if you do it long enough. This is an important reason why walking can decrease inflammation in your body, which is vital to mitigate the aging process. This generalized inflammation increases with age and is characterized by small inflammatory substances (cytokines) that continuously circulate in all areas of the body and damage the cells ("inflammaging"). Additionally, exercise makes the cells more sensitive to insulin and better able to process sugars. All of this has healthy effects even as far away as in the brain, given that our brain is very sensitive to too many sugars and inflammation. Middle-aged people who begin to exercise, such as by walking half an hour per day twice a week, had a 62 percent lower risk of getting Alzheimer's disease, according to one study.[182] In another study, people between age 55 and 80 went for a 40-minute walk three times per week. After one year, researchers observed on the brain scans that the hippocampus, an important structure in the brain that is responsible for storing memory, had increased in size.[183] Professor Kirk Erickson reported, "We think of the atrophy of the hippocampus in later life as almost inevitable. But now we've shown that even moderate exercise for one year can increase the size of that structure." Plenty of exercise can decrease the risk of all kinds of aging-related diseases. An important reason is that exercise forces our cells to work harder and longer. The damage they suffer makes them stronger for the future.

In addition to metformin and exercise, the temperature in the environment can also play a role in hormesis. When you expose fruit flies to a high temperature for a short period, they live longer.[184] That could also be a reason why an occasional sauna or cold shower can have a healthy effect on the body. Heat is infrared radiation, but there is another kind of radiation that may have a hormetic effect too; namely, radioactivity. When crickets and mice undergo a small amount of radioactive radiation, they live longer.[185] Something similar may be true for people. A report of the Atomic Energy Commission in the United States found that people living in the six states with the *most* radioactive background radiation had a 15 percent *lower* risk of dying of cancer compared to the other states.[186] The people in the three states with the highest background radiation—Idaho, Colorado, and New Mexico—had a 24 percent lower risk of dying of cancer than people living in states with three times lower background radiation, such as Mississippi and Louisiana.

This background radioactive radiation originates from the soil and rocks, more specifically from radium, a naturally occurring radioactive element found in rocks. More radium is found in some regions than in others. One of those regions with higher natural radioactivity is the Greek island of Ikaria. On this island there are surprisingly many old people: ten times more people aged 90-plus than in the rest of Europe.[187] This prompted the American National Institute of Aging, together with the *National Geographic*, to conduct a study on Ikaria to find out why the life span is so long there. Some researchers believe that the high radioactivity on the island plays a role because of its hormetic effect. There is even a spring on the island that the locals call "immortal water." This spring contains a lot of radioactive radium, even so much that people who drink from the spring run the risk of a radiation overdose.[188] Continuous exposure to a small amount of radioactivity can be healthy in theory because radioactivity slightly damages the cells, so that they arm and protect themselves against this as well as other kinds of damage. However, I am not recommending that readers go and live near a nuclear plant or move to a radioactive Greek island. After all, there can be many other reasons that people on Ikaria live longer, such as healthy nutrition, less stress, and more exercise. And since radioactivity is very dangerous, even a little bit too much can have a harmful effect. The concept of hormesis, however, shows that the line between healthy and harmful things is not always clear. Sometimes harmful things can be healthy and healthy things can be harmful. The latter is nicely illustrated by antioxidants. We think that antioxidants are healthy but is that really true?

Antioxidants are vitamins, such as vitamin A, vitamin E, and beta-carotene, but also substances, such as co-enzyme Q10 and acetylcysteine. Numerous magazines, websites, and TV programs proclaim that antioxidants slow down the aging process (and when you buy two bottles of antioxidants you get a third one free). Scientist and physician Denham Harman introduced his oxidation theory of aging around the 1960s. It is one of the best known and most popular theories of why we age and it goes as follows: Our cells continuously produce free radicals as side effects of the metabolism, in the same way as smoke comes out of the chimney of a coal plant. Free radicals are small, very reactive molecules that react with proteins, DNA, and fats in our cells, which damages them. According to Harman, we age because we are constantly exposed to free radicals that slowly but definitely cause irreparable damage to our cells. An interesting aspect of this theory is that, if aging is caused by free radicals, antioxidants can then come to our rescue, since antioxidants react with free radicals and thereby make them harmless. Antioxidants wipe up those free radicals, as it were, so that they cannot do their destructive work in our cells. They are the bodyguards that catch the bullets. This, of course, was music to the ears of the manufacturers of dietary supplements, who began to promote antioxidants as a remedy for free radicals and therefore aging as well.

This was too good to be true, however. In the past decades, scientists have administered various dosages and combinations of antioxidants to lab animals, but the animals did not live a day longer. Of course, there are also studies showing that a certain antioxidant does make lab animals live longer, but these often turned out to be poorly executed or very small studies with genetically abnormal or diseased animals, the promising results of which were later refuted in larger studies. It is the same for research with humans. A study with more than 230,000 people shows that antioxidants do not extend life span, with the possible exception of selenium.[128] Some antioxidants, such as vitamins A and E, actually increased mortality to some extent. Other studies show that, when athletes take antioxidants after training to promote recovery, they actually undo the benefits of exercise.[189]

Yet other studies show that too many antioxidants can even be harmful; for example, antioxidants increase the pace of lung cancer in mice and in humans.[132, 190] It is quite logical that taking antioxidants when you have cancer is not a good idea because cancer cells grow uncontrollably and are therefore unable to adequately maintain their metabolism. As a result their metabolism produces many free radicals, in such large quantities that they can damage the cancer cells. Cancer cells actually profit greatly from antioxidants that wipe out the free radicals for them. That is why it might not be advisable to take antioxidants during treatment for cancer, as is sometimes suggested.

Even stranger things have happened: Some studies show that exposure to *more* free radicals causes lab animals not to live shorter but actually *longer*. Worms that had been genetically manipulated in such a way that they produced more free radicals lived 32 percent longer than regular worms. When you give worms a weed killer that increases free radical production in their cells, they live 58 percent longer (although I do not advise sprinkling weed killer on your breakfast).[191]

How is it possible that many antioxidants do not slow down aging, or even accelerate it, and that free radicals can slow down aging? This can be explained by hormesis. Free radicals are not always bad. They set off all kinds of alarm bells in the cells, and in response the cells begin to produce proteins that repair the cell, maintain it better, and neutralize free radicals. These antioxidant proteins made by the body itself are a thousand times stronger than any antioxidant supplement from the supermarket. Hormesis makes the cells healthier. If you take antioxidant supplements, your cells think that there are plenty of antioxidants already and that there is less need to protect themselves, which in the long term can even increase your risk of dying.

Of course, this is not to say that antioxidants are completely unnecessary or unhealthy, because a lack of antioxidants is also unhealthy and in the long term can damage the body. If you have a deficit of vitamin A or co-enzyme Q10, for example, it may be useful to take these supplements to remedy that deficiency. But unfortunately, in the case of most antioxidants, taking extra-high doses to slow down the aging process is not successful. Nevertheless, many people decide to give it a try. They take dozens of different kinds of antioxidants and other substances daily so as to live longer. However, an excess of many antioxidants actually can speed up the aging process.

If most antioxidants cannot slow down the aging process, nor decrease your risk of many aging-related diseases, why is it that certain foods, such as vegetables, fruit, coffee, and herbs, can? These foods are often said to be healthy because they contain antioxidants, but as we have seen, that is not a good explanation. An important reason these foods are healthy is that they are mildly toxic: They have a hormetic effect on the body.

Take coffee, for instance. All too often we are told that coffee is not good for you, but many studies show that coffee can lessen the risk of various aging-related diseases, such as Alzheimer's and Parkinson's disease, type 2 diabetes, clogging up of the arteries, and several types of cancer.[192–195] Of course, coffee may also have negative effects: If you drink too much, it can increase your risk of osteoporosis, heart arrhythmias, and insomnia. The advantages of coffee outweigh the disadvantages, though, and it can be healthy if you drink it in moderation. Most guidelines recommend drinking a maximum of three to five cups per day. One reason coffee is healthy is because it contains mildly toxic substances that activate an alarm-protein, called Nrf2, in our cells. When Nrf2 detects these mildly toxic plant substances in the coffee, it travels to the DNA in the cell nucleus, where it starts up the production of our own body antioxidant and detoxification proteins. Detoxification proteins are activated because the cells want to eliminate these mildly toxic substances as quickly as possible. The liver, in particular, starts producing these detoxification proteins. At the same time, the liver then cleans up other substances that are much more toxic than those in coffee. These substances would otherwise harm the body, increasing our risk of cancer and aging-related diseases.[196] Hence, coffee has a detoxifying effect.

This is interesting because the concept of detox often generates a lot of discussion. *Detoxing* means "freeing the body of poisons." Opponents of it consider detoxing nonsense; proponents think that detoxing is very healthy, but they often do not know what they are talking about and think that detoxing means removal of "stored waste materials," or "removal of poisons from the body." Sometimes far-out treatments are suggested, such as rigorous liquids-only diets, colonic cleanses, intravenous chelation therapy, or electrolytic footbaths. Many of these treatments are not supported by science and can sometimes even be dangerous.

All this does not mean that we should throw out the baby with the bathwater and call detoxing nonsense. Detoxing can be explained scientifically and can have a noticeably healthy effect. Only, you do not need a clay bath or colonic cleanse: A cup of coffee or a piece of broccoli is all you need, because ingesting hormetic substances via healthy foods promotes the production of all kinds of detoxification proteins (including cytochrome P450 enzymes, glutathione-S-transferases, and UDP-glycosyltransferases) in our cells and particularly in the liver. These detoxification proteins enable the body to break down all kinds of toxic substances faster, so that they can cause less harm to the body. In studies with lab animals where these detoxification systems are activated, we see that these animals live longer. However, to achieve a real health effect, you have to detoxify on a regular basis. A detox diet of one week on an exotic island does very little if you then fall back into your usual, unhealthy eating habits. For a real, long-term effect, we have to eat healthy foods all the time, so that our liver and cells are continuously hormetically activated.

Another example of hormesis is vegetables. Take broccoli, for instance. This vegetable contains mildly toxic substances, such as sulforaphane, which activate proteins in the body that protect and detoxify. This can decrease the risk of all kinds of diseases, such as Parkinson's and cancer. One study shows that when sulforaphane was given to fruit flies, their nerve cells were better protected against Parkinson's disease.[197] The researchers concluded:

> Remarkably, sulforaphane and allyl disulfide robustly suppressed neuronal loss in both of our models of PD [Parkinson's disease]. Our findings raise the possibility that these and perhaps other chemical inducers of the phase II detoxification pathway represent potential preventive agents for PD.

This detoxifying ability could play an important role in slowing down the aging process. Researchers are becoming more and more convinced that it is not so much free radicals that are harmful, but in particular the toxic substances in our body, such as those that are produced as by-products of our metabolism or come from our food or drugs (xenobiotics). The better organisms are able to clean up these toxic substances, the more slowly they age. Studies in which the detoxifying ability of lab animals is increased (via genetic manipulation or by giving them substances from vegetables, garlic, or herbs) show that these animals live longer and age more slowly.[198–200]

Broccoli is again a good example. The mildly toxic substances in broccoli activate the production of more detoxification proteins in the liver, so that many more toxic substances are broken down than would otherwise cause mutations of the DNA in our cells, causing cancer to develop or making it mutate and evolve faster. Rats with prostate cancer that were given broccoli powder had a 42 percent reduction in tumor growth. If, in addition, they were given tomato powder, the growth was reduced by 52 percent. In the other rats, which were given finasteride, a medication that slows down the production of a certain form of testosterone, tumor growth was reduced by very little.[201] A study that followed men with bladder cancer for eight years found that men who regularly ate broccoli had a 43 percent lower risk of dying compared to men who did not eat broccoli.[202] Women who ate more than 2 pounds of broccoli per month, had a 40 percent lower risk of breast cancer than women who ate only 10.5 ounces of it or less.[203] A study in which smokers ate about 9 ounces of steamed broccoli per day, shows that their DNA mutated less and was damaged more slowly than in the group of smokers who did not eat broccoli.[204] Broccoli and other vegetables can even protect against sunburn. We know that the UV radiation of the sun damages the DNA in our skin cells, which causes sunburn and makes the skin darker as a protection against this DNA damage. Certain substances in broccoli can reduce this DNA damage or even prevent it.[205] This study and numerous others are why large cancer organizations worldwide recommend a diet rich in fruit and vegetables, to reduce the risk of cancer.

Green tea also contains mildly toxic substances that are healthy. People who drank three or more cups of green tea per day had a 21 percent lower risk of a stroke.[206] Among the mildly toxic substances in green tea are catechins. In one study, men with "high-grade prostate intraepithelial neoplasia," a precursor of cancer (30 percent of men with this high-grade growth will develop cancer after one year), were divided into two groups. One group was given catechins from green tea and the other group was given a placebo (a pill that has no active ingredients). After one year, 30 percent of the placebo group developed prostate cancer, as was to be expected. In the group that was given the green tea extract, only one of the 30 patients (3 percent) developed prostate cancer. The men who took the green tea extract had a ten times lower risk that their high-grade prostate tissue growth would evolve into a prostate tumor.[207]

Cacao contains even more catechins than green tea. Cacao is an ingredient of chocolate. The darker the chocolate, the more cacao it contains, and the healthier it is. A large study with 114,000 participants found that those who regularly ate a piece of chocolate had a 37 percent lower risk of a heart attack and a 29 percent lower risk of a stroke.[208] Cacao can also slow down the aging of the brain. Old people with mild cognitive impairment—often a precursor of Alzheimer's—were given a drink with cacao extract daily. After eight weeks, they performed significantly better on various cognitive tests and their cognitive decline had slowed down. Their blood pressure had also improved, as well as their sugar metabolism.[209] A study that followed more than 400 men over fifteen years, found that those who ate the most cacao had a 47 percent lower risk of dying than did those who ate little cacao.[210] Companies are currently busy extracting these mildly toxic materials from cacao and putting them in a pill to reduce the risk of cardiovascular disease or dementia. However, it is not necessary to take a chocolate pill, which will probably be very expensive, when eating 10 grams of dark chocolate (about one fifth of a chocolate bar) is sufficient to ingest enough of these substances that are good for your heart and blood vessels, as well as your brain. The dark chocolate should contain at least 70 percent cacao.

Fruit also contains healthy, mildly toxic substances. Blueberries, for example, contain anthocyanins, which give the berries their characteristic blue color. According to a Harvard study with more than 186,000 participants, people who ate these berries three times per week had a 26 percent lower risk of getting type 2 diabetes.[211] People who regularly eat blue fruit can slow down brain aging by several years.[212] It is not surprising that the more fruit and vegetables people eat per day, the longer they live. For each portion of fruit people ate, their risk of a heart attack was reduced by seven percent, according to a study that included more than 220,000 people.[213] Another study that followed 65,000 people found that people who ate five portions of fruit or vegetables per day had a 29 percent lower risk of dying during the almost eight years of the study. Those who ate seven or more portions had a 42 percent lower risk of dying. Vegetables proved to be even more effective than fruit. The following figure illustrates these results.[214]

How eating fruit and vegetables can decrease the risk of death

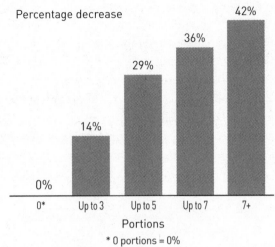

Percentage decrease

- 0% 0*
- 14% Up to 3
- 29% Up to 5
- 36% Up to 7
- 42% 7+

Portions

* 0 portions = 0%

source: *Journal of Epidemiology and Community Health*

People who ate seven or more portions of fruit and vegetables per day had a 42 percent lower risk of dying during this study that followed 65,000 people for an average of eight years. Vegetables were found to have the greatest health benefit.[214]

Of course, coffee, broccoli, or blueberries are healthy not only because they contain mildly toxic substances; they also contain fiber, for example, which can slow down the release of sugars, or they may contain other substances that reduce inflammation, activate specific genes or cell receptors, or have epigenetic effects. However, the mildly toxic substances they contain are an important reason why healthy foods can decrease the risk of all kinds of aging-related diseases and why antioxidants are overrated. But if vegetables, fruit, green tea, and coffee are healthy because of their mild toxicity, is it then not harmful if you eat too much of them? Not really, because these foods contain only *mildly toxic* substances and in small amounts. If you eat many of these healthy foods in a varied diet, you cannot consume too many of them. Furthermore, we should not forget that today's healthy, mildly toxic food is much less toxic than in prehistoric times. Our body has been adapted by nature to an environment that was much more toxic than is the case today. Our ancestors consumed huge amounts of plant-based foods. Plants in prehistoric times contained much larger amounts of toxins than they do today, because most plants do not want to be eaten, so they use toxins to defend themselves. Our vegetables in the supermarket are really only very watered-down versions of the prehistoric vegetables that grew in the wild. Today's broccoli does not remotely resemble a wild broccoli of 30,000 years ago. Wild broccoli looks like a measly plant with a few yellow flowers. Our typical broccoli, brussels sprouts, and cauliflower were bred from this wild broccoli; in fact, when you eat broccoli or cauliflower, you are actually eating flowers. These vegetables are descendants of the same prehistoric plant, but via long-term plant breeding (selection of plants with characteristics that make them more edible or easier to grow), they became separate varieties that look completely different—and contain much fewer toxins.

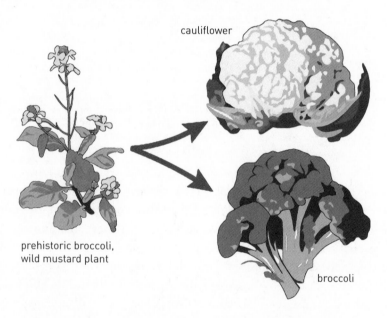

Broccoli, cabbage, brussels sprouts, cauliflower, and kohlrabi are all descendants of the prehistoric broccoli, a measly mustard plant.

The same is true for carrots. A prehistoric carrot looked like a plant root: small, thin, and white instead of large, thick, and orange. A prehistoric carrot tasted bitter because it was full of toxins. Or take fruit. A wild apple, for instance, was a small, shriveled little thing that looks completely different from the large, shiny apples in the supermarket that have been bred for taste and durability. Prehistoric almonds contained much more cyanide than do almonds today. In short, in prehistoric times, humans were much more often exposed to toxins and our body is designed for that. That is why the liver is the largest organ in the body (not counting the skin): because the liver is working 24 hours a day to break down toxic substances. These days however, it is particularly busy breaking down the excessive amounts of sugars it is flooded with daily in the form of soft drinks, baked goods, bread, or pasta. It is mainly an excess of sugars—and not an excess of natural toxins—that our liver today has to contend with.

You can tell from the taste that our current healthy foods contain fewer toxins. Many of today's vegetables and fruits taste much less bitter than the prehistoric or wild varieties. It is the toxins in foods that give them the bitter taste. Many toxins taste bitter because it is a taste that most people do not like. That is not a coincidence: Our taste buds have evolved to such an extent that we dislike toxic substances, so that we will not eat foods that contain too many toxins. You want to spit out a toxic plant because it tastes bad. That is also why many people do not like certain vegetables, because they contain mildly toxic, bitter substances. It may also explain why some people, who have a mutation that makes their taste buds work differently, live longer. With that mutation, they do like the bitter taste, so that they automatically eat more vegetables, mild toxins and all. People who like brussels sprouts live longer. In short, we do not need to worry that vegetables, fruit, and legumes contain too many toxins. However, some foods can be bad for your health when consumed in excess. They are not just mildly but very toxic, such as alcohol.

Alcohol is a human invention, or more likely, an incidental human discovery. Alcohol may have been discovered by chance about 9,000 years ago, probably when some honey or berries were left out in the open too long and began to ferment: The yeast they contained converted the sugars into alcohol. This gave people the idea to produce alcohol, and in large quantities. In the past, various studies showed that drinking alcohol in small amounts may be healthy, particularly for the heart and blood vessels. For example, one study with 85,000 women found that women who drink one to three alcoholic beverages per week have a lower risk of a heart attack.[215] Other studies showed that already one glass of alcohol per day can increase the risk of breast cancer in women (but of course, many more women die of a heart attack than of breast cancer). A recent large study with almost 600,000 participants published in the medical journal *The Lancet* showed that even consuming one glass of alcohol per day is associated with an increased risk of dying. However, this increase in risk is very small. The mortality risk is increased substantially starting from two glasses of alcohol per day. So it is important to keep in mind that when you drink even a little too much, your risk of all kinds of aging-related diseases increases dramatically. This is because alcohol is not just mildly toxic, it is very toxic. Of all the types of alcohol, ethanol is the only one people can drink—if we drink, for example, methanol, we become blind or we die. Since alcohol is so toxic, even a small amount of it can be harmful.

How much is too much? The recommendations vary from country to country. Often a maximum of one serving for women and two servings for men is recommended. Some countries have reduced this maximum to one serving per day for both women and men. It is also recommended to skip drinking alcohol a few days per week, so that the liver has time to recover. When people drink more than is recommended, their risk of cancer, heart disease, and stroke increases. The toxicity of alcohol causes thousands of people annually to end up in the hospital with alcohol poisoning, whereas it is very rare to find someone in the emergency department with broccoli poisoning. One more thing to remember about alcohol is that it can also make you gain weight. Often people have a healthy diet but they still do not lose weight; this may be because they still drink too much alcohol. People often forget that alcohol is the fourth macronutrient, after sugars, fats, and proteins, and it, too, can therefore be converted into fat.

Just like too much alcohol, too much coffee can also be unhealthy, although the effects are not as serious. As we have seen, coffee has more advantages than disadvantages, and a moderate consumption (a maximum of three to five cups per day) can decrease the risk of all kinds of aging-related diseases, like cardiovascular disease, type 2 diabetes, and cancer. In short, people who have a varied, healthy diet, with a moderate amount of alcohol and coffee, do not need to fear that they are consuming too many mildly toxic substances. The liver of prehistoric man had to work much harder every day to be able to metabolize all the wild broccoli, toxic berries, and moldy nuts than does the liver of people today with their shiny apples and pre-washed lettuce from the supermarket.

The second step of the longevity staircase showed us the importance of hormesis and how hormetic principles can slow down the aging process. Let's now take a look at the third step, which is about growth stimulation and to what extent too much growth can result in accelerated aging.

SUMMARY

Step 2: **Stimulate hormesis**.

Hormesis is the process whereby **mild damage or toxicity** can bring about healthy effects, because it activates repair, protection, and detoxification mechanisms in the cells.

Examples of hormesis are

- Mildly toxic substances in medications (metformin) and food (flavonoids, sulforaphane, phenolic acids, stilbenes, alcohol)

- Long or short intensive exercise (walking or HIIT)

- Radioactivity (possibly)

- Temperature (heat or cold)

Hormesis also explains why many **antioxidants** do not slow down the aging process and sometimes even shorten the life span. The antioxidants that can slow down the aging process often do so via hormesis and not because of their antioxidant activity.

Detoxification often works via hormesis.

Examples of **food with hormetic properties** are green tea, coffee, vegetables, dark chocolate, and fruit.

Step 3: Reduce Growth Stimulation

Often people see aging as wear and tear. A classic example are free radicals damaging our cells. But what if, in addition to wear (which does not have to be inevitable, as we have seen in chapter 1), another process also plays an important role in aging? A process that is not well known; namely, growth stimulation? This growth stimulation continuously spurs on the aging process.

Growth stimulation is caused by the bombardment of our cells with growth-stimulating substances, such as insulin, IGF, growth hormone, testosterone, glucose, and amino acids. These substances prompt our cells to produce lots of energy, proteins, and other substances, which makes them age faster: The proteins start to coagulate, the mitochondria (the energy generators) must work at top capacity, all those sugars create cross-links, and so on. This is a reason why growth-stimulating substances, such as insulin, IGF, and growth hormone, accelerate aging and why larger lab animals (that have grown a lot) die earlier. It is also why dwarfs, supercentenarians, and lab animals with fewer of these growth-stimulating substances live longer. These growth-stimulating substances activate all kinds of switches in the cells that make them age faster.

The problem is that in people who follow a Western diet, these aging switches are in the on position all the time. They are continuously activated by our excess of unhealthy foods. We consume lots of foods with fast sugars, amino acids (from animal protein), and unhealthy fats, which activate the growth switches in our cells, make us gain weight, and make our body age faster. The most common and obvious result is overweight. An overweight person is someone whose cells are continuously in growth stimulation mode, which spurs on the cells and results in overweight and accelerated aging. That explains why overweight people are at a higher risk of cancer and various aging-related diseases, such as type 2 diabetes, cardiovascular diseases, and dementia.

In short, if you want to slow down the aging process, you must also reduce growth stimulation. Furthermore, if you are overweight, this reduction in growth stimulation will also cause you to lose weight. That is interesting, certainly in view of the current epidemic of obesity. Between 50 and 65 percent of people in the West are overweight, so let's first look at why so many people weigh too much, and why the official recommendations about overweight are outdated. Then we will automatically find out what is the best diet or dietary pattern for losing weight. It is not a coincidence that such a diet also slows down aging.

LOSING WEIGHT: EASY OR NOT?

Losing weight is not easy. To begin with: What diet should you follow? There are hundreds of diets, one more outlandish than the other. There are the well-known classics, such as high-protein diets (Atkins, Dukan, and paleo diets). In these diets, you must eat a lot of protein from meat, eggs, or expensive protein products. There are the usual low-fat diets, in which you need to avoid unhealthy—but unfortunately also healthy—foods with a high fat content. Another popular weight loss method is the low-calorie diet—simply eating less. Then, there are hundreds of other strange or nonsensical diets and fads you can follow, such as the blood group diet (eating according to your blood group), the seven-color diet (you eat a different color of food every day), or the fish-facelift diet (eating salmon three times a day to achieve a nutritional facelift. This works especially well for movie stars who have already had a facelift). There are also dangerously monotonous diets, such the apple diet, the soup diet, or the egg diet (one egg in the morning and two in the evening). Some movie stars and photo models opt for only tea or vegetable juices or a feeding tube for a while. There are even people who ingest the eggs of a tapeworm to lose weight—you always eat for two: yourself and the yards-long tapeworm that lives in your intestines.

It is interesting to know that no matter which diet you try, during the first weeks or months, you do indeed lose weight in most cases. Soon, however, the weight simply comes back on, usually because you are unable to stay on that weird or difficult diet. Most diets do not work in the long term and are often unhealthy as well.

It is difficult, not only for the public but also for physicians and dietitians, to choose the best diet. Many hospitals use a high-protein diet, a low-fat diet, or a low-calorie diet. As we shall see, these diets are not very effective and may even be unhealthy in the long term. You can also get nutritional advice from the government and official institutions. Their advice is based on what they see as the main cause of overweight: We consume too many calories and get too little exercise. You hear this explanation from most health experts in the media. According to the government, eating too much and exercising too little is why so many people are overweight. Could it really be that simple?

TOO MANY CALORIES, TOO LITTLE EXERCISE?

Eating too much and exercising too little is even the official answer of the World Health Organization (WHO) to the question of why people are overweight. The problem is this explanation is outdated and oversimplified. Let's begin with the latter. The explanation of too many calories in, too few out, would suffice if our body were a steam engine. Like an engineer, using a few simple formulas, you can calculate up to a few decimals how many calories or heat are lost or converted in the body. However, the body is not a steam engine; it is much more complex, as we will see later on. That means that this oversimplified explanation for the current obesity epidemic falls very short.

Furthermore, this explanation is not really an explanation in itself; it is a pseudo-explanation. Compare obesity or the accumulation of calories with a room that fills with people. The room is the body and the people who fill the room are the calories. Like the WHO, you could say that the room fills up (like we fill up with calories) because more people enter the room than exit (we take in more calories than we use up). However, this does not explain why the room fills up; it only describes what happens. But why does the room fill up so easily? Does it fill up because there is something special to see inside, so that people tend to hang around? Maybe the floor has glue on it, so that people cannot leave? Or maybe people cannot leave because they cannot find the exit or the exit is too narrow?

It is clear that this official explanation for overweight is inadequate. It is an oversimplification and a pseudo-explanation that does not fully clarify the real causes of overweight. Many studies show that this explanation is insufficient. If we become overweight because we eat too many calories, then we should lose weight by simply eating fewer calories. However, numerous studies have shown that low-calorie diets (that require you to eat less) do not work. To achieve substantial weight loss, the number of calories would have to be reduced so much that the diet would become a starvation diet. An adult needs about 2,200 calories per day. But even if you let people follow a starvation diet of 800 to 1,000 calories per day for many months, even then only one in four participants loses a mere 22 pounds.[216, 217] Furthermore, people cannot keep up such a starvation diet for long. As soon as the diet is finished or they stop, they will start eating more again. The simple explanation of why low-calorie diets do not work is that when you force people to eat less, they only become hungrier. Due to this simple feedback mechanism, even when people change from a starvation diet to a somewhat less restrictive diet, but one that still has hundreds of calories fewer than what they need per day, they immediately start gaining weight. Usually people lose about 11 pounds in the first six months, but after one year the large majority weigh at least the same as they did before the diet. Eating fewer calories simply does not work for long-term weight loss, as has been shown time after time by numerous research studies.[218]

In addition to diets, there may also be circumstances that force people to eat less. One example is poverty. In the past, physicians observed that children from poor families were often thin and malnourished, as is to be expected when they eat less. The mothers, on the other hand, were often overweight. Why? Not so much because they ate too many calories (the fact that their children were thin shows that there were not enough calories to go around in the family), but because they ate the wrong calories; namely, calories from cheap and unhealthy carbohydrates, such as bread, baked goods, sandwiches, chips, and soft drinks, plus cheap, processed red meat: the foods of choice for people who have little money or time. The children often stay thin in spite of this unhealthy diet because their body is young and their cells are still able to process this excess of sugars. Their mothers, by contrast, whose metabolism after age 30 is already aging, become overweight. Research and clinical practice show that eating less rarely works to achieve weight loss, certainly in the long term. That is the first hint that the too many calories in, too few out theory fails.

Let's also take a look at the second part of this hypothesis: the explanation of too few calories out. It is often said that people are overweight because they get too little exercise. If obesity is only the result of too little exercise, then moving more—in other words, burning more calories—should make you lose weight. But it is not that simple. There are many people who exercise regularly and do not lose weight or even gain weight. Studies show that exercise is a very inadequate method for preventing obesity. An international team of world experts in the area of exercise and health who analyzed the existing scientific literature concluded that exercise does not really result in weight loss.[219] Another analysis found that exercise had only a modest influence on prevention of obesity.[220] According to a large, long-term study at Harvard University, exercise was not an adequate method for preventing weight gain in people who are already overweight.[221] According to the researchers, once people were overweight, it was actually too late to prevent further weight gain by exercising. Other researchers found that regardless of whether you exercise a little or a lot, you steadily gain weight as you grow older.[222] Professor Eric Ravussin, who conducts research in the area of exercise and overweight, summarizes it as follows: "In general, for weight loss, exercise is pretty useless."

It is also interesting that overweight often occurs more often in people with jobs where they get lots of exercise: road workers, gardeners, miners, factory or construction workers. These people move much more on a daily basis do than white-collar workers who are stuck behind their desks, but strangely enough, they are often more overweight. Could it be that they gain weight mainly because of the cheap, unhealthy food they eat?

In spite of these insights and numerous other scientific studies, people are constantly told that they should make sure they exercise if they want to lose weight, and that they are overweight because they sit on the couch and watch too much television. But consider that it also may be the other way around: Do they often sit on the couch because they are overweight? We will come back to this later.

Of course, all this is not to say that exercise is not healthy. Exercise is very good for the body: It can drastically reduce your risk of chronic illness, such as cardiovascular disease or dementia. But studies show that, for losing weight or preventing weight gain, the effect of exercise (burning calories) is disappointing. There is a simple explanation for this: When you exercise more, you get more hungry. Everyone has experienced that after an hour of working out or jogging, you are ready to grab a snack, cookie, or sandwich, so that the calories you lost through exercise immediately come back. This simple feedback mechanism makes exercising a disappointingly difficult way to lose weight.

We have seen that eating less and exercising more has very little effect on losing weight in the long term. That seems to suggest that the too many calories in, too few out approach is inadequate. But why is it inadequate? The most important shortcoming is that it makes people believe that overweight is only a matter of the *amount* of calories and not the *nature* of the food that supplies these calories; that is, the idea that whether you eat 300 calories in the form of a hamburger or 300 calories in the form of broccoli, you will gain the same amount of weight. However, that is not the case. Numerous studies show that not all calories are made equal.[223] This must sound like blasphemy to many food experts, who for decades have accepted without questioning the dogma that a calorie is always a calorie.

Let's look at a few examples showing that a calorie is not always a calorie. Take walnuts, for example. Walnuts are chock-full of fats (two thirds of a walnut are fats). Fats contain many calories. This makes many people think that it would be best not to eat too many walnuts, since they are bad for your waistline. But a study found that women who ate two handfuls of walnuts per day (which amounts to an extra 300 calories—of the 2,000 calories a woman needs daily) did not gain weight.[224] Several other studies show that a few hundred calories per day of nuts do not increase your weight. In some studies people even lost weight.[225, 226] Researchers call this the "mystery of the missing calories." How is this possible if a calorie is always a calorie?

Looking at it from the traditional approach that says that a calorie is always a calorie, this is indeed strange. Suppose you would take the fats out of the walnuts and burn these fats in a lab beaker. Then, 100 grams (3.5 ounces) of walnut fats would yield 900 calories. That is a lot indeed. (Burning things in a lab beaker is the method used to measure the number of calories in foods. Food is burned in the vessel and the amount of heat generated [expressed as calories] is measured. For the scientists among us, 1 calorie is the amount of heat, or energy, that you need to heat 1 liter of water by 1°C [and to make it even more complicated, in some countries one calorie is considered as 1,000 "small" calories, so kilocalories and calories can be used interchangeably]. An average woman uses about 2,000 calories per day; a man, 2,500 calories. That is the amount of energy you need to keep your body temperature steady and keep your body functioning.)

A calorie is always a calorie. That is true for a lab beaker, but the human body is not a lab beaker; it is much more complex. That explains why women who eat hundreds of calories of walnuts extra per day did not gain weight. The fats in the walnuts are not completely burned up as is the case in a lab beaker. Some fats are used to build up the body, such as cell membranes, which consist mainly of fats. Other fats from the walnuts are not burned for energy, but converted to substances that control all kinds of processes in the body, such as inflammation and cell maintenance. The fats in the walnut can also turn all kinds of switches in the cells on and off, which influences numerous processes in the body, such as sugar metabolism, hormone production, and fat burning.[227] In contrast to an inert lab beaker, which simply burns all the food completely, food interacts with the body in numerous ways, before it is, or is not, burned up. Food is not just calories. Food is information that continuously programs and influences the body, right down to the level of the DNA in our cells. Walnuts contain thousands of substances that influence and build up our body, so that we do not gain as much weight despite the many more additional calories per day.

Thus, it is not only the amount of calories that makes a food unhealthy or causes weight gain. All fats in our food contain an equal number of calories (900 calories per 100 grams of fat). But omega-3 fats are very healthy and may even boost weight loss, whereas trans fats clog up your blood vessels and drastically increase your risk of a heart attack.[228] Glucose and fructose are two kinds of sugars that contain equal amounts of calories (400 calories per 100 grams). Both are unhealthy in large amounts, but fructose even more so than glucose. Glucose can be processed by all organs in the body, whereas fructose is processed mainly in the liver. Consequently, fructose causes an even greater risk of fat accumulation in the liver, resulting in a potbelly, more fats in the blood, and insulin resistance. In addition, fructose creates cross-links with proteins much faster than glucose does. Fructose also sends fewer saturation hormones to the brain than does glucose, making you eat more of it and gain more weight. In short, although all these substances contain equal amounts of calories, they have completely different effects on your metabolism and your health, certainly in the long term. Professor David Haslam, president of the British National Obesity Forum, states in this regard:

> It's extremely naïve of the public and the medical profession to imagine that a calorie of bread, a calorie of meat and a calorie of alcohol are all dealt with in the same way by the amazingly complex systems of the body.

And he continues:

> The assumption has been made that increased fat in the bloodstream is caused by increased saturated fat in the diet, whereas modern scientific evidence is proving that refined carbohydrates, and sugar in particular, are actually the culprits.

There are many other reasons why a calorie is not always a calorie. The digestive system is one of them. In contrast to a lab beaker that always neatly burns all its contents, our intestines do not absorb all calories. Some foods are not completely digested or are simply not absorbed by the gut cells. The way in which you digest and absorb food depends on many factors, from the amount of digestive enzymes you produce to the length of your intestines. For example, researchers compared the intestines of Russian populations to those of Polish people. It turned out that the intestines in some Russian population groups was on average more than twenty inches longer than in certain population groups in Poland. These Russians with their long intestines will absorb more calories from the same amount of food because their intestines are longer, hence they can better digest and absorb food. This puts them at greater risk of becoming overweight, even though they may eat the same number of calories.

Furthermore, it also takes energy to digest food. Take proteins, for example. Thirty percent of the energy a protein can produce (if you would burn it completely in a lab beaker) is lost by digesting the protein (breaking it up into pieces, so that it can be absorbed by the gut). When the body then wants to "burn up" these pieces (convert the amino acids into calories), it first needs to convert them into other substances, which also takes energy. Hence, the proteins can actually deliver only half of their energy (200 calories per 100 grams of protein instead of the standard 400 calories per 100 grams of protein). The immune system of the intestine also plays a role: If your food contains lots of bacteria or is full of foreign substances that the intestinal immune system does not recognize, the immune system will start to fight these food components, which again takes energy, and therefore calories.[223]

Your microbiome—that is, the composition of the bacteria in your gut— also influences how many calories certain foods actually deliver. It is often claimed that our gut contains about 300,000 billion bacteria, about ten times as many bacteria as there are cells in our body. However, a recent study estimates the number of gut bacteria to be about 40,000 billion, by and large the same amount as the number of human cells that make up our body. Anyhow, the composition of the gut microbiome can determine how much food (calories) we absorb. Some Japanese people have bacteria in their intestines that are specialized in breaking down seaweed. Thus, the seaweed is better absorbed and will deliver more energy in the form of calories than it would for Europeans who do not have this type of bacteria in their gut.

It is only recently that scientists are becoming aware of the importance of the microbiome in relation to overweight. Researchers have raised mice in a completely sterile environment so that they had no bacteria in their gut. These mice weighed very little and were very slim. They had 42 percent less body fat, even though they ate 29 percent more than did mice in a control group with gut bacteria. This in itself already shows that being overweight or underweight is not just a matter of calories. Next, the scientists introduced bacteria into the guts of the sterile mice. These mice suddenly became much fatter, with a 57 percent increase in body fat, even though they ate the same number of calories per day as before the intervention.[229] Other research shows that mice with a certain type of bacteria in their guts have an increased tendency to get fat. When these bacteria are transplanted from a fat mouse to a thin mouse, the thin mouse will also get fatter. Something similar may be true for humans as well.

More and more research points to the importance of the composition of our gut bacteria in relation to overweight and to our health. This composition is strongly influenced by how healthy or unhealthy our food is. The microbiome can also be influenced by medical interventions, such as the use of antibiotics or fecal transplantations. One woman is thought to have become overweight due to a fecal transplant. This is a procedure whereby fecal matter from another person is introduced into the gut of another person (via a tube inserted rectally), with the goal of changing the microbiome; the bacteria in the fecal matter spread throughout the gut. This treatment is sometimes performed in people who have had chronic diarrhea for many years, caused by an overgrowth of certain harmful bacteria. This growth may have been started, for example, by long-term use of certain antibiotics that killed too many beneficial gut bacteria, so that one harmful type of bacteria can take over and cause chronic diarrhea. This woman who had chronic diarrhea received fecal matter from a woman who happened to be overweight. Before the intervention, the first lady weighed 150 pounds. After the transplantation, she gained a total of 44 pounds. It is possible that she gained weight because the chronic diarrhea had disappeared. Before her diarrhea, however, she had a normal weight. Another possibility is that the composition of her gut microbiome changed, which made her gain weight much faster.[230]

From walnuts that do not make you gain weight to bacteria that help you digest food, numerous studies show that a calorie is not a calorie. Actually, you do not even need studies to tell you this. Anyone with a basic knowledge of biochemistry knows that the human body is no simple lab beaker. Why is it, then, that we so often hear the claim that we get fat because we eat too many calories and get too little exercise? There are several reasons. One is that this explanation is music to the ears of the food industry. They very much like the dogma that a calorie is always a calorie. That way, there is no "fattening" food. That you get fat or unhealthy is only a matter of too many calories and not the nature of the food: You can still have soft drinks and hamburgers; you just need to eat fewer of them. With this dogma, one can also shift the blame for being overweight from food to exercise: We become fat not because we eat too much unhealthy, fattening food, but because we do not exercise enough. The food industry employs and deploys all kinds of nutrition experts and key opinion leaders who keep communicating this message to the media, dietitians, and physicians.

WHY DO WE GAIN WEIGHT?

If we want to know why people gain weight, we should not look only at calories. To focus only on calories ignores the complexity of the human body and the reason that so many people are overweight. Of course an excess of calories plays a role in excessive weight, but that is only part of the story. Nonetheless, in the West, it is very easy to take in too many calories. One can of soft drink contains 330 calories and about ten teaspoons of sugar. In prehistoric times, if you wanted to eat that much sugar, you would have to consume three feet of sugar cane. That would keep you busy for quite some time. Now you can consume a can of soda in one minute and get the same amount of pure sugar. We all know that calorie-rich soft drinks, fast food, candy, and baked goods are not healthy and make you fat. That is the first elephant in the room.

The second elephant is not as well known yet, however: Even when people stop consuming soft drinks, fast food, and candy, and eat lots of whole grain bread and pasta, they may still lose little or no weight. They may even gain weight, certainly when they are getting older and their body loses its ability to process large amounts of carbohydrates. In other words, the obesity epidemic cannot be stopped simply by asking people to consume fewer soft drinks, fast foods, and sweets. They must also eat fewer starchy foods, such as bread, pasta, potatoes, and rice. Only then can they achieve significant effects in terms of weight loss and health parameters. Therefore, we need to pay more attention to this second elephant in the room.

These starchy foods also have a large influence on our metabolism. They can *reprogram* our metabolism, and this bring us to another explanation for overweight, one that goes far beyond calories and that also points to another well-known phenomenon: constant hunger. Often people become hungry again very soon after they have eaten. Within an hour or two after eating a whole plateful of potatoes or pasta, they are hungry again and open the fridge to quiet these gnawing feelings. Then, they eat some more and so they gain more weight. How is this possible? They just ate carbohydrate-rich food with more than enough calories, and now they are hungry again?

As discussed earlier in the book, carbohydrate foods, such potatoes, bread, rice, and pasta cause high sugar peaks in the blood because starch is made up of sugar. This creates high insulin peaks, because the insulin wants to chase all these sugars from the bloodstream into the cells to be processed. The insulin has an additional effect: It prompts the fat cells to store fats. That is logical—a high insulin peak means that the body has received lots of energy in the form of sugars; therefore, your fat cells are wise to hold on to the fats (fatty acids) they already have, as fats are not needed now for energy, because lots of energy was delivered already in the form of sugars. As a result, in the hours following a meal, the fat cells keep their fats to themselves and do not release them into the bloodstream. That becomes a problem because sugars deliver energy only for a short time (they are processed quickly by the body). In the first few hours following a meal, the sugar level begins to decrease because the sugars are processed by the body; in particular, by the liver cells, muscle cells, and fat cells. However, when the sugars in the blood decrease, and the fat cells do not release fatty acids into the bloodstream (because they have been programmed by the insulin peaks to hold off doing so), then the body runs out of energy, since there are neither sugars nor enough fatty acids it can use for energy.

When our cells do not have sufficient energy to be able to do their work, it gives us an intense feeling of hunger, particularly a strong desire for carbohydrates, because these are the fastest source of energy. This becomes a vicious circle. Following a carbohydrate-rich meal, people quickly become hungry again. Then, they have a strong desire for more carbohydrate-rich products, which again makes their fat cells hoard more fats (because the insulin peaks programmed them to do so), which makes them hungry again (because in the hours after a meal one cannot rely on fats for energy) and fatter (because the fat cells store more and more fats), while craving more and more carbohydrates. Our insulin-producing food reprograms our body, so that we get hungrier and fatter meal after meal.[118, 231–233] This explanation goes a lot further than that we become overweight simply because we eat too many calories.

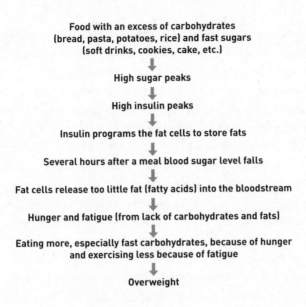

Food with an excess of carbohydrates
(bread, pasta, potatoes, rice) and fast sugars
(soft drinks, cookies, cake, etc.)
↓
High sugar peaks
↓
High insulin peaks
↓
Insulin programs the fat cells to store fats
↓
Several hours after a meal blood sugar level falls
↓
Fat cells release too little fat (fatty acids) into the bloodstream
↓
Hunger and fatigue (from lack of carbohydrates and fats)
↓
Eating more, especially fast carbohydrates, because of hunger
and exercising less because of fatigue
↓
Overweight

Excess carbohydrates reprogram your body.

This insight turns the traditional explanation for overweight on its head. According to the traditional explanation, the cause of overweight is eating too much and exercising too little. But the explanation discussed above reverses that: Eating too much and exercising too little are not so much the *cause* but can also be the *effect* of a faulty eating pattern. Thus, you can no longer simply say that people become overweight only because they eat too much. They also eat too much because they are overweight. Their body has been reprogrammed by the continuous insulin peaks, making them hungry more often (and by other changes in their bodies and brains, as we will see), so that they have to eat more. Also, the more overweight you are, the more calories you need per day, because you are carrying dozens of pounds in extra body weight, and all these extra pounds of body tissue (particularly fat tissue) need energy to function. Therefore, overweight people must eat much more because on a daily basis they use up more calories than thin people do.

You often hear that people are becoming more overweight because portions have become larger; in the 1960s a hamburger weighed on average 1.75 ounces and a soft drink was on average 7 ounces. Today, hamburgers may weigh as much as half a pound and soft drinks may be as large as 32 ounces. Rather than wonder why portions have become supersize, we should also ask why people's appetites have become supersize. It is because the nature of the food we consume reprograms our metabolism so that we have an increasing craving for giant portions.[233] That is why decreasing portion size has such a disappointing result in the long term. Many health experts advise eating smaller portions, for example, half a portion of french fries instead of a whole portion. But they are still french fries, which cause high insulin peaks and program your fat cells to store fat. The result is that you simply become hungry again very soon after eating that small portion and wish for increasingly larger portions.

If that were not enough, today's foods also make us very tired. The high insulin peaks cause sugars to be processed faster and fats to be stored more, so that we have too little energy to keep our body running. That is one reason why people feel tired after eating a plate of potatoes or whole grain pasta. No wonder they do not feel like exercising. That is a different explanation from being too lazy or not having enough will power to lose those calories by exercising.

We also often see that when people consume fewer soft drinks and baked goods but also less bread, potatoes, rice, and pasta, they will be much less tired after a meal. And, yes, that also applies to whole grain bread. It is not without reason that people complain about an afternoon energy dip after eating a whole wheat bun with lettuce and tomato for lunch. Another reason we are often tired after a meal is that Western meals are so rich in sugar, fat, and proteins, which takes a lot of energy for our digestive system to process.

Some researchers have even noted that people who exercise a lot and are slim, are not slim only because they exercise, but they also exercise so much because they are slim. Their good metabolism gives them enough energy to be able to exercise regularly. This makes it much easier for a fit fitness guru to say to an overweight person, "Just get off the couch more!" However, the metabolism and healthy food habits of the fitness guru works in such a way that he simply has much more energy and feels like exercising, whereas the metabolism of overweight people is caught in a vicious circle of fatigue and hunger.

Furthermore, today's approach to overweight mistakenly saddles people with guilt feelings: If overweight is simply a matter of too many calories and too little exercise, then it is mainly people's own fault that they are over-weight—they do not have enough willpower to eat less and exercise more. The food industry, of course, plays into this belief. To put it in the words of Harvard professor David Ludwig:

> The food industry would love to explain obesity as a problem of personal responsibility, since it takes the onus off them for

marketing fast food, soft drinks, and other high-calorie, low-quality products.

Apart from the fact that today's food programs our metabolism to store lots of fat, it is also addictive. If you keep concentrating on the influence of calories, you ignore the addictive aspect of unhealthy nutrition, which causes us to eat ever more calories. Food manufacturers do their utmost to make our food addictive: It tastes delicious; it stimulates and overrides pleasure and rewards centers in our brain; and it satiates little, so that you keep eating more. When you start eating a bag of chips, it is hard to stop. Chips, baked goods, french fries, pizzas, and even bread (often with added salt and sugar) play on age-old mechanisms in our brain. Our brain is programmed to love sugar, fat, and salt. Sugar and fat provide energy to the body, which in prehistoric times was always more than welcome, since food was very hard to come by. Salt also plays an important role in the body; among other things it regulates the water balance and allows cells to send signals. In the prehistoric savanna there was very little sugar, fat, and salt to be found, let alone all three together. But now you can ingest all three in one bite, in the form of a pastry, a bag of chips, or a snack bar. These are completely new inventions that our ancestors did not experience for thousands of years. That is why this type of food is very good at circumventing the satiety mechanisms in our brain. Everyone has experienced this. In a restaurant or at a family get-together, you have eaten from the main course till you are full; you cannot eat another bite. But then the desserts are brought in and chances are that you suddenly will still find a spot for them after all, which, after hundreds of years of refinement have been elevated to such a height of culinary enjoyment that they can easily defeat the satiety systems in our brain. This is because nature had never foreseen that we would invent such things as desserts.

Modern food can even stimulate the pleasure centers in our brain to such an extent that it can be addictive. Studies show that sugar-rich food can have an addictive effect similar to that of cocaine and heroin, and that it can even cause withdrawal symptoms. For example, if at four in the afternoon you eat a piece of marzipan and you repeat that several days in a row, you can be sure that the next day at four, you will begin automatically salivating and thinking of marzipan. You may even be doing that right now.

Researchers at Yale University therefore have created an addiction scale of foods.[234] The more you answer yes on this scale, the greater your risk of being addicted to food. These are a few examples: "I notice that when I eat certain foods, I eat more than I had planned"; "I often feel sluggish or lethargic after I eat certain foods"; "After a while I need to eat more of certain foods to achieve the same effect, such as fewer negative emotions or enjoying myself more"; "I had withdrawal symptoms when I ate less of certain foods or stopped eating them, such as feeling irritable or anxious." Did you answer yes often? Then, there is a chance that you are addicted to food, and that the food you crave will rarely or never be broccoli or apples but preferably something in a brightly colored package. Focusing too much only on calories ignores the tastiness and addictiveness of many unhealthy foods that are so delicious that one almost cannot stop eating them.

Another factor that plays a role in the epidemic of overweight is a poor ratio of macronutrients. Macronutrients are carbohydrates, proteins, and fats. In the West the ratio between these macronutrients can be better: We eat too many carbohydrates and thereby automatically too little fat. That is regrettable because fats are important for our health. An important reason that this ratio between carbohydrates and fats became skewed is again the too many calories in, too few out dogma. That contributed to the fact that for decades, fats were eschewed because they were considered the most important cause of overweight. If you approach overweight from a simple calorie point of view, you are quickly inclined to discourage people from eating fats because they contain many calories. All over the world, millions of people were advised to eat less fat and go on low-fat diets. However, low-fat diets are disappointing in terms of weight loss. A study of 20,000 women who for eight years ate a low-fat diet that on average contained 360 calories fewer per day (with many fiber-rich carbohydrates, such as whole grain bread), showed a mere pound of weight loss at the end of those eight years! Furthermore, these women on average had gained a larger waist circumference, which suggests that they had actually lost mainly muscle mass and gained unhealthy belly fat instead.[235] The women also did not have a lower risk of heart attack, cancer, or other diseases. In another study three types of diets with the same number of calories (1,600 per day) were compared: a low-fat diet, a low-glycemic diet (a diet with food that has a low glycemic index [GI] and therefore causes fewer high sugar peaks), and a low-carbohydrate diet (a diet that contains few carbohydrates). The low-GI and low-carbohydrate diets yielded much healthier body parameters—reduced fats in the blood, improved insulin sensitivity, lower blood pressure—than the low-fat diet. It is counterintuitive that a diet that is most effective in decreasing the fats in your blood is not a low-fat diet but a diet with fewer sugar peaks and carbohydrates. This study also showed that a calorie is not always a calorie. Even though all three diets had the same number of calories, the people on the low-GI and low-carbohydrate diet burned 125 to 325 calories more per day than did the people on the low-fat diet, and their blood vessels and metabolism were much healthier.[118]

Another large study (a meta-analysis) that compared several types of diets found that the best and healthiest diet was not a low-fat diet but a diet with a low glycemic index or low glycemic load (which causes fewer high sugar peaks or contains fewer carbohydrates).[236] The researchers concluded: "A dietary pattern with a lower glycemic load is an efficient method to lose weight and decrease the fats in the blood, and can easily be integrated into a person's lifestyle." What is noteworthy in this analysis is that the people who followed a low-glycemic diet were still allowed to eat as much as they wanted but nevertheless lost more weight than did those who followed low-fat diets in which they also had to reduce their calories (food intake).

This conclusion need not surprise us when viewed from the perspective of aging, nor is it anything new. As far back as 1956 the well-known medical journal the *Lancet* published a study in which participants were put on three types of extreme diets to make an extreme point. People were put on a diet consisting of 90 percent fats, 90 percent proteins, or 90 percent carbohydrates, respectively. The people on the high-fat diet lost the most weight (!), followed by those on the high-protein diet, whereas those on the high-carbohydrate diet actually gained weight.[237] People who care for animals have known this for a long time: Their animals often develop diabetes or fatty livers when they are given food with many and fast carbohydrates, like sugars and starches, whether they are gorillas in the zoo or house cats. It is also well known that the best way to fatten up geese, so that they develop a fatty liver (foie gras), is to feed them a carbohydrate-rich diet, particularly starch. A fatty liver is also one of the most frequently occurring diseases of our Western civilization: 30 percent of the population suffers from it and the percentage is steadily increasing. If the liver becomes too fatty, it can even result in chronic inflammation of this organ. In this respect we are not that different from geese and their foie gras livers.

The healthiest and most effective diets are diets that contain fewer carbohydrates and more healthy fats. These are the dietary patterns that have a better ratio of macronutrients.

Now we have discussed several causes of overweight. Of course, numerous other causes play a role. These include, for example, sleep deprivation (people who do not get enough sleep gain weight faster), heat (the higher your thermostat, the more risk of overweight), your family background (how often there was fast food on the menu), or the fact that we live in an obesogenic (weight-gain-promoting) environment (food advertising, fast-food restaurants, and snack dispensers). Not all these factors contribute equally; some are more or less important. There is that one large elephant (sugar-rich foods) but also that other, less well-known elephant (too many starchy foods, such as bread, potatoes, pasta, and rice). These high-carbohydrate products reprogram our metabolism so that we are often hungry; they are not filling, and are often addictive; they contain few healthy micronutrients; and they make us eat fewer other healthy macronutrients (such as healthy fats).

Why is it, then, that we still so often hear that we gain weight from too many calories and too little exercise? Why is it that the nutrition models of so many countries still consider carbohydrates such as bread and potatoes the basis of a healthy nutrition pattern, rather than vegetables, fruits, legumes, or mushrooms? As mentioned earlier, it is important for the food industry that the message is kept alive that overweight is caused by too many calories and too little exercise. That way, there is no unhealthy food, and you can blame overweight on eating too much, exercising too little and on laziness and lack of willpower in general (it is not because the food we eat reprograms our taste buds, brain chemistry, and metabolism, making us continuously hungry, tired, and addicted). This old dogma persists for several reasons, which leave the general public in the dark about what really are the important causes of the obesity epidemic. Often, outdated insights, little effective advice, or confusing information is given. Providing confusing information is also a tactic followed for tens of years by the tobacco industry. Doubt is spread by saying that "This is not the scientific consensus" or "Everything is unhealthy when you consume too much of it" (as the director of the tobacco company Philip Morris said to a government committee). The food industry has been doing the same for decades. Studies that showed that sugar, soft drinks, or red meat are unhealthy have for many years been trivialized, or criticized, or swept under the rug, and the investigators discredited, so that official advice against them came decades too late, and at the cost of a lot of disease, suffering and deaths that could have been prevented.

Besides spreading doubt and confusion, another favorite tactic of food companies is to sponsor health organizations or physicians and dietitians associations to push their own opinions about food and health. Not very long ago, a national association of dietitians launched a large *pro-sugar* campaign, with ads proclaiming, "Sugar can be part of a healthy eating pattern. Healthy food and enjoyment can perfectly well be combined. Sugar or sucrose tastes good and provides energy." As it later turned out, this campaign was sponsored by Coca-Cola. Such campaigns spread a confusing and ambiguous message to the public. The food industry often collaborates with official health organizations. Food companies pay about $7,000 annually to the American Heart Association in exchange for a sticker with the association's logo on their products. That logo tells the consumer that the product has been approved by the American Heart Association, because it contains little fat, saturated fat, or cholesterol—despite studies which for years have shown that many fats and cholesterol do *not* play a role in the risk of heart attack. Finally, the food industry ensures that its representatives are members of advisory councils, or government and other official organizations, to promote their own interests and water down health recommendations.

In addition, the food industry may object directly and openly to new health guidelines and nutrition advice. An example is a health report by the WHO, composed by a panel of 30 experts from 22 countries. The conclusions of that panel were fairly obvious: Too much sugar and fast food are unhealthy, and advertising of unhealthy food to children is not a good thing. Despite this obviously being sensible advice, a huge protest by the food industry ensued. A deluge of letters and protests followed, both addressed to the panel and to the government, from the Snack Food Association, Wheat Foods Council, Corn Refiners Association, International Dairy Foods Association, the Sugar Association, US Council for International Business, and many more. They suggested that this report was trash and not based on scientific consensus. This is a frequently used tactic: referring to the scientific consensus (which can often be reached only by making too many concessions) and scientific studies that fit their own opinions or have been funded by the food industry. There were even calls for stopping financial support of the WHO by the United States. Developing countries were urged to protest against this report, which they did, since many developing countries produce sugar and oils. Finally all this controversy resulted in withdrawal of the director of the WHO, Gro Harlem Brundtland, from reelection because, according to her explanation, her policies were too contrary to the interests of the food and tobacco industry.[238]

Usually the influence of the food industry is more subtle and less direct. One way is by sponsoring research at universities and research institutes. A large part of the income of certain universities comes directly from the food and agricultural industry. Sometimes entire university departments or teaching chairs are established by food companies. Another way is creating all kinds of scientific research centers with scientific and neutral-sounding names, such the "Nutrition Foundation," created jointly by the National Biscuit Company, the Corn Products Refining Corporation, and General Foods. It is a good thing to conduct nutrition research, but one must be very wary of conflict of interest, since the industry that pays for this research also earns money with the products that are being investigated. We should not be naive about this. Research shows that when a study is paid for or sponsored by the food industry, there is an eight times' greater chance that the results are positive for the food industry.[239] It is always possible to have research done that puts your food product in a good light. For example, you can conclude that your food product is healthy by comparing it with something that is *less* healthy (like comparing whole grain bread with white bread), or you can ignore findings that do not fit your purpose, or analyze them in such a way that they still show a positive effect, which is sometimes referred to as "torturing the data."

These institutes and centers that are sponsored by the food industry employ or train scientists and then often present them to the media as nutrition experts. These experts in turn influence physicians, nutrition scientists, dietitians, and the public at large. Often these experts truly believe what they say. That is not difficult if you work in an environment where you are constantly told that people gain too much weight because they simply eat too much and exercise too little. Or that sugar is OK in moderation—of course it is, but what is in moderation? Or that everything is OK as long as you have a varied diet—another one of those platitudes that is of little help. Or that there is no such thing as unhealthy food; that it is all a matter of the amount you eat, whether it comes from a hamburger or cauliflower. If you are bombarded with these outdated ideas and this dubious and inefficient advice for many years, it is understandable that eventually you begin to believe yourself that eating less calories and a varied diet are sufficient to keep people healthy.

If you begin to doubt these dogmas, then the food industry is always there to help you out. It organizes lectures and congresses where scientists keep on proclaiming this outdated knowledge. I once saw an invitation for a scientific meeting organized by a large food company, with lectures about nutrition and health given by a professor. One of the lectures was on the topic "How to communicate an understandable nutrition message to the public." In short, the food industry wanted to explain to dietitians and physicians what to tell people about healthy nutrition! The meeting would be concluded with a visit to the factory and an interactive workshop on making margarine, followed by a happy hour with healthy food and drinks. I have no complaints about this last item.

Of course, it also not necessarily the case that nutrition experts are brainwashed by the food industry. Usually that is not necessary because nutrition is a very complex and comprehensive scientific field. There are few nutrition scientists who have a broad view of nutrition and health and who approach nutrition from scientific fields other than only nutrition, such as aging, evolution, medicine, pathology, biochemistry, nutrigenetics, neurology, psychology, and so forth. Also, nutrition science and human health is a very complex area, so many nutrition specialists take for granted what they are being told by famous experts, "key opinion leaders" or the government ("*eminence* based medicine" instead of "*evidence* based medicine"). Furthermore, many nutrition scientists are chemists, food technologists, or biologists who have never seen a patient up close and have no real idea what kind of damage an unhealthy nutrition pattern can do to the body. They get their knowledge mainly from the scientific literature and research that often has many shortcomings. As a university professor and physician once remarked to me, "There is a huge difference between scientific studies and practice." Many nutrition experts have never seen or treated patients who are becoming blind or whose foot needs to be amputated due to diabetes. These experts should think twice before proclaiming to the public that a varied diet is enough, or that eating lots of whole grain bread and potatoes is good for diabetes patients. This kind of advice will not reverse diabetes, whereas much better advice is available that can reverse diabetes and prevent patients from becoming blind or losing a foot. Patients have a right to know that.

There are, of course, also many experts who do have a broad perspective of nutrition but they are often careful to voice their opinions about it. When a university professor advises us to eat fewer potatoes or drink less milk, he may be harshly criticized and not only by the food industry but also by his colleagues. Many professors with more up-to-date insights prefer to avoid these controversial discussions in the media to not to harm their career or reputation.

Ultimately the food industry can always put forward its own experts (university professors, dietitians, and other spokespersons), who persist in creating doubt, who keep hammering on the old dogma of too many calories, and who give a different slant to studies that show certain foods to be unhealthy,

sometimes to an absurd degree. Charles Baker, biochemist and scientific director of the Sugar Association, responded to new recommendations to eat less
sugar that this was "not practical, unrealistic, and not scientifically supported."
Meanwhile, the WHO has made these recommendations even stronger. Dr.
Richard Kahn, scientific and medical director of the American Diabetes Association, commented: "There is not an iota of proof that sugar has anything to
do with developing diabetes." According to Dr. Kahn, prevention of diabetes
is a waste of money. Meanwhile, professors at top universities, such as Harvard and Yale, have stated that 90 percent of the risk of type 2 diabetes can be
prevented, primarily by healthier nutrition. Studies show that diabetes can be
reversed in only a few weeks via healthy nutrition.[49]

Therefore, we must be critical about the official nutrition recommendations.
Dr. Richard Smith, editor of the *British Medical Journal* and one of the leaders
of the Cochrane Collaboration (the famous institute that reviews thousands
of scientific articles so as to draw conclusions from them), wrote a well-known
article with the title "Are Some Diets Mass Murder?" In this article he refers to
various errors of the government and official organizations in regard to nutrition recommendations, in part because these organizations rely too much on
dubious science and are influenced by the food industry and other interested
parties. Dr. Smith writes, "In short, bold policies have been based on fragile
science, and the long term results may be terrible. . . . It's surely time for better
science and for humility among experts."

Needless to say it is not all to blame on the food industry. It would be too
easy to blame it for everything. Some companies are sincerely concerned about
public health or want to make their products healthier. For those companies, it
is frustrating that in doing so they are bound by very conservative government
guidelines. Companies are not allowed to say that their broccoli can decrease
the risk of cancer, or that their green tea can reduce the risk of stroke, or that
kale may slow down the development of macular degeneration. Government
organizations overseeing the food industry still operate with the outdated principle that every health claim about food must be supported by almost the same
strict scientific evidence as the claims about prescription drugs. If you want to
make a health claim for broccoli, you (not the government) better conduct a
clinical, randomized, placebo-controlled study, in which you let 20,000 people
eat broccoli for ten years, and another 20,000 eat a placebo broccoli for the
same number of years, and then check whether less cancer has occurred in the
broccoli group. Such research is virtually impossible to do (how would you

make a broccoli placebo?) and would cost tens of millions of dollars. Pharmaceutical companies can afford to pay for such studies only because they can earn millions with their patented drugs, but this is not an option for broccoli farmers. As a result, the consumer is stuck with a government that permits very few claims about healthy nutrition.

In addition, the government often operates based on old guidelines or knowledge, of which major nutrition scientists worldwide have said for years is outdated. It often takes a very long time before new scientific knowledge works its way into government recommendations. We have known since the 1980s that trans fats are unhealthy, but it took until 2003 for Denmark to impose a ban on them, and more than ten years later the United States was still considering it. How many thousands of deaths could have been prevented if these insights had been implemented much earlier?[240] This example also shows that official guidelines can differ from country to country, and that one country is sometimes more than a decade faster to adopt "new" insights.

Many government recommendations, as well as those of official institutions, could be better and healthier. That is shown in research again and again. There was a study, for example, in which participants could follow one or the other of two types of diets: the official recommendation of the American Heart Association (a classic low-fat diet) or an unofficial Mediterranean-inspired diet with vegetables, fruit, nuts, healthy fats, and white meat. After two years, the results showed that the group on the higher-fat Mediterranean diet had a 70 percent lower risk of death compared to the group that followed the official low-fat diet of the American Heart Association, an organization that issues all kinds of health recommendations.[241] The study was halted prematurely because it would be "unethical" to allow people to continue following the American Heart Association diet.

Not only are official recommendations often outdated but they are also oversimplified: good fats and bad fats? That is too difficult for the public to understand, so let's tell them to cut down on all fats. The same with sugars. The glycemic index and glycemic load are much too complicated for people to understand, so we will not include them. In addition, many official recommendations are based on watered-down consensus science, in which statements are issued that everyone can agree with, including experts from the food industry (or from universities sponsored by the food industry) or experts who adhere to outdated knowledge. They often acquiesce to the demands of the food industry and the cultural food practices of a country:

They can't take people's potatoes away or advise healthy foods that are too expensive, difficult to prepare, or unknown, like walnuts, quinoa, blueberries, and oyster mushrooms. Furthermore, the government must serve two masters: the people and the industry. A government that recommends eating less meat, dairy, or grain products also damages its own economy. The result is that many recommendations are too weak and ineffective.

Another thing that does not help is that medical students learn very little about nutrition, health, and preventive medicine. Their education is focused primarily on curing (insofar as possible) and not on prevention. Physicians are trained mainly to intervene when it is already too late: when your blood vessels are so clogged up that you have a heart attack, or when your tumor has spread to such an extent that you find blood in your urine or stool. Physicians could play a large role in the debate around healthy nutrition. They have a thorough scientific background and, very importantly, an extensive knowledge of how the human body works and how diseases arise. They can also see how good (or bad) official health recommendations work in practice because they actually see patients. They can also remain more independent, since they have their own practice and are often not tied to a university or company and they can therefore be more outspoken. Furthermore, they are practical and they do not live in an ivory tower but are in daily contact with patients and their chronic lifestyle diseases.

Finally, we should not forget the role of the media. We are continuously bombarded with conflicting health headlines. Many journalists are constantly trying to meet deadlines. They do not have much time to do a thorough investigation and sometimes unquestioningly accept the opinions of so-called experts, who still proclaim outdated or plain wrong insights.

In summary, because of a complex interplay of the food and agricultural industry, nutrition experts, the government, physicians, journalists and many other parties, we live today in a kind of "health vacuum." As a result, for many years now we often receive outdated, weak, inefficient, and conflicting health and nutrition recommendations. Given ever increasing healthcare costs, and the tsunami of obesity and "chronic" diseases that are sweeping the world, we cannot afford to be so lenient about health advice, and we cannot continue to underestimate the power and great importance of healthy nutrition and a healthy lifestyle in general.

As a society, we need to realize that it is ultimately the consumer who has the power. As consumers, we need to be critical: of the nutrition experts, the industry, the health gurus, and the government. Patients have the right to know—certainly when they may become blind from diabetes, or when their coronary arteries have become more than 80 percent clogged—that their dietary recommendations could be much better.

But how then can we see the forest for the trees with all those contradictory recommendations? We can base our choices and decisions on large, well-conducted, independent scientific studies and on the opinions of internationally recognized nutrition experts who have no ties to the food industry and who are not afraid to discuss their findings, even if they are contrary to many economic interests. These experts often work at top universities, they have a very broad view of nutrition, and they approach the topic from different professional perspectives. We can also base them on the recommendations of new associations that have split off from the official organizations so as to be able to provide more independent and up-to-date guidelines. The only problem is that when these associations become larger, they automatically come to the attention of the food industry again and, for example, are offered sponsorship. Then, they, too, will perhaps start to be more careful about what they say and do and make compromises.

Ideally, we should have an organization with physicians, dietitians, and scientists with a broad background who are independent of the food industry, or not from universities or departments that are sponsored by the industry, and who approach nutrition from multiple angles, such as aging, evolution, medicine, biochemistry, and psychology. It would be best if these nutrition experts came from different countries, so that it could include top experts from across the world and not only those from the homeland, as is often the case.

Physicians should also be better educated with respect to healthy nutrition and prevention. This is important, as physicians are usually the first medical professionals people turn to. Some US universities already offer their medical students courses in nutrition and even culinary medicine. In an ideal future, physicians will be able to prescribe not only medication but also specific foods for people who are overweight or have prostate cancer or diabetes. Physicians should not base their advice for such important and serious applications on outdated, oversimplified, or watered-down health recommendations.

SUMMARY

The **general recommendation** to lose weight and prevent overweight, namely, **eat less and exercise more**, is mostly not effective, especially in the long term.

A **calorie is not always a calorie** because

- Not all food substances we eat or drink are completely absorbed by the gut.

- Some food substances are not converted to calories but are used to build up the body or to perform tasks in the body.

- The bacteria in our gut also use up food substances or, conversely, release them.

- It also costs energy (calories) to digest and convert food substances before they can be burned into calories.

- Many food substances can affect the metabolism, so you consume or burn more or less calories.

- Etc.

Regarding **overweight**, there are two important causes or elephants in the room:

Elephant 1 (very well known): an excess of fast sugars, in the form of soft drinks, candy, chips, baked goods, and fast food

Elephant 2 (not so well known): an excess of starchy products such as bread, potatoes, pasta, and rice.

These foods

- Cause high **sugar and insulin peaks**, which reprogram out metabolism so that we quickly become hungry again and tire easily (so that we eat more and exercise less)

- Are **addictive** and not **filling**

- Make us eat **fewer** other **macronutrients** (such as healthy fats and healthy proteins)

- Are empty calories that contain very **few** healthy **micronutrients** (vitamins, minerals, flavonoids, omega-3 fatty acids, etc.).

Other elephants are

- **Too much animal protein** (particularly in red processed meat)

- **Too many unhealthy fats**, such as trans fats in industrially prepared baked goods and oils high in omega-6, such as corn oil and sunflower oil.

Also important:

- An **abundance** of (usually carbohydrate-rich) products and a **lack** of healthy alternatives (for example in food dispensers or in restaurants)

- **Lack of time** to prepare healthy, tasty food

- **Marketing** of unhealthy food, even addressed to young children (for example, so-called whole grain cereals or baked goods that contain 75 percent carbohydrates)

- **Lack of knowledge** about the importance of healthy nutrition

- Disruption of sleep and day-night rhythm (night shifts or irregular shifts increase the risk of overweight and diabetes), temperature (the warmer it is, the more easily you gain weight), emotion (stress, fear, or unhappiness can lead to overeating), or an unhealthy diet during pregnancy (reprograms the metabolism of the fetus, so that it later has a greater risk of overweight).

Outdated, weak, and ineffective **health recommendations** contribute to the **difficulty** for many people to **lose weight**.

REDUCING GROWTH STIMULATION WITH SPECIFIC NUTRITION

It is not a coincidence that overweight people are at greater risk of various aging-related diseases, such as heart attacks, diabetes, dementia, and stroke. The reason is that both accelerated aging and overweight are the result of growth stimulation, a continuous bombardment of growth signals in the form of sugars, amino acids, and unhealthy fats. Fortunately there are dietary changes and nutritional substances that can slow down this growth as well as its results, such as that nasty protein agglomeration that plays such an important role in aging.

The first recommendation has already been dealt with in detail: Consume fewer fast and starchy carbohydrates, such as soft drinks, candy, baked goods, bread, pasta, rice, and potatoes. As a result, you will get less stimulation of aging switches, such as insulin and IGF, as well as less sugar cross-linking. Eating less meat and replacing animal proteins with vegetable proteins from nuts, legumes, tofu, or mushrooms is also healthy. This results in less activation of growth and aging switches[242] that, for example, stimulate protein production. This in turn results in less agglomeration of proteins.

It should not surprise us that various healthy nutrition plans already contain these recommendations. These diets have in common that they are all primarily plant-based. They contain lots of vegetables, legumes, nuts, and mushrooms—all foods that all contain few fast sugars, animal proteins, or other growth-inducing substances. In addition, these diets contain all kinds of substances that tone down those specific growth-stimulating aging switches. These include, for example, quercetin, a substance that is found in vegetables, fruit (particularly apples), and capers. Quercetin can reduce atherosclerosis (narrowing of blood vessels) and the risk of cancer.[243] Green tea and coffee contain substances such as EGCG (epigallocatechin gallate) and caffeine, which inhibit important growth and aging switches.[244, 245] A study that followed 82,000 Japanese people between the ages of 45 and 74 over an average of thirteen years found that those who drank several cups of tea a day had a 35 percent lower risk of stroke.[246] Another study that followed 1,400 people over 21 years shows that people who drink three to five cups of coffee per day have a 65 percent lower risk of Alzheimer's disease.[192] It is the caffeine in coffee, among other things, that slows down the protein agglomeration, one of the causes of aging.[247] Therefore, it is best to drink regular rather than decaffeinated coffee. Some people should be careful not to drink too much coffee, though, because it can irritate the mucous membrane in the stomach and intestine and cause indigestion. Of course, these foods and drinks are healthy not only because they inhibit growth-stimulating mechanisms in cells but also because of various other reasons, for example, because they contain many micronutrients or induce hormesis, which results in decreased inflammation, better DNA protection, improved detoxifying capabilities, and so on.

Besides caffeine, there are many other substances that can slow down protein agglomeration, such as curcumin, which is found in turmeric.[248, 249] Curcumin is responsible for the typical yellow color of curry sauce, a favorite food in many Asian countries. Mice that were fed curcumin had 43 percent less protein agglomeration, which causes Alzheimer's disease.[250] Some researchers speculate that Alzheimer's occurs less among elderly people in Asia because they use a lot of curcumin in their food, among other things.

Olive oil is another product that is often used in healthy diets, especially in Mediterranean countries. Olive oil contains oleocanthal, a substance that has the characteristic bitter taste of olive oil. Studies show that oleocanthal can also slow down protein agglomeration.[251, 252] This may be one reason that diets rich in olive oil protect against aging-related diseases, such as Alzheimer's. Cinnamon also contains substances that can specifically slow down protein agglomeration. Cinnamon extracts slow down cognitive decline in mice with Alzheimer's disease and improve the blood sugar levels in diabetes patients.[253, 254]

Healthy diets also contain much fiber, fats, and sour foods, such as vinegar and lemon juice (used in salad dressings, for example). These substances reduce the high sugar peaks that accelerate aging. Fibers package the sugars, so that they are released into the bloodstream more slowly. Fats and vinegar slow down the emptying of the stomach, which also results in lower sugar peaks. In the Middle Ages, vinegar tea was one of the treatments used for diabetes patients. Taking vinegar before a meal—for example, one tablespoon in a half or full glass of water—can lower sugar peaks and even promote weight loss.[255, 256] Do not overdo it, however, because in large quantities vinegar can cause bone loss and osteoporosis.

It is noteworthy that in areas where people on average live longer, many people often deliberately eat less. Eating less is an excellent way to turn off all those growth-stimulating switches on our cells. In Okinawa, for example, an island off the coast of Japan where there are five times more centenarians than in the West, it is common for people to stop eating when they are only about 80 percent full.

Calorie restriction goes one step further, eating about one quarter less than what you need. For example, if a woman needs 2,000 calories per day on average, she consumes 1,500 calories per day under calorie restriction. Studies show that calorie restriction has many beneficial effects on people: They have healthier blood vessels, less atherosclerosis, and a heart that is more elastic and flexible.[256-259] Fasting is also a form of calorie restriction. This involves eating nothing or very little for one or more days (but you do need to drink fluids). This temporarily turns off the growth switches in our cells. A lot of research is being done on fasting and it looks like fasting has a number of health benefits, such as improving the insulin sensitivity of the body.[260, 261] Fasting can be done in many different ways. Some people skip evening meals (so they fast from noon to the next morning) or fast one or two days in a week. Others fast one day every month or a few days every three months. Some people eat completely nothing during a fast, others eat one or two small meals (about 300 calories per meal) per day. I would recommend not to fast too strictly, meaning: eat one or two small meals or a bit of food during the day instead of completely nothing. If you eat nothing during several days, you have the risk of breaking down your own muscles too much, which taxes your body, and you will also produce all kinds of stress hormones, like noradrenaline, while often feeling very bad. But just skipping evening meals, or having a very light dinner, can be already a great way to lose weight and maintain your health. And you will often sleep better, because you are not suffering from a full stomach or acid reflux.

Vegetables, fruit, legumes, mushrooms, olive oil, spices, coffee, tea, and vinegar and not overeating—there are many reasons why these are part of a healthy diet. Thanks to insights about the aging process, we are getting to understand better why such foods are healthy. For example, they slow down growth stimulation of our cells, or protein agglomeration, or they have a hormetic function (whereby they reduce inflammation and induce repair, protection, or detoxification mechanisms).

To condense this knowledge and make it easy to apply, I have created a model that I call the food hourglass. It consists of two triangles: The top triangle contains less healthy foods of which we should eat less; the bottom triangle, healthy foods of which we should eat more. The two triangles are each other's counterpart. That means that it is easy to see how you can replace the

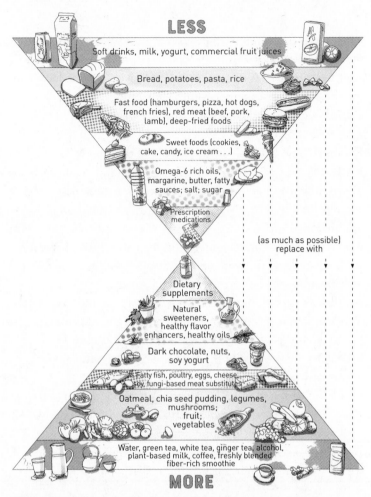

LESS

Soft drinks, milk, yogurt, commercial fruit juices

Bread, potatoes, pasta, rice

Fast food (hamburgers, pizza, hot dogs, french fries), red meat (beef, pork, lamb), deep-fried foods

Sweet foods (cookies, cake, candy, ice cream . . .)

Omega-6 rich oils, margarine, butter, fatty sauces; salt; sugar

Prescription medications

(as much as possible) replace with

Dietary supplements

Natural sweeteners, healthy flavor enhancers, healthy oils

Dark chocolate, nuts, soy yogurt

Fatty fish, poultry, eggs, cheese, soy, fungi-based meat substitutes

Oatmeal, chia seed pudding, legumes, mushrooms; fruit; vegetables

Water, green tea, white tea, ginger tea, alcohol, plant-based milk, coffee, freshly blended fiber-rich smoothie

MORE

Smart dietary supplements: vitamin D, iodine, magnesium, selenium, B vitamins
Note: Never change medication without consulting with your health-care provider.

Natural sweeteners: stevia, tagatose, erythritol, applesauce, banana mash
Healthy flavor enhancers: herbs and spices (turmeric, parsley, thyme, rosemary, basil, oregano, marjoram, mint), garlic, onion, lemon juice, vinegar (balsamic or raspberry), potassium salt
Healthy oils: olive oil, flaxseed oil, walnut oil, canola oil, perilla seed oil
Unhealthy oils rich in omega-6: corn oil, sunflower seed oil, palm oil, sesame oil

Fatty fish: salmon, mackerel, herring, anchovies, sardines
Meat replacements: soy (tofu, miso, natto, tempeh) and fungi-based meat substitutes
Organic meat and dairy products (from free-ranging, grass-fed cows and chickens)

Legumes: beans, peas, lentils, soybeans

Water can be flavored with lemon, sage, or thyme
Plant-based milk: soy milk, almond milk, hazelnut milk . . .
Alcohol: a maximum of one drink per day, including alcohol-free days
Coffee: a maximum of three to five cups per day
Tea: white tea, green tea, ginger tea, black tea . . .
Smoothie: preferably made from low-sugar fruit like blueberries, blackberries, and strawberries, as well as vegetables

Calorie restriction: Eating 25 percent less can extend life span.
Exercise: It is not the intensity that counts but the regularity.
Relaxation: Do meditation, yoga, self-hypnosis, deep-breathing exercises.
Social contacts: Spend time with family, friends, join clubs, and do volunteer work.

less healthy foods in the top triangle with healthier alternatives from the bottom triangle. For example, you can replace red meat from the top red layer with healthier alternatives in the bottom red layer, such as fatty fish, white meat (poultry), tofu, or fungi-based meat substitutes.

The food hourglass represents seven simple principles:

1. Eat much less bread, potatoes, pasta, and rice.
2. Replace bread with oatmeal or chia seed pudding made with plant-based milk (soy, hazelnut, almond milk). Potatoes, pasta, and rice are replaced by (extra) vegetables (mainly), legumes, mushrooms or quinoa.
3. Replace animal milk or yogurt with plant-based (soy, hazelnut, almond, cashew) milk or yogurt. Cheese and eggs are allowed in moderation.
4. Eat little or no red meat (beef, pork, and sheep) and more fatty fish (salmon, mackerel, herring, anchovies, and sardines), poultry (chicken, turkey), tofu, or fungi-based meat substitutes.
5. Vegetables are the base of the food hourglass. Fruit, legumes, mushrooms, and quinoa are healthy additions.
6. Drink lots of water, several cups of green or white tea per day, and one glass of freshly pressed fiber-rich fruit or vegetable smoothie. Coffee and alcohol are allowed in moderation.
7. Take smart dietary supplements, such as selenium yeast, vitamin D3, vitamin K2, B vitamins, magnesium malate, and iodine.

The goal of the food hourglass is to slow down aging and reduce the risk of aging-related diseases. The model is based on the latest research into aging. The food hourglass has been shared with many physicians and scientists, such as Harvard professor Walter Willett, one of the most renowned and cited nutrition experts in the world. He wrote that the food hourglass model "does seem very consistent with scientific evidence."

A Few Clarifications on Milk, Cheese, and Butter

Why is cheese permitted but milk is not, since cheese is made of milk? There are several reasons. Cheese is like a partially digested, fermented form of milk, so you cannot compare them. For example, in contrast to milk, cheese contains a lot of vitamin K, probiotics, less immunogenic (immune system–provoking) proteins, and less galactose (a milk sugar that accelerates aging). Studies show that not all dairy products are equally healthy and that cheese is healthier than milk.[166, 262] Meanwhile more and more scientists warn against the long-term effects of milk.[263] An important reason to be wary of long-term milk consumption, is that milk was created by nature to make calves grow as fast as possible. Therefore milk contains many growth-inducing substances. We have extensively discussed in this book that more growth means faster aging, and that growth-stimulating substances, like insulin and IGF, accelerate aging and shorten life span. If you drink milk, you exactly increase the production of these substances in your body and activate all kinds of growth switches and mechanisms, which can in the long term accelerate aging (the growth-promoting effects of milk are the reason why the Thai government for example, wants to promote milk intake in its population, to boost the height of its citizens—of course with the aid of the milk industry). Also, milk contains galactose, a sugar that accelerates aging. Galactose causes inflammation, glycation, cross-linking, and oxidative stress (damage to cell components), among other things. Scientists even use galactose to induce or accelerate aging in their lab animals to study aging.[264-266] They do not need very high doses to do that, a comparable human dose can be found in a few glasses of milk (an average glass of milk contains already five grams of galactose).[267]

Based on these and many other insights, it is therefore not really surprising that many studies point to an increased risk of cancer, aging-related diseases, and mortality from drinking milk.[267-270] One Swedish study found that women who drank three or more glasses of milk per day, had almost double the risk of dying compared to women who drank less than one glass of milk per day.[267] This study was interesting, because it is one of the few studies that are so large (more than 100,000 participants), long enough (the average duration was 20 years), and look at *mortality* instead of a specific disease. Of course, there are also studies that show that milk can have healthy effects, but they are all too often sponsored by the milk industry and their science institutes, and their duration is also mostly too short—for example, a few years at best (while it takes decades to discover aging-accelerating effects in humans), or they look only at *a specific disease* that is decreased in milk drinkers while ignoring the most important clinical outcome, *death* (though the Swedish study looked into this), or ignoring other diseases for which milk increases the risk. The milk industry is always happy to point to studies that milk perhaps decreases the risk of colon cancer, but they ignore the many studies that show that milk consumption is associated with an increased risk of Parkinson's disease,[270] prostate cancer (an effect demonstrated in more than a dozen studies),[271] various other diseases, and most importantly, an increased risk of dying.[267] And did I already tell you that milk does not protect against osteoporosis or bone loss, despite what the milk industry has told us otherwise for decades?[267, 272] Of course, you do not often hear about these studies. Every time a study that questions milk appears in the media, it is harshly criticized or "must be interpreted with extreme caution," and when a daring scientist or physician publicly questions the long-term effects of milk, she or he often gets a flood of critique and comments, which is one reason why many researchers avoid publicly criticizing milk.

Anyway, viewed from the science of aging and from a long-term perspective, animal milk consumption is not advisable. However, keep in mind that it is always important to get enough calcium. Luckily, most vegetable milk drinks (like hazelnut and almond milk) are fortified with calcium. Many vegetables contain lots of calcium, especially leafy green vegetables like broccoli, spinach, and kale, of which the calcium is much better absorbed than calcium in milk. This is one reason why people who eat lots of vegetables have less risk of osteoporosis. But to really make sure you get adequate amounts of this important mineral, you can opt for daily calcium supplements. However, do not take calcium in too high doses in one go, because this will cause a lofty calcium peak in your blood, which can accelerate the calcification of your arteries, and increase your risk of a heart attack.[273] Make sure your supplement does not contain more than 400 mg calcium per dose, and spread different doses throughout the day.

Also, keep in mind that cheese and eggs contain animal proteins, and they should be consumed in moderation.

In the food hourglass, butter is still listed under foods to be reduced, although we have seen that various saturated fats, such as in butter, are not as unhealthy as first thought. Butter can be consumed in small amounts, such as to cook with, but there are healthier alternatives to butter, such as olive oil, flaxseed oil, and walnut oil for cold dishes, and avocado oil, olive oil, and coconut oil for cooking.

The food hourglass also forms the basis for a new field of science that I have introduced: *nutrigerontology*.[274] Nutrigerontology is the scientific discipline that studies the role of nutrition in the aging process. More specifically, it investigates how certain foods, food substances, diets, and dietary patterns can accelerate or slow down the aging process and influence the risk of aging-related diseases, such as heart disease, diabetes, and dementia. The more we know about why we age, the better the nutrition recommendations we can provide, because most diseases in the West are aging-related diseases. By studying aging, we can also provide better *long-term* recommendations and, as such, dispel many myths about food. We know that much advice on nutrition is based on short-term studies and effects, such as weight loss or lowering cholesterol. This is problematic, because in the short-term almost every diet or intervention works, while this is not the case in the long-term. Even worse, lots of diets or interventions that show healthy effects in the short-term, can have negative effects in the long-term. Take high-protein diets for example. In the short-term they improve glucose levels, blood fats, blood pressure, weight loss, and so on. But thanks to research into the aging process, we now know that protein agglomeration plays a role in aging and many aging-related diseases. This then allows us to predict that high-protein diets are not healthy in the long-term. More and more studies confirm that, even though many earlier, short-term studies showed healthy outcomes.

Nutrigerontology can also be very useful in the prevention of aging-related diseases, since it focuses on the mechanisms that cause aging. Readers who want to know more about the food hourglass and about the influence of specific foods on the aging process can read my book *The Food Hourglass*.

Now we are ready to go to the next, and last, step. This step involves even more powerful methods to slow down the aging process. It is about new technologies, which in the future will change aging and the lives of all generations.

SUMMARY

Step 3: Reduce growth stimulation.

Growth stimulation is caused by growth-stimulating substances, such as glucose, amino acids, insulin, IGF, growth hormone, and testosterone, which

- Activate aging mechanisms and switches in the cell

- Deactivate repair, protection, and maintenance mechanisms in the cell

This leads to more protein agglomeration, formation of sugar cross-links, mitochondrial damage, etc.

Growth stimulation can be reduced by

- Eating fewer **carbohydrates**, both fast carbohydrates (soft drinks, candy, chips, baked goods, commercial fruit juices) and slow carbohydrates (bread, potatoes, rice, pasta)

- Reducing intake of **animal proteins**

- **Slowing down** the **emptying of the stomach** and the **release of sugars** into the bloodstream via
    - Fibers (in vegetables, fruit, mushrooms, etc.)
    - Healthy fats (olive oil, flax seed oil, walnut oil, olives, avocados, nuts, etc.)
    - Vinegar (or other sour foods, such as lemon juice)

- **Specific substances** that reduce growth stimulation (flavonoids, curcumin) in apples, capers, turmeric, blueberries, coffee, tea, broccoli, etc.

- **Exercising** after a meal (cycling, walking, weightlifting), which lowers the sugar peaks

- **Calorie restriction**: eating about one quarter less than what you need

- (Intermittent) **fasting**, such as one to two days per week or at the end of every season.

The **food hourglass** is a nutrition model that integrates all these points.

Step 4: Reverse the Aging Process

What if we could reverse the aging process? Not simply slow it down but really reverse it, so that people would become younger, and a wrinkly skin becomes smooth and radiant, a previously weakened heart can again force-fully pump blood through elastic arteries, and Alzheimer's patients could remember everything just as clearly and exactly as when they were in their twenties. Reversing the aging process would be the ultimate breakthrough in medicine. Not only would we live longer but we would not be afflicted with debilitating aging-related diseases and stay healthy much longer. Is this possible?

Some researchers think it is. That is why this fourth step of the longevity staircase is special. Whereas the previous steps were designed to *slow down* the aging process, this step goes one step further: The methods described here are meant to *reverse* aging. I make a point of discussing only methods that are already reasonably concrete and far advanced, not those that exist only on paper or are a far-fetched fantasy of a daydreaming science fiction writer. Some methods have already been successfully tested on animals. Others are currently being tested in clinical studies with humans and have already cost billions of dollars to develop. Yet others are already used in humans, albeit for other reasons, such as to cure fatal diseases. All have the potential to make people younger. Let's take a look at some of them.

CLEANING UP THE PROTEIN DEBRIS

As mentioned earlier, protein agglomeration in and around our cells is an important cause of aging. This protein debris strangles our cells, so that they cannot function as well and may even die, as is the case in Alzheimer's disease, a typical disease of old age. If we could clean up this protein debris, our cells could become younger, as it were. How? One method is by vaccination.

Usually vaccines are developed against viruses that cause measles or influenza or against bacteria that cause whooping cough or tuberculosis. The principle of vaccines is actually very simple but very effective: A vaccine contains a neutralized virus or bacterium, or parts of it, which is injected into the body. The immune system will attack the virus or bacterium parts, in the process learning to recognize these viruses and bacteria, so that if in the future we are infected with the real, complete virus or the living bacterium, the immune system can quickly attack and destroy it, even before we become sick.

This attack takes place via antibodies. Antibodies are proteins produced by white blood cells, which are part of the immune system. These proteins have a specific form, which makes them stick only to the virus or bacterium that the immune system wants to clean up. If a bacterium is studded with antibodies, it can no longer function and it disintegrates, or it is cleaned up by white blood cells; the antibodies work like fishhooks or anchors for the white blood cells.

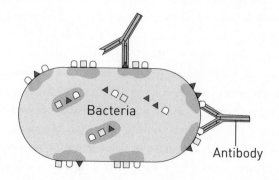

Antibodies (proteins) attach themselves to bacteria and thereby damage and hamper them.

Vaccines are one of the greatest medical breakthroughs ever—they have saved the lives of hundreds of millions of people. Take the polio vaccine, for example. Polio was caused by a virus that made children seriously ill and in some cases could paralyze part of the body, or even the entire body, which put them in a wheelchair, or if their breathing muscles were paralyzed, in an iron lung for the rest of their lives. The polio vaccine was invented in 1952, and since then, the disease has virtually disappeared in the West. The greatest success story, however, is the eradication of smallpox. Smallpox afflicted humankind for thousands of years and it was a horrible disease. If you contracted smallpox, you had a considerable chance of dying. Even in the twentieth century, smallpox killed 350 million people. More than two thirds of those who survived the infection often had long-term complications, like arthritis or blindness or ugly scars on their face or body as a result of the blisters, or they remained fatigued and weakened for years following the disease. Since 1978, after a worldwide intensive vaccination campaign, smallpox was completely eradicated. The last smallpox death was a British researcher who was infected because she worked above the lab where research on smallpox was still ongoing and the virus reached her lab on the higher floor via the ventilation system (the woman's superior also subsequently committed suicide presumably because of this).

Vaccines have played a very important role in medicine. Could they do this again in the case of aging, that final, terminal disease with a 100 percent risk of death? Scientists are working on it. It is possible to develop vaccines against the proteins that agglomerate in the body and drive aging. Such a vaccine contains a specific protein (that accumulates in the body as we age) or pieces of it. If you inject this into the body, the immune system will learn to make antibodies against this aging-related protein, just as it would against any virus or bacterium. These antibodies attach themselves to that aging-related protein, and the white blood cells in the immune system will then recognize these proteins and clean them up, so that they cannot accumulate in the body.

Various large pharmaceutical companies are currently working hard to develop such vaccines, among other things to treat one of the most feared aging-related diseases, Alzheimer's disease. Some of the vaccines can clean up the proteins that accumulate in the brain of Alzheimer's patients. In one study, people who had produced sufficient antibodies against these Alzheimer's proteins, showed less cognitive decline in the years following vaccination.[275] These studies do not always go smoothly, however. In one study, in one in fifteen patients the brain became inflamed after vaccination by a massive overreaction of the immune system (a condition called "encephalitis," or inflammation of the brain). Thus it is important to develop vaccines that do not cause a too strong reaction to the protein debris and thereby damage the brain.

Unfortunately, some studies show that their specific Alzheimer's vaccines do not work. They do not show sufficient improvement in cognition. Some researchers suggest that this is because these so-called amyloid vaccines target only one protein that clusters *around* the brain cells, whereas Alzheimer's disease is caused by a different type of protein (tau protein) that clusters *inside* the brain cells and thus the vaccine is ineffective. Another possibility is that these vaccines are given too late, after billions of brain cells have already been damaged and died. In that case it might be better to give the vaccines many years earlier, so that the proteins do not get a chance to pile up.

However that may be, various studies do show that it is possible to develop vaccines that clean up the protein debris. Pharmaceutical companies are spending billions of dollars on this kind of research. They want to develop vaccines not only against Alzheimer's disease but also against other aging-related diseases, such as Parkinson's disease and against the transthyretin protein, which accumulates and causes protein agglomeration everywhere in the body, a process that fells even the toughest supercentenarians. These aging vaccines are able to remove the protein debris from the body and thereby make it younger. Maybe in the future, people will get an aging vaccine every ten years, to clean up the protein debris from their blood vessels, brain, and other organs, so that they can stay young.

Vaccines that target proteins only outside our cells are not enough, however. Proteins also accumulate inside our cells, not only around the cells. Those are more difficult to clean up, because antibodies usually do not get into the cells; they circulate outside them. To get around that problem there is the possibility of using another method: lysosomal enzyme therapy.

We have talked about lysosomes before. Lysosomes are small bags that float around in our cells. They are the incinerators of the cell; they break down debris into smaller pieces, as such digesting it. The debris that is broken down includes proteins, fats, and sometimes parts of the cell, such as mitochondria. The problem, however, is that the more we age, the less effective the lysosomes become. They, too, fill up with proteins and other debris, which they can then no longer break down. As a result, more and more proteins and debris fill up the lysosomes and subsequently the cells, so that they age. We need to find ways to help the lysosomes, and that is indeed possible. It is possible to inject people with lysosomal *enzymes*—specific proteins that are specialized in breaking down other proteins and substances. Once injected, these lysosomal enzymes automatically travel to the lysosomes and help them break down the accumulated debris. Better yet, we can smuggle enzymes into the lysosomes that they never had before so that they can break down even the toughest debris and thereby prevent the lysosomes from filling up.

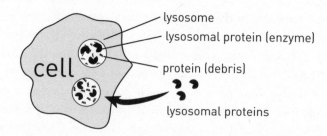

Additional or more potent lysosomal enzymes are injected into the bloodstream and find their way to the lysosomes, where they break down the toughest debris.

This is not as far-fetched as it seems. Researchers have indeed found such proteins, sometimes in the strangest places, such as cemeteries. When someone dies of old age, the lysosomes of that person contain a lot of "indestructible" debris that has accumulated in the body for decades and contributed to its aging and death. That body ends up in a cemetery and starts to degrade. That raises the question, what happens with all that indestructible lysosomal debris in nature? In nature, everything is used, so there must be bacteria somewhere that are able to break down this lysosomal debris. There is no better place to find them than in a cemetery, where there is a lot of lysosomal debris from dead bodies. Thus scientists took their shovels and went to cemeteries, hoping to find these bacteria, and indeed, after some digging, they found bacteria that contained unique enzymes capable of breaking down even the toughest lysosomal debris (to convert it to food for themselves). This goes to show how inventive nature is. Most often, nature is light years ahead of us in finding solutions for certain problems.

The only thing left to do was to find a way to introduce these bacterial enzymes into human lysosomes. That is possible: One can hang a small molecule (a kind of tag or flag) onto the bacterial enzymes, which ensures that these enzymes are automatically transported to the lysosomes. Upon arrival, they can help break down even the toughest, unbreakable proteins and other debris, which would otherwise accumulate in the body and cause aging. With this method, it could be possible not only to slow down aging but even partially reverse it. That way the dead—and their cemetery-soil-dwelling bacteria—could help the living postpone death.

Lysosomal enzyme therapy seems like a far-out treatment that may become reality sometime in a distant future. But this is not so. Just like the protein vaccines, some lysosomal enzymes are already used today to treat certain metabolic diseases. There are often deadly diseases whereby the lysosomes do not work efficiently—these are called *lysosomal* storage disorders. They occur when debris accumulates in the lysosomes because certain lysosomal enzymes are not functioning or are absent. A well-known example is Gaucher's disease, in which a certain lysosomal enzyme is not functioning. Normally that enzyme breaks down a specific substance in the lysosomes. When this does not happen, this substance accumulates in the lysosomes and in the cells as well. This affects specifically the cells that produce much of this substance, such as the liver, spleen, bones, eyes, brain, and lungs. These cells become more and more filled up and incapacitated, causing severe bone pain, bruising (because the liver normally produces clotting proteins), a swollen abdomen (because the poorly functioning liver swells up), a greater risk of infection (because the bone marrow, where white blood cells are produced, does not function well), or epileptic seizures (because the brain cells cannot function properly due to the accumulation of debris). Until recently, this disease was always fatal. However, scientists have succeeded in producing the defective lysosomal enzyme in the laboratory. These enzymes are injected into the patient's bloodstream, where they automatically travel to the lysosomes and begin to break down the offending substance. This lysosomal enzyme therapy shows that defective lysosomes can be repaired.

The problem is that this therapy is still very expensive. One vial of lysosomal enzymes costs about $1,400. A Gaucher's patient needs a dose of twelve vials every two weeks, which comes to about $400,000 per year. The patient needs this therapy for the rest of his life, or he will die. Treatment for twenty years would cost $8 million per patient. In the future, newer, cheaper production methods and expiration of the patents will make this treatment cheaper. The same thing happened with antibiotics. The first antibiotic was developed around 1942 and it was so difficult to make and expensive that the first patient, who initially responded successfully, still died because the antibiotic was no longer available. Physicians collected the urine of their first antibiotics patients to filter out the antibiotics, which could then be administered again. Today, antibiotics are produced by tons at a time and the cost is down to almost zero.

Thus, the possibility exists that in the future you will get an intravenous lysosomal enzyme infusion every other year or so to keep you young and healthy. The lysosomal enzymes will travel to the lysosomes to break down all that cellular debris and rejuvenate your cells. At this time, an infusion still requires a needle in a vein, but in the future those painful needles may be replaced, for example, by patches that contain hair-thin injection needles so you will not feel any pain at all. You simply apply a rejuvenation patch to your arm before you go to work in your self-driving car.

CROSS-LINK BREAKERS: CLEAN UP THOSE TENACIOUS SUGAR-LINKS

Earlier in the book, we discussed in detail how sugars also accelerate the aging process. One of the ways they do this is via cross-links. Cross-links are made from sugar and link the proteins that make up our body together. This causes stiff and wrinkly tissues, hardening of the blood vessels (high blood pressure), loss of elasticity of the lungs (more risk of pneumonia), creaky joints (from cross-linking in the cartilage), and cataracts (from cross-linking in the lens of the eye, which makes it cloudy). The formation of these cross-links seems inevitable because we need sugar as fuel, but it is not inevitable per se. Birds are a good example: A lot of sugar is circulating in their bloodstream because they need a lot of energy to be able to fly. The level of sugar in birds' blood is four times higher than in people and would quickly become fatal for a human being. Nevertheless birds live three times longer on average than you would expect for their size. They must have found ways to drastically slow down the cross-linking. Blood sugar levels in birds are only one example of how nature can outwit aging if it wants to.

How can we get rid of these cross-links? We can do that by developing cross-link breakers. These are substances that can break or cut the cross-links. The proteins that build up our tissues can then break loose from one another, making our tissues less stiff. Wrinkles could lessen or disappear, the lungs could become elastic again, and the heart and blood vessels become unclogged and flexible. One of the first cross-link breakers to be developed was a substance by name of N-phenacylthiazolium bromide (PTB). In rodents that were given this substance, the cross-links were broken. Their aging blood vessels became elastic, and their stiff hearts became supple and were better able to pump blood around their body again. What most surprised the researchers was that PTB did not only slow down the aging process but actually reversed it—the heart and blood vessels rejuvenated.

The problem, however, was that PTB did not work well in humans: The human body broke down this substance too fast. Subsequently a variation of this substance was developed, called alagebrium (also called ALT-711). In test animals, alagebrium was even more effective than PTB and rejuvenated not only the heart and blood vessels but also the kidneys, which had fewer cross-links as well. In dogs that were given alagebrium, the heart became 40 percent more flexible, which improved its ability to pump blood around the body. The heart of these dogs became almost as elastic as when they were young.[276] In rhesus monkeys that were treated with alagebrium, the results were even more spectacular. The monkeys' heart and blood vessels rejuvenated and became 60 percent more flexible.[277] Scientists were extremely excited about these results. For the first time, they had succeeded in reversing the aging process in test animals.

Needless to say, the first experiments with humans soon followed. Hundreds of patients were given alagebrium and the results were . . . quite disappointing. The patients' blood vessels became only slightly suppler, their blood pressure did not go down, and there was very little improvement in their heart function. In the best cases, the experiments showed only a slight improvement, but the results were not as impressive as in the experiments with rats, dogs, and monkeys.[278, 279] How is that possible? One possible explanation is that people have a different type of cross-links than dogs or monkeys. Monkeys have mainly alpha-diketone cross-links, whereas people have more pentosidine and glucosepane cross-links. Glucosepane, in particular, accumulates in the human body and this cross-link is very difficult to break. It is likely that humans have different cross-links from most animals because humans live so long. Since humans can live 80 years or more, our body has more time to form very resistant cross-links that are more difficult to break than the cross-links in animals that have a life span of only a few years (mice) or a decade (dogs).

What these experiments did show was that cross-links can indeed be broken and that we can break the chains of aging. Old animals can be rejuvenated. Their heart pumped more vigorously, kidney function improved, and their blood vessels became more elastic. Scientists are currently searching for substances that can break the tough glucosepane cross-links in humans. Recently researchers succeeded in producing glucosepane in the laboratory. That is an important step forward, because if you can make as many glucosepane cross-links as you want, you can use these to test various substances to see which of them are best able to break these cross-links. According to some researchers, it is only a matter of time before the first effective cross-link breakers are developed that work in humans. We will then be able to take it in the form of a pill or have it injected into our bloodstream. This medication would almost immediately take effect and could rejuvenate the body: Blood vessels and lungs would become more elastic, cartilage would become supple, lenses with cataracts would become more transparent, and wrinkles would lessen or disappear.

REPAIRING OUR ENERGY GENERATORS

Another reason we age is that our mitochondria, the energy generators in our cells, decline. We have discussed this process earlier in this book: The DNA in the mitochondria (which contains the building instructions for mitochondria) really gets a hammering from the free radicals that are continuously produced as a by-product of our energy metabolism. With too much damaged DNA, the mitochondria cannot maintain and repair themselves, and they deteriorate. Their energy production decreases, which causes various aging symptoms, such as fatigue, concentration problems, or muscle weakness.

How can we keep our mitochondria healthy? Often antioxidants are proposed as candidates. Antioxidants are substances, such as vitamins A and E, that neutralize free radicals. Studies show, however, that most antioxidants are not effective: They do not extend the life span of lab animals or of humans. One reason is that these antioxidants do not get into the mitochondria in large enough quantities, where they are most needed. Researchers have therefore tried to increase the number of antioxidant proteins (proteins that our own body produces to clean up free radicals) in the mitochondria, so that the free radicals in the mitochondria can be cleaned up. The results are contradictory, however. Sometimes test animals live longer, sometimes not. To really reverse the aging process, the damaged DNA in the mitochondria would need to be repaired.

So researchers tried a different approach. Instead of trying to prevent damage with ineffective antioxidants, they attempted to repair and rejuvenate the damaged mitochondria directly. That is possible by replacing the aged, damaged mitochondrial DNA with fresh new mitochondrial DNA. That was done by injecting pieces of mitochondrial DNA directly into the bloodstream, together with a marker that leads the DNA to the mitochondria. That new DNA can then replace the damaged DNA and rejuvenate the mitochondria. With this method, researchers were able to repair aged cells with Parkinson's disease and make them healthy again.[280]

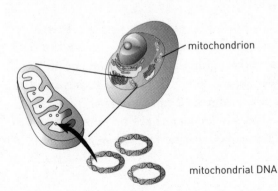

mitochondrion

mitochondrial DNA

The mitochondrial DNA (the circles) contains instructions to build up the mitochondria and gradually becomes damaged as we age. New mitochondrial DNA can be transported into the mitochondria to rejuvenate them.

Another method is to move the mitochondrial DNA to the safer and quieter cell nucleus. As we have seen, the mitochondrial DNA is damaged precisely because it is located in the mitochondria, where is it continuously exposed to the harmful free radicals that are produced as a by-product in the mitochondria. This problem can be solved by injecting mitochondrial DNA that does not travel to the mitochondria (where it is damaged by the free radicals) but that settles in the safer cell nucleus. Thus, our cells get a backup of mitochondrial DNA that stays safely in the nucleus of our cells.

This may sound improbable or impossible, but researchers have already accomplished that. They have used this method to cure cells from mitochondrial diseases that were thought to be incurable. One of these is called Leber's hereditary optic neuropathy, which causes blindness in young people and can also cause movement disorders because the brain gets damaged as well. The disease occurs because a certain protein in the mitochondria is not functioning well. Researchers have succeeded in inserting DNA (which contains the building instructions for the mitochondrial protein) into the nucleus of cells. Then the mitochondrial protein is produced inside the cell nucleus and travels automatically to the mitochondria, where it can replace the defective protein. The result was that the mitochondria of the cells functioned several times better than previously.[281]

This and other research shows that aged mitochondria can be rejuvenated. Perhaps in the future, people will get treatments whereby mitochondrial DNA or other substances are injected that rejuvenate the mitochondria.[282] You will get these substances on a regular basis, so that the mitochondria function just as well as when you were young: You can walk around for hours without getting tired, just like a child; your concentration and thinking speed stay optimal; and your vision and hearing remain sharp (this of course in combination with other treatments that work on other aging mechanisms).

OTHER METHODS

The methods we discussed for reversing the aging process are not futuristic dreams but are already being developed and tested. Some are already standard treatment for certain diseases that used to be incurable or fatal. Today, scientists all over the world are working on development of yet other methods to slow down or reverse aging. One method that has received much attention in the media is stem cell therapy.

Stem cells were discussed earlier in the book. They are cells that make other cells. Stem cells divide and split into two cells; one remains a stem cell and the other becomes a specialized cell, such as a skin cell, white blood cell, or gut cell. Stem cells continuously renew and maintain the cells that make up our tissues. Just like most other cells in our body, stem cells age (because of protein agglomeration, mitochondrial deterioration, shortening of the telomeres, etc.). As a result, when our stem cells no longer function well, we wilt, as it were: Insufficient healthy skin cells are produced to keep our skin from becoming weak and wrinkly, insufficient white blood cells are produced to maintain our immune system, and insufficient muscle cells are produced and maintained to keep our muscle cells young.

It is possible to inject people with young, healthy stem cells that nestle in our tissues and produce new cells there. The problem, however, is how to get stem cells. Researchers cannot easily find them in the human body, because often only one in tens of thousands of cells is a stem cell, which also looks very much like any other cell. In the past, stem cells could be obtained from young embryos, whereby the embryo itself was lost. This met with a host of ethical concerns because embryos had to be sacrificed for stem cells. Furthermore, these stem cells come from a foreign embryo and not from your own body, so that they could be rejected by your body. Fortunately, Japanese scientist Shinya Yamanaka found a solution. He discovered a method to transform regular body cells into stem cells. This was a phenomenal breakthrough. It is now possible to take, for example, a skin cell, add four substances to it, and the skin cell changes into a stem cell, which can then in turn form heart muscle cells, brain cells, or stomach cells. These stem cells are not rejected because they are made from your own body cells. It is not surprising that it did not take long for Yamanaka to receive the Nobel Prize, which some scientists have to wait 50 years to get.

Thanks to Yamanaka's method, it became much easier to make stem cells, without having to use embryos. Such easily obtained stem cells can then be used to build new tissues and organs, both in the body, by injecting them, or in the laboratory. Researchers have succeeded in growing a complete heart from stem cells in the lab. To do this, they took a heart from a mouse and removed all cells, leaving only the framework, which consists mainly of collagen proteins. You could compare this with a concrete apartment building (the framework) from which you remove all the people (the living cells). The stem cells then began to cling to the framework and automatically started making heart muscle cells, which together formed a new, beating heart.[283]

In the future, it may be possible to take a heart from a pig (because it is very similar to a human heart) and remove all the pig's heart cells. Next, the framework is filled with your own stem cells (made by transforming a few of your skin cells to stem cells). Then, you can grow a new heart in the laboratory, which is later implanted in your body. The big advantage is that this heart will not be rejected by your immune system (as happens with a transplanted heart from another person and certainly with that from a pig) because the heart is made using your own stem cells. With this procedure, entire organs can be created in the laboratory to replace your worn and aged organs and tissues. Young stem cells can also be injected, to settle into your tissues and build lots of new, healthy cells that build up and maintain your tissues and organs. Creaky joints? Your family doctor can inject stem cells into your knee to make new cartilage. Memory loss? Stem cells can be injected into your brain to make new brain cells. Had a mild heart attack? Stem cells can be injected into the damaged area to repair the heart muscle.

Another promising technique is CRISPR proteins. Currently, most people have never heard of this, but the eyes of scientists shine brightly every time they hear that term. CRISPR proteins are a recent discovery that enables researchers to rewrite genes (pieces of DNA that contain the building instructions for proteins). With this method you can quickly, easily and accurately change people's DNA. Until recently this was a very laborious and time-consuming process. A certain gene had to be made in the laboratory (a piece of DNA that could cure a disease caused by absence of that gene or a poorly functioning gene). This gene had to be inserted into a virus and that virus was injected into a person. The virus then infected cells and planted the gene somewhere at random in your DNA. Since this is a completely random process, it could, for example, cause cancer if the gene was planted in an area of DNA that controls cell growth; uncontrolled cell growth can cause cancer.

Via CRISPR proteins this can now all be done very fast and very precisely. They are designed to search out and rewrite specific genes in the DNA. Scientists have succeeded in curing mice of a genetic metabolic disease simply by injecting CRISPR proteins into the tail. These proteins rewrote the DNA of the mice so that they no longer suffered from this genetic disease.

In the future, it may be possible to rewrite genes that play a role in aging. Some people may object that this would be very difficult, since they believe that many thousands of genes are involved in the aging process. It would be difficult to change all these genes. But that does not seem to be necessary; often only one gene needs to be changed to extend the life span, as has been shown in numerous experiments with lab animals. Changing only one gene, such as the gene that controls insulin metabolism, could allow a mouse to live, for instance, 50 percent longer. These genes are often master genes that can influence the activity of hundreds of other genes. You would need to change only these master genes. In the words of Professor David Gems, who has been studying aging all his life:

> One of the most remarkable discoveries in biology in recent decades is one that surprisingly few people know about: it is possible to slow down aging in laboratory animals. In fact, it is easy.

CRISPR proteins and similar DNA rewriting techniques can play an important role in rewriting or reprogramming the body to make us age more slowly. We are entering a whole new era in which we can rewrite the code for our own body as we can already do with our computers. And it seems that rewriting this code is actually fairly easy, because we have already identified important master genes that extend life span. Finally, for the reader who is curious what CRISPR means, it's "clustered regularly interspaced short palindromic repeats" (the description of the DNA that has been used by bacteria for millions of years to recognize undesirable viral DNA and attack it via CRISPR proteins).

There are other interesting techniques for reversing aging. One of these may look somewhat like a cheap vampire movie, namely, giving old people young blood. Scientists have discovered that when old mice are given young blood, they rejuvenate.[284] That was done by sewing an old mouse onto a young mouse, in such a way that they share the same bloodstream.

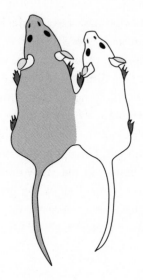

Heterochronic parabiosis is sewing
together an old mouse and a young mouse,
so that they share each other's blood.
The old mouse becomes younger
and the young mouse, unfortunately,
becomes older.

After having been sewn together for a few weeks, the tissues in the old mouse have rejuvenated. Muscles and organs, such as the heart, brain, and liver, can renew and repair themselves better.[285] Muscle cells heal themselves just as well as in young mice, and liver cells can multiply at the same rate as when they were young. The reverse is also true: The younger mouse that was exposed to the blood of the older mouse, aged faster. The cells of the young mouse lost some of their ability to renew and heal.

These experiments show that certain substances circulate in the bloodstream of young animals that can reprogram old cells to make them younger again. Or that old blood contains substances that induce aging (scientists are still debating which mechanism is most important). This confirms once again that aging is not inevitable and that existing damage can be repaired. It is ironic that, for many ages, shamans, quacks, and eminent healers have advised their patients to bathe in blood or to drink blood of younger people (preferably young virgins) so as to rejuvenate themselves. Many legends originated in the supposed rejuvenating effect of blood, such as that of vampires who must drink human blood every night to stay immortal. Of course, such methods do not work because, when you bathe in blood or drink it, the blood does not enter into your bloodstream—it does not go through the skin and is broken down in the digestive system.

Currently experiments are under way whereby Alzheimer's patients get a weekly infusion of young blood to see what happens. The question is whether these vampirish experiments will have any effect because exposure to the young blood is only very brief. In the studies with mice, the old mice were exposed to the blood of younger mice 24 hours a day for many weeks since they were sewn together. In the experiments with people, they are given a shot of young blood only once a week and only for a total of four weeks. Fortunately, other scientists have meanwhile identified several of the rejuvenating substances in young blood. When you inject these substances into mice, their tissues, such as the heart and brain, revitalize.

What these studies show is that cells in the body can be rejuvenated by exposing them to a young environment, such as young blood. In the future, it may be possible for people to regularly get an infusion with young blood or specific rejuvenating substances, so that their body stays young and healthy. The advantage is that these substances can then rejuvenate the entire body, not only one specific organ. To quote Professor Amy Wagers from Harvard University, "Instead of taking a drug for your heart and a drug for your muscles and a drug for your brain, maybe you could come up with something that affected them all."

Finally, another interesting method that could partially reverse aging involves the epigenetic clock. Remember from earlier in the book how a 30-year old fertilized egg cell from a 30-year old mother can reprogram itself to be zero-year old again, so that the baby born from this fertilized egg cell is zero years old and not 30-years old? One way egg cells achieve this is by epigenetically reprogramming themselves after fertilization by a sperm cell. As we have seen, the epigenome is the complex molecular machinery that surrounds the DNA and that regulates which genes (parts of DNA) are active and which are not. The older we get, the more this system gets messed up: genes that should be inactive are active (like genes that promote cancer growth), and vice versa. Scientists were able to epigenetically reprogram the cells of old mice, so that the aging process was partially reversed in them. Muscle and pancreas cells were rejuvenated, and the life span of mice with an accelerated aging syndrome was increased by 30 percent.[286] It was quite spectacular to see pictures comparing the muscle cells of old mice with the ones of rejuvenated mice: the muscle cells of the old mice were small, shriveled, and surrounded by fibrous tissue, while the muscle cells of the rejuvenated mice looked young again—fresh, bulky cells in great numbers and clear from fibrous strands entangling them. In the words of Harvard University professor David Sinclair: "This work is the first glimmer that we could live for centuries." Studies like these go much further than just trying to slow down aging. They try to reverse it.

In conclusion, in this chapter we briefly discussed some interventions that could reverse aging. There are many other methods, but what they all have in common, is that they show that aging is not a one-way ticket toward debility or an inexorable, always advancing march into decrepitude but that aging is a plastic process, amenable to reversal.

SUMMARY

Experiments in animals and medications for humans show that it is possible to not only **slow down** the aging process but also to **reverse** it.

Rejuvenating people can be done via

- **Vaccines** against protein agglomeration

- **Lysosomal enzymes**, which help the lysosomes digest the waste in the cells

- **Cross-link breakers**, which break the cross-links, so that our tissues become flexible again

- **Pieces of mitochondrial DNA**, which replace the damaged mitochondrial DNA and thereby make the mitochondria younger

- **Stem cells**, which can replace old or lost stem cells

- **CRISPR proteins**, which can accurately repair or reprogram DNA

- Transfusions with young **blood** or specific **blood substances** that can make the body younger

- **Epigenetically reprogramming** cells

- Etc.

Conclusion

We have discussed a few methods that go beyond only slowing down the aging process to reversing it. These methods look promising, but there is one problem. It will take many more years before they become available to everyone. To date, none of these methods is currently being used to slow down aging in healthy people.

That makes our lifestyle the most powerful instrument we currently have available to slow down aging. Nutrition is the most effective way to slow down the aging process. Exercise is also important, as well as other healthy lifestyle habits, such as not smoking, having a positive outlook, and sleeping well.

A healthy lifestyle is the best way to slow down aging and will remain so for many years to come. Numerous studies have demonstrated how powerful the influence of our lifestyle is on our life span. One study, which followed more than 20,000 men for eleven years, found that men who lived according to five simple guidelines (they ate healthy, had no potbelly, did not drink too much, did not smoke, and exercised regularly) had an 86 percent lower risk of having a heart attack compared to men who did not.[287] Professor Agneta Akesson, who was the principal investigator of that study, said about these results, "It is not surprising that healthy lifestyle choices would lead to a reduction in heart attacks. What is surprising is how drastically the risk dropped."

Renowned scientists like Professor Walter Willett and Professor David Katz have been saying for years that 80 percent of the risk of heart attack and 90 percent of the risk of type 2 diabetes can be prevented. The EPIC study, which followed 23,000 people for an average of eight years, showed that people who followed four simple guidelines (they did not smoke, exercised at least 3½ hours per week, followed a healthy diet, and were not overweight) had a 93 percent lower risk of diabetes, an 81 percent lower risk of heart attack, a 50 percent lower risk of stroke, and a 36 percent lower risk of cancer compared to people who did not.[288]

Another well-known study is the NHANES III study, which followed more than 16,000 people over an average of eighteen years, found that those who had a healthy lifestyle (not smoking, eating heathy, getting enough exercise, drinking alcohol in moderation) had a 63 percent lower risk of dying during the eighteen years of the study.[289] The investigators concluded that "following four simple lifestyle factors had a strong influence on the prevention of chronic illness." And for anyone who is still not convinced there is the INTERHEART study, which had 30,000 participants. According to this study, lifestyle factors are 90 percent responsible for the risk of heart attack.[290] A similar study, which followed 81,000 women for 26 years, found that women who were not overweight, did not smoke, exercised regularly, and had a healthy diet, had a 92 percent lower risk of heart attack than women who did not.[291] This and other studies leads some scientists to believe that almost every heart attack or stroke that takes place before the age of 80 could have been prevented (at least in people who are not seriously genetically predisposed).

However, if you have a healthy lifestyle, you may still die from heart attack, stroke, cancer or dementia . . . but the difference is that this will happen at a much later age. A healthy lifestyle enables you to not get a heart attack at age 64 but maybe when you are 82. A healthy lifestyle dramatically increases the chances not only that you will live many years longer but also that you will stay healthy longer. Scientists call this "compression of morbidity" (*morbidity* means "illness," *mortality* means "death"). People in the West are often already chronically ill when they are in their early forties. Chronic illness does not necessarily mean that you are in a wheelchair or continuously attached to a drip. It also includes symptoms that many people do not even notice, such as high blood pressure, (pre)diabetes, narrowing blood vessels, and lung fibrosis.

That people are often already chronically ill in their forties is an important point because a classic argument against a healthy lifestyle is that we continue to live longer in spite of our unhealthy diet. True, in the past hundred years, the life expectancy has almost doubled, from 40 to 80 years. However, this increase is mainly due to better hygiene, better food supply, better housing, fewer physically demanding jobs, and the invention of antibiotics and vaccines, which drastically reduced the risk of infection and child mortality. A further increase in life expectancy is due to medical developments, such as heart surgery and drugs (aspirin, blood pressure–lowering drugs, and chemotherapy), which allowed people who would otherwise have died, to still pull through.

Thus, we live longer but we are less healthy. Just 25 years ago, people did not get chronically ill until they were in their fifties—ten years *later* than people do today. We get older but we are sick longer. According to scientists, such as Harvard University professor Daniel Lieberman, this is primarily to blame on our numerous *diseases of civilization*, which occur due to our unhealthy food and lifestyle and actually are not part of the normal course of aging, in the sense that they should not be appearing tens of years before we eventually die. He refers to afflictions such as type 2 diabetes, narrowing of the blood vessels, many cancers, a fatty liver, Alzheimer's disease, high blood pressure, hemorrhoids, osteoporosis, constipation, emphysema (smoker's lung), and the metabolic syndrome—and this is only a short list.

According to Professor Lieberman, not only older people but increasingly more young people and children are suffering from these civilization diseases. These include flat feet, back problems, gastric reflux, depression, asthma, inflammatory intestinal diseases (Crohn's disease, ulcerative colitis), insomnia, gout, irritable bowel syndrome, hammertoes, lactose intolerance, malocclusion, and impacted wisdom teeth. We consider these diseases almost normal because they are so common, but in the past, before the industrialization of our food, and even earlier, before the development of agriculture, they were not so common. A good example is tooth problems, such as impacted wisdom teeth and malocclusion (the upper teeth do not fit well on the lower teeth). Many young people get braces to correct this or they may have to have their wisdom teeth pulled because they do not have enough room to grow. We consider this normal, but in prehistoric times this would not have been possible. Then, an impacted wisdom tooth would have been a death sentence. Problems with wisdom teeth and malocclusion were very rare in those days. So why are today so many braces placed and wisdom teeth pulled? This is because the jawbone of children develops abnormally. It is the result of eating too much soft foods with not enough fiber. White bread with jam, cookies, and sugary breakfast cereals do not require much chewing, so that the jaw bones cannot develop properly—resulting in a lot of work for dentists, orthodontists, and dental surgeons.

In any case, all these civilization and aging diseases, which affect both young and old, are not an elegant way to grow old. Ideally, older people should be independent and healthy for almost their entire life and die after a brief period of dependence and illness—usually less than one or two years. Not only do people become chronically ill much earlier but in some areas the life span is decreasing, for the first time in centuries. Studies show that in some regions in the United States children will have a shorter life expectancy than their parents do. It is not surprising that this happens in the United States, a country with one of the worst dietary patterns in the world.

In other words, the argument that our unhealthy diet is not terribly important because life expectancy has always been increasing does not hold water. We live longer but we are also sick longer, particularly people with an unhealthy lifestyle.

Another argument against a healthy lifestyle—usually brought up by people who want to continue to smoke or do not want to give up their fast food—is that there are centenarians who smoke, drink soft drinks, and eat hot dogs but still make it to age 100 or more. Indeed, such centenarians do exist. An example is Elizabeth Sullivan, who at the age of 104 still drank several cans of Dr Pepper every day. On her 104th birthday, she even received from the company a birthday cake in the shape of a soft drink can, as well as a large supply of her favorite drink. However, it would not be a good idea to compare yourself with centenarians, because they have exceptional genes that allow them to grow very old (and we should not forget that if they did adhere to a very healthy lifestyle, perhaps they might have gotten even older). Unfortunately, most people with a normal, average life span do not have such protective genes. Studies show that for most people, life span is 75 percent dependent on lifestyle and 25 percent is genetically determined.[292] But that is not true for those very rare centenarians. Their long life span is mainly genetically determined. This explains why close family members of centenarians, who have many genes in common, also have a twelve times greater chance of reaching that 100th milestone. To quote Professor Steven Austad, who does research on aging, "If you want to become a healthy 80-year-old you need to live a healthy lifestyle; if you want to become a healthy 100-year-old, you need to inherit the right genes." Therefore, unless you have parents who have just celebrated their 100th birthday, you would be wise to eat healthy, not smoke, and get enough exercise.

A healthy lifestyle is currently our most powerful instrument to stay healthy and live longer. The latter is important if you want to benefit from LEV. This stands for "longevity escape velocity." It means that you continue to live long enough each time to benefit from a new medical breakthrough, which then allows you to live even longer, long enough to profit again from a new advance. Suppose that healthy eating allows you to live ten years longer. That may be just enough for you to benefit from a new therapy, such as a new cross-link breaker or lysosomal enzyme therapy, that extends your life span by another fifteen years. That in turn may be long enough to benefit from the next therapy that can extend your life span by another ten years, and so on. In short, many people living today may in the future be able to benefit from the great breakthroughs that will take place in the coming hundred years. Each time, they may live long enough to benefit from the next innovation, to ultimately reach the escape velocity that propels them into a very long life.

Unfortunately, there will also be many people who die before these new technologies become available. Some researchers claim that this applies to everyone alive today; others believe that the first people who will live to be 1,000 have already been born. Whatever will happen, in the coming decades many people will still die of the aging-related diseases we are faced with today. There is nothing we can do about it. Or is there one last straw one can cling to?

There are companies that claim to offer such a straw. They provide the option to have your body cryopreserved. Your body can then be stored until science has advanced far enough to bring you back to life and to heal or rejuvenate you. This method is called cryonics. Immediately following death, your body temperature is rapidly brought down. Your blood is replaced with a cooling fluid containing an anticlotting agent and an anti-freezing agent. When the body is cooled to –320°F (–196°C), it is stored in a large tank filled with liquid nitrogen. Both in the United States and in Russia, a number of companies offer this service.

People who plan to have their body cryopreserved hope that at some time in the future science will have advanced sufficiently to allow reviving the body and restoring it to full health. In the event that this is not successful, some people hope that their consciousness can still be simulated in a kind of virtual reality after scanning their preserved brain; hence some people choose the cheaper option to have only their brain or their head preserved.

Cryonics has fascinated scientists for centuries. The scientist and philosopher Francis Bacon, while on the road in his horse-drawn carriage in the cold winter of 1626, came up with an idea: Would it be possible to preserve animals by using snow? He saw a chicken by the side of the road and had the carriage stopped. He had the chicken slaughtered and filled up with snow and ice, in what was probably his first and only experiment with cryonics. Unfortunately, this cost Bacon his life because he contracted severe bronchitis in the cold and died shortly thereafter. Nonetheless, scientists remained intrigued. In 1967, the first real cryonics experiment took place, when the first person had his body cryopreserved. This first *cryonaut* was James Bedford, a psychology professor who was 73 years old at the time. His well-preserved body is still floating in a tank of nitrogen today.

Although cryonics has often been fodder for science fiction writers and scientific optimists, it is wrought with some difficult problems. First of all, you have to be dead before you can be cryopreserved—preserving a living person would be equal to murder or assisted suicide. Often several hours, and sometimes days, pass between the death and the cryopreservation. The problem is that when you die, your cells become heavily damaged at the molecular level; your DNA disintegrates, parts of your cell components break apart, calcium atoms enter the cells and stick to everything, the acidity in the cells changes, which causes the structure of the proteins to change, and so on. Your cells become a mess when you die; hence in the future you would not only have to be thawed (which is not a big problem in itself), but you would also have to be restored and your damaged cells repaired, a difficult hurdle to overcome. A solution is to cryopreserve people while still alive, such as an 85-year-old who has terminal cancer and knows that he has only a few weeks or days to live. By cryopreserving someone alive, you prevent the damage caused by death. But this is forbidden by law. Furthermore, even if you cryopreserve someone alive, you still have the problem of the damage caused by the freezing itself. When you freeze living beings, minuscule ice crystals will form in and around the cells. These ice crystals damage the cells. You can partly solve this problem by injecting large quantities of antifreeze and by very rapidly lowering the temperature, but even then it is very difficult to prevent the formation of ice crystals, which can damage the cell walls, DNA, and proteins.

Still, there are animals in nature that are able to freeze and thaw out again months later, without dying or even suffering any damage. An example is the wood frog (*Rana sylvatica*). When winter approaches, the frog hides under some leaves and allows itself to freeze. Its heartbeat stops, there is no longer any brain activity, and the frog becomes a solid clump of ice. Come spring, the frog thaws and he is alive and kicking again. To survive this freezing, the frog fills its blood vessels with an antifreeze agent, namely, glucose. Glucose is a very effective antifreeze agent because it prevents the formation of ice crystals. Some scientists think that this can explain why diabetes is more prevalent in very cold areas, such as Finland and Siberia. Because it is colder there, a natural antifreeze agent like glucose could prevent freezing of the fingertips and the nose, for example. So, perhaps the people living there have on average more glucose circulating in their bloodstream to protect them against the cold. This protection has the side effect of increasing the risk of diabetes.[293]

In any case, cryonics still has a lot of obstacles to overcome. Proponents believe that in the future science will solve them. They also argue that if you die and do not have your body cryopreserved, you currently have a zero percent chance of ever coming back. But if you are cryopreserved, you have at least a chance, however small (and we will not even mention a potential future earthquake which would destroy your liquid nitrogen tank, or what if the cryonics company that froze you goes bankrupt in 200 years?). Another obstacle for many people is the price. Cryopreserving your body costs about $150,000 (and it is not covered by your health insurance). However, the cryonics companies have a solution for that: You can make small monthly payments while you are still alive.

Cryonics is the final, last desperate act of people who wish to live longer. Others hope that they will still live to see breakthroughs that can significantly slow down the aging process. So far, however, our diet is still the most important trump card we have for a long and healthy life. But it is certain that in the future we will live longer and healthier. Such a future is the topic of the next chapter.

SUMMARY: THE LONGEVITY STAIRCASE

AVOID DEFICIENCIES: Many micronutrients are necessary for the proper functioning of the body

Vegetables, and not bread, pasta, potatoes, or rice, ("empty calories") should be the **basis of your diet.**

Eat a healthy, very varied diet that contains lots of micronutrients, such as vegetables, fruits, legumes, mushrooms, nuts, seeds, omega-3-rich fish, olive oil, white meat (poultry), herbs, and spices.

Take smart food supplements (in the right form and dosage):

- For example, vitamin D_3, vitamin K_2, selenium yeast, B vitamins, magnesium malate, iodine

- Consider a calcium supplement if you do not consume enough calcium-fortified vegetable milk and calcium-rich vegetables (but do not take more than 400 mg calcium per dose to avoid excessive calcium peaks in the blood).

STIMULATE HORMESIS: To induce repair, maintenance, anti-inflammatory, and detoxifying mechanisms in the body

Consume foods that contain hormetic substances: tea (preferably white and green tea), coffee (preferably with caffeine), green leafy vegetables (broccoli, kale, cabbage, spinach, brussels sprouts), tomatoes, blueberries, strawberries, raspberries, pomegranate, dark chocolate, spices (oregano, turmeric, rosemary, ginger, garlic, parsley, thyme, basil)

Exercise: high-intensity interval training (HIIT), walking, weight lifting, etc.

Heat and cold exposure such as cold showers, sauna

REDUCE GROWTH STIMULATION: So that cells age less quickly and maintain themselves better

Replace animal protein (meat, fish, eggs, cheese) **more with vegetable protein,** like vegetables (broccoli, kale), legumes (peas, beans, lentils), soy (tofu, miso, natto, tempeh), fungi-based meat substitutes, nuts (walnuts, almonds), and seeds (flaxseeds).

Replace animal milk with low-sugar vegetable milk (such as soy, hazelnut, almond milk).

Consume less sugary foods like soda, sweets, pastry, snack bars, high sugar-loaded yogurt, sauces, and condiments.

Replace sugar more with natural (nonartificial) sweeteners that do not cause sugar peaks like stevia, erythritol, and tagatose.

Replace starchy foods (bread, pasta, potatoes, rice) **more with vegetables, legumes or mushrooms.**

- For breakfast: replace bread and cereals with oatmeal, nuts, seeds (chia seed pudding, flaxseed), fruit, dark chocolate, a dish of vegetables with tofu or lentils, etc.

- For lunch and dinner: replace pasta, potatoes, and rice with vegetables (cauliflower or broccoli mash, a second portion of other vegetables), legumes (peas, beans, lentils), mushrooms (oyster, chanterelle, shiitake, cremini mushrooms), etc.

Use vinegar, fats (olive oil, nuts, dark chocolate), **and fiber to reduce the sugar peaks after a meal.**

Consume tea, coffee, herbs and spices (such as turmeric), **vegetables, and fruit** to reduce growth-stimulation pathways and protein accumulation.

Eat less: smaller meals, skip or downsize the evening meal, practice caloric restriction or (intermittent) fasting.

REVERSE AGING WITH NEW TECHNOLOGIES

Live healthy so you can live long enough to **profit from new biotechnologies** that can extend life span further (longevity escape velocity).

Examples of new technologies: aging vaccines, lysosomal enzyme therapy, cross-link breakers, mitochondrial rejuvenation, substances derived from young blood, gene editing (CRISPR proteins), and epigenetic reprogramming.

Anticipate big changes in education, jobs, retirement, and personal finance when life spans will—drastically—increase in the coming decades and **plan** for it.

OTHER

Sufficient restorative **sleep, be happy** (have goals, meaning, social contacts, engage in lifelong learning, do not retire, help others), **reduce mental stress and worries** (meditation, yoga, cognitive behavioral therapy, deep breathing exercises, self-hypnosis), maintain a **good posture** (Pilates, yoga, Alexander Technique, physiotherapy).

4

Some Thoughts About Aging, Longevity, and Immortality

We will all experience aging and therefore many people consider aging normal; however, an increasing number of physicians and scientists are beginning to see aging as a disease, or at best an "abnormal" normality.

Most people will object that aging cannot be a disease because aging is natural. But is that really true? In nature, life-forms exist that age very little or not at all, such as certain polyps, jellyfish, turtles, lobsters, and cancer cells. This shows that immortality or very long life spans can also be natural. Second, that aging is a natural process is not necessarily of concern to humans. Humans are a very unnatural species, with their unnatural newspapers, table manners (eating with knife and fork), airplanes (people were not made to fly), and contact lenses. Since its early beginnings, the human species has been developing ways to outsmart nature and to live longer: We invented fire, clothing, and footwear, and also antibiotics, vaccines, diabetes medication, and heart surgery. All of these unnatural interventions were aimed at prolonging life. Very few people would argue that we should let nature take its course and let people die from an infection, cancer, or a heart attack, which are all very natural things. Third, aging might actually not be very natural, for it seems that nature does not really want you to age. Or at least it would prefer you to live much longer. Mother Nature—or the process of evolution—is interested only in one thing: reproduction. The longer you live, the more offspring you can produce. Immortality, or at least a very long life span of thousands of years or more, would be ideal for nature because you could produce offspring indefinitely. Yet, nature is forced to let you age because there is no other way. In prehistoric times, the world was full of danger in the form of diseases, predators, aggressive tribesmen, lightning strikes, and famines. Our ancestors had no use for the kind of genes that could have made them thousands of years old because they would long since have perished from causes unrelated to aging, such as the claws of a saber-toothed tiger or a fall into a ravine. But if nature could choose, it would love to let people live much longer. That is easy for us to observe. As soon as an organism develops a way to survive longer in the wild, such as a shield, wings, or a safe society, its life span increases significantly (because spontaneous mutations [changes in DNA] that extend the life span are selected: Every mutation that makes you live longer gets the time to be expressed and exert its effect). You could, therefore, consider aging a kind of makeshift measure of nature because, after all, the world was not a safe haven where you could pet lions and where flesh-eating bacteria did not exist. But such a world is coming because our world has become a very safe place, with its heated homes, antibiotics, and leopard-free streets. Every mutation that allows you to live a hundred years will now be useful because now people will actually have a chance to survive that long. Then, they can reproduce more and longer, so that this mutation will also be passed on to their children. This means that the average age will increase generation after generation. From a biological point of view, there does not really have to be an end to it; as long as energy and building blocks are available in the form of food, in principle a body can continue to repair and maintain itself indefinitely. If nature can let an entire body grow from one tiny fertilized egg cell, surely it can also find a remedy for a little bit of protein agglomeration in our cells. Via this mechanism each new generation will not only grow older but also remain healthy longer. The same mechanisms that make us live longer also lowers the risk of aging-related diseases after all, as long as we do not ruin this effect with our unhealthy lifestyle.

In short, the argument that aging cannot be a disease because it is natural is not convincing. Immortality also occurs in nature and longer life spans are often desired by nature. Furthermore, since its beginning, the human species has invented various unnatural ways to live as long as possible, from spears and footwear to antibiotics and artificial heart valves.

Yet many people will still not agree that aging is a disease. Do we not all grow older? This is in contrast to a specific disease that not everyone may get. One person gets meningitis and another gets arthritis. Some people have multiple sclerosis (a neurological disease), whereas others never get any serious disease at all. Aging affects everyone. However, this is not a very convincing argument because, even though everyone ages, in the end everyone also gets aging-related diseases.

There is really no fine line between aging and aging-related diseases. The same mechanisms that cause normal aging, such as protein agglomeration and sugar cross-links, also cause aging-related diseases, such as Alzheimer's, cataracts, and narrowed blood vessels. Aging and aging-related diseases are two sides of the same coin. That means that actually everyone becomes sick as a result of aging, and the processes leading up to it already starts at a young age. Autopsies show that eighteen-year-olds already have the first signs of atherosclerosis (hardening of the arteries). This process occurs in everyone; ultimately everyone gets narrowed arteries and one in three people will die of a heart attack. The same is true for Alzheimer's disease. The agglomeration of proteins in the brain happens to each of us. That explains why from age 65 up, the risk of Alzheimer's doubles every five years, so that one in three 85-year-olds has the disease. In other words, if you grow old enough, everyone will have a form of Alzheimer's *disease* or vascular *disease*. It is therefore ironic that we do not call aging itself a disease, but that we do call aging of specific organs a disease, such as heart disease, Alzheimer's disease, and cataract. Aging organs are sick but an aging person is not sick and therefore normal.

Another argument why aging is thought not to be a disease, is because a disease usually affects one specific organ or part of the body, whereas aging affects the whole body. Crohn's disease affects the gut, osteoporosis affects the bones, multiple sclerosis affects the nerves, psoriasis affects the skin, and so forth. Aging affects everything. Yet many diseases affect more than one organ or body part. We call such diseases multisystemic diseases. An example is rheumatoid arthritis. This disease usually affects the joints, but also many other body parts. The heart muscle can become inflamed as well as the lung membrane, the eyes, the artery walls, the nails, and the skin. The lungs can develop sclerosis, the liver can enlarge, nerves can stop functioning, and the kidneys can get damaged leading to kidney failure. In short, in such a disease as rheumatoid arthritis, almost no organ or body system is unaffected. The same is true for many genetic disorders, which can affect the entire body.

That is why some researchers call aging a multisystemic disease. Professor David Gems, a researcher of aging, calls aging a special kind of disease, namely, a "multi-factor disease that is 100 percent inherited and 100 percent fatal." It is a disease that affects virtually every organ, and of which you do not know exactly how you will die from it. Just as a rheumatoid arthritis patient can die of kidney failure or a heart attack, an aging person can die of a stroke or lung infection, because virtually all organs are affected and one of these organs will have to be the first to fail.

Now, we finally come to what for many people is actually the most important reason that they do not want to call aging a disease; namely, the potential stigmatization of older people and the inevitability of aging. If you say that aging is a disease, you might offend older people, since you could then label them as sick. It is a disease that everyone will get, however, and therefore nothing to be ashamed of or indignant about. Another reason is the inevitability of aging. That is why people do not want you to call aging a disease: because that creates the impression that you could and should do something about it; it could encourage people to search for a cure for aging and to fight a disease that is inevitable and incurable in any case. Thus, for our own peace of mind, we do not want to face the fact that aging is a disease and we consider it something that we must accept and submit to.

Some people may be of the opinion that you should not give false hope by saying that aging is a disease, which would imply that something can and should be done about it. According to some researchers, however, it is important to put this emotional wish—which actually should not play a role in a scientific discussion—aside and consider aging a disease. This would be a big step forward for research on aging, and thereby automatically also for aging-related diseases. Officially, aging is not a disease and as a scientist or pharmaceutical company you cannot officially develop drugs or treatments for it. Medications and treatment against aging cannot be covered by insurance either because it is not considered as a disease. For a researcher, it is also difficult to obtain research grants for trying to treat or cure something that is considered natural and normal. This is why research on aging has been badly underfunded for decades, which is actually an absurd situation because most diseases that plague people in the West arise from aging. They are aging-related diseases, such as cardiovascular diseases, type 2 diabetes, and Alzheimer's. By studying aging, you actually study all these diseases in one fell swoop, for they all have the same underlying causes as aging itself. Some researchers and companies try to get out of this dilemma by testing their aging-targeting medications in specific aging-related diseases, such as a cross-link breaker in high blood pressure or heart disease. In short, because aging is officially not a disease, is has been difficult to finance research on it for decades.

What has not helped, either, is that for many decades aging research was also taboo among scientists. Why do research on curing something that is natural? You would be better off putting your time and money into *real* diseases. But even if you would find a spectacular remedy that could cure all heart disease at once, the average life span would increase by only 2.8 years because people would still die from other aging-related diseases.[294] If you found a miracle cure for heart disease, your patient would still die two years later from a broken hip or frontotemporal dementia. That is why it is so important to study aging itself.

In addition, many scientists believed that aging was too complex to study, let alone find a solution for it. This changed around 1990, when the first studies appeared showing that the life span of test animals could be dramatically extended by simple mutations. Since then, everything has started moving very rapidly.

Thanks to pioneers and scientists who no longer avoid the taboo around aging, more and more attention and money is spent on research, whereby it is stated openly that the search is on for medications or treatments to slow down or reverse the aging process. Some play a pioneering role in this, both at a scientific as well as at a thought-provoking level. The scientist Aubrey de Grey argues that the first human to become 1,000 years old has already been born. In 2013, Alphabet, the mother company of Google, founded a new company called Calico in collaboration with eminent aging researchers and large pharmaceutical companies with the goal of fighting aging. *Time* magazine quickly published a cover with the question "Can Google solve death?" Scientific institutions and universities organize conferences where renowned biochemists, molecular biologists, and physicians give talks about aging and ways to extend life span. Gradually, awareness is growing in the scientific world that fighting aging-related diseases really also means fighting aging and vice versa. More and more scientists predict that in the future we will experience breakthroughs in life extension and health, and that we may even be able to reverse aging. The question is: Do we really want all that?

SUMMARY

Aging can be seen as a **100 percent fatal, 100 percent genetic, multifactorial, multisystemic disease that is the result of evolutionary neglect**.

Many people do not want to see aging as a disease because it could **stigmatize** older people and because it would imply that aging can and should be **cured**.

Yet, most diseases that plague the Western world **are the result of aging**: Cardiovascular disease, type 2 diabetes, Alzheimer's disease, Parkinson's disease, macular degeneration, sarcopenia (wasting away of muscles), osteoporosis, and stroke are all aging-related diseases.

The same mechanisms that cause **aging** are involved in **aging-related diseases**.

Slowing down the aging process also dramatically decreases the risk of **aging-related diseases**, because they are essentially the same.

Do We Really Want to Grow That Old?

Many people would hate to be 120 years old. If you ask them why, the usual answer is that they would not want to be in a wheelchair, incontinent, bald, half-blind, deaf, and toothless, with a nurse beside them to feed them some liquid food. That is the classic image people have of becoming very old. But if you would instead ask, "Would you like to be 120 years old if you could still be alert, fit, and healthy, and able to independently perform all your usual activities?" the answer likely will be a lot more positive. And if you were to ask, "Would you want to be 120 and still look like you are 30, with the same level of fitness, health, and vigor as a 30-year-old?" then the reply would be even more positive. As we have seen, the latter scenario may not be as far-fetched as it seems, when cross-link breakers, antiaging vaccines, telomere therapies, stem cell therapy, lysosomal enzymes, and other therapies become available. In short, the thought that old age goes hand in hand with a loss of physical and mental capacities, is why many people simply do not want to be very old. But if they could be old and healthy, people have a more positive attitude toward it.

Even so, many do not want to become 100 years old or more. The thought of having to stay in the same job for several more decades, or to be forced to live with an ever-rejuvenating mother-in-law, or visiting the same museum or coffee shop for the umpteenth time out of sheer boredom, makes many people think that with so much time on their hands they would become bored and tired of living. Of course, that is very well possible, but there are many other people who find life so fascinating and challenging, that they are worried that 80 years may not be enough. They still want to read many more books, learn things, visit countries, meet people, and develop ideas. Furthermore, there are solutions for the problem of boredom. Maybe in the future there will be medication against boredom, for example by making you produce more dopamine or endorphins so that you are always motivated and happy. New technologies, such as virtual reality, may ensure that you are never bored and immersed in new worlds and experiences all the time. Research also shows that the activities that almost never bore us are also the ones that make us happiest, such as friendships, supporting good causes, exercising, or having sex—all activities that do not cost anything (usually anyway).

It is interesting that particularly young people would like to live as long as possible (in good health, of course) and that older people often say that living longer is not something they really want. That may be because older people have experienced enough of life. However, there may also be an important biological reason that they think that way. Older brains work differently from young brains. For example, the older you get, the fewer neurotransmitters, such as dopamine and serotonin, your brain cells exchange to activate one another. Dopamine is particularly important because it ensures pleasure and motivation in life; 70-year-olds make less dopamine than 25-year-olds do. It is not surprising that many older people are not that interested in prolonging life. That does not mean that they lack motivation. On the contrary, older people are often very satisfied with their life. But older brains think differently about old age, and one reason for that is precisely because they are old. They have different neurotransmitter ratios and produce fewer neuropeptides and neurohormones. That can explain why for many older people enough is enough, whereas younger people are full of enthusiasm, fire, and motivation to change or discover the world. But suppose that an 80-year-old would still have a brain that is exactly as fit, healthy, and young as a twenty-year-old, that person may still have that typical youthful enthusiasm and motivation for life.

Some people are very much against research into prolonging life and reversing aging. They think that aging and death should remain as they are, otherwise life would lose much of its appeal. Death and the short span of our existence enable us to live more intensely, to enjoy our short moments more, knowing that it will not last and even go by fairly quickly.

Is that really true? Do we need a continuous awareness that life is finite in order to be happier in life? That is actually a strange way of reasoning because most people prefer to think of death as little as possible. Most people live as if they were immortal. They must, because otherwise why would you get out of bed if you knew that you are going to die anyway? It would be quite unbearable to continuously think about the fact that your life will end. This makes me think of a patient who was admitted to a psychiatric hospital because she could not bear to be mortal. The thought of dying someday was so abhorrent to her that she wanted to commit suicide. Fortunately, most people have a cognitive defense mechanism against their mortality: to think about it as little as possible. They pretend that an unlimited number of days lie ahead, even though they are only one of the thousands of billions of short-lived, mortal life-forms on the crust of a congealed planet that turns around a star, of which there are no less than 300 billion in our galaxy. To put it in the words of Belgian novelist Walter van den Broeck, "We know that we will die but every morning but we act as if that is not true. . . . Whatever else we do—the fuss about who will win the Oscars or Paris-Roubaix—they are simply diversionary tactics in order not to think about that awful ending—death. As long as we are collecting stamps or writing books, we push that thought away."

Of course, we do think about death, maybe many times a day, but we push that thought away to quickly focus on the order of the day. We need to do that, because otherwise such a heavy load would quash our motivation and zest for life. Only when we are suddenly confronted with a terminal illness, do we realize how relative and brief our existence is and how death is now knocking on the door.

Another argument against the idea that death makes our life better is that we are happiest when we are focused on something completely other than our mortality. Scientists who study happiness use the term *flow*. This is the moment when people are very happy or really enjoy themselves, such as in the grip of a spellbinding movie or a riveting book or when we are painting, sculpting, writing, or cooking and are so immersed in the experience that we forget we exist. We are swept along in the flow of the moment. Time does not seem to exist. These are the kind of experiences where at the end we look at the clock and think: Is it that late already? We are often happiest when we forget about ourselves and time and thus also how our own time slowly ticks away and how finite our existence is. This is in direct contrast to the words of philosopher Bernard Williams, who said, "If we as people would no longer be able to die, what sense would it make to lead a happy life?" However, our happiest moments are often those in which we forget time and our mortality, and live completely in the here and now.

These insights also refute the notion that death is necessary to be able to plan our life. For many people, life has a fixed pattern, which usually looks as follows: childhood, study, find a partner, start a family, work, retire, enjoy yourself a little bit, and then you die. Without the prospect of a finite life that takes about 80 years, we would wander about aimlessly on our life's path, not knowing when to start or stop each of our life phases. Death serves as a guiding light that gives our life direction and to which we are attracted as moths to light. However, because we are trying to ignore death as much as possible, and we are often happiest when we are no longer aware of time, that also means that all this planning is relative. If people would grow 200 years old, life could still always have a lot of meaning and beauty, particularly because it is mainly the experiences of the moment that make us happy.

That we need to have a normal life span and death to be happy is not true. Even Bernard Williams, the philosopher who viewed death as giving meaning to life, realized at the end of his life that he found it difficult to accept that he was sick and about to die. He admitted, "Maybe I deny that truth more often than I want to face it." Maybe we need to stop convincing ourselves that without finality and mortality our life is less valuable and simply recognize that death and aging are not pleasant but that we must try to give them a place in our lives.

In addition to boredom and death as sources of meaning, there is another often-heard argument against living longer: overpopulation. If everyone would become very old, the world would become even fuller than it already is. Of course, you can make this same argument against vaccination, antibiotics, and health care in general: By keeping people alive longer through these inventions, you contribute to overpopulation. Nevertheless, most people will not object to doctors and antibiotics.

We do indeed have a population problem. That problem, however, is perhaps not *over*population but *under*population, because people are having fewer children. At no time in the history of our species was the birth rate this low. As a result the population will shrink, which in most industrialized nations is already happening. There, the birth rate is around two. A Western woman, on average, will give birth to two children, which is too few to maintain the population—as not all these children will in turn have children. In various Asian countries, the birth rate is even lower than in Europe. For example, a woman in Singapore on average has only one child in her life. The authorities in Singapore would like to do whatever it takes to raise the birth rate. They even subsidize every baby that is born. The authorities give couples a baby bonus of $12,000 for each firstborn child and as much as $20,000 from the third child on. Nevertheless, these premiums are having little effect.

Even in developing countries, fewer children are born as the population becomes more affluent and better educated (education is one of the most powerful measures to reduce family size). The average birth rate in developing countries hovers around four, which is a lot less than the clichéd notion of eight or ten children for every woman. The average worldwide birth rate (including developed and developing countries) is 2.36 children for every woman, which is dangerously close to 2.1, the number that is required to maintain the population. Africa is the only continent where a substantial growth can be expected in the coming decades, but from the moment this continent becomes prosperous enough, the birth rate will see a dramatic decline there as well; this has already happened in such countries as Iran and Brazil.

This worldwide decline in birth rate has been going on for several decades. This is due to the increased affluence (you do not depend anymore on only your children to take care of you in old age); the abolition of child labor (in the past, children helped out on the farm or in the factory, so that the more children you had, the more helping hands there were); education; birth control; and the fact that women also stay in school longer and get jobs, so that they have fewer children and have them at a later age. These are all very good evolutions but the result is that people get far fewer children than in the past.

As a result, we are headed toward a demographic revolution. According to some estimates, by the year 2300 the number of Europeans will decline from 455 million to 59 million, and in such countries as Russia and Italy, the population will decrease by a factor of ten. Some scientists are of the opinion that underpopulation is a much greater threat to the extinction of humankind than meteorite impacts or a super volcano eruption. Maybe that was also the cause of the extinction of the Neanderthals, another human-like species that once roamed the earth. The Neanderthals were also an intelligent species that had language and created music and jewelry. Nevertheless they became extinct about 30,000 years ago, possibly because they simply did not have enough children, and as a result, they slowly but surely disappeared into oblivion.

In the short-term, meaning in the next hundred years, the population will continue to increase. However, in the long term, looking at periods of 300 years and longer, we should not fear a population *explosion* but a population *implosion*. Extending the life span can slow down this massive population implosion. The argument that a longer life automatically leads to overpopulation is not so straightforward, because we need to consider the declining birth rate as well. Of course, if everyone lived a thousand years or more, this could in the long term result in overpopulation. However, even if everyone would suddenly become immortal, the population would still increase very slowly and there would be no explosion.[295] Our society will have enough time to find solutions. Overpopulation can be avoided by better control of births and deaths to keep the population in balance, and may be compensated by new developments, like better farming and food production methods, more recycling, and other environmentally sustainable technologies.

In short, overpopulation is not the serious problem it was thought to be. An extended life span can offer a buffer for the decline in population, and managing the birth rate is an important tool to prevent or slow down overpopulation. A potentially more thorny issue is that long-lived people could stay in power much longer. Such people as murderous dictators, corrupt ministers, conservative professors, or incompetent directors would no longer make way for younger people with new, fresh, and progressive ideas. The well-known physicist Max Planck already pointed out that science progresses "funeral by funeral." No one would like it if a Hitler or Stalin could stay in power for centuries, but you could look at the other side of the coin: Such geniuses as Mozart or Einstein would continue to amaze us with their intellect and creativity for a very long time.

As far as cruel dictators, corrupt ministers, and incompetent CEOs are concerned, we could think of solutions for this problem, such as limiting the time people in higher ranks can keep their positions. This is already the case for many presidents, who are elected only for a maximum of two terms. They are forced to make way for others. A similar policy can be established at universities, companies, and other organizations. University professors or

CEOs would not be able to keep their position indefinitely; at a certain time they would have to make room, regardless of whether they are old and wrinkled or still look like a 30-year-old. In regard to the fear that dictators would never voluntarily step down, that is already often the case. There have already been dictators who remained in power far longer than is justified. Most of the time, they are removed by force, long before they die of old age, be it with the aid of Molotov cocktails or offensive cartoons.

We have discussed some pros and cons of an extended life span. Some people have no desire to live longer—that is for them to decide. Some are against living longer because of arguments such as boredom, death as giving meaning to life, and overpopulation. But as we have seen, these doomsday scenarios are not as self-evident as they may seem, and for many of these problems there are also solutions.

SUMMARY

Many people do not want to grow very old even if they were healthy, often bringing forth arguments such as **boredom**, **loss of purpose in life**, **intellectual stagnation**, or **overpopulation**.

Solutions can be found for many of these problems.

Population predictions that look far enough into the future (300 years or more), show that not overpopulation but **underpopulation** is a potential scenario, which could ultimately even mean the extinction of humankind.

A New Society

Humankind has an enormous problem. Never before in the 200,000 years that our species has existed, have we been able to create a civilization that is so affluent and safe. This allows almost everyone to stay alive and die of old age. Old age did not exist in nature. For hundreds of thousands years, most of our ancestors died from external causes; they were eaten, succumbed to an infection, or became lost in wide-open spaces or forests without phones, hospitals, or supermarkets. Nature could never have foreseen that people would establish such a successful civilization that most of us can die of old age. That is why we now face an increasing epidemic of age-related diseases, such as Alzheimer's disease, heart disease, diabetes, and stroke, all diseases that can last for decades, reduce the quality of life, and cost millions in health care. On the one hand we can regret this; on the other, we can be happy that thanks to our advanced civilization we finally can become old enough to develop Alzheimer's disease or a heart attack. Governments are not so happy: 86 percent of health-care costs is spent on aging-related diseases, and those costs will rise and take an increasing bite out of the government budget.

Whether we like it or not, our life span will continue to increase. Not only because of the increasing prosperity, better medicine, and the new technologies we discussed earlier but also for evolutionary reasons: Every spontaneous mutation that increases the life span can now survive because people live longer. Life span has been increasing by six hours every day, which means that every week you gain an extra weekend. This evolution has been going on for some time. In a little over a century, the life span has doubled. In 1900 people's average life expectancy was about 40, now it is 80. In that time, the chance of becoming age 65 has tripled, from 30 to 90 percent. The number of centenarians is increasing even more. A person born in 1932 had a 4 percent chance of becoming 100. A child born in 2011 has a 30 percent chance of becoming 100. Thus, a baby born in 2011 has a seven times greater chance to become a centenarian than does her great-grandfather. The first children who will live to be 135 have already been born.

We are approaching a world in which people will live longer and longer. Our society will change drastically because of this. The first thing to go will be the retirement age. Since people become older, the number of retired people will increase. In 1970, there were thirteen people working for every retired person (65 years or older); by 2030, in many developed countries there will only be two working people for every retiree.

Two working people supporting one retired person; it is obvious that this is unsustainable. Inevitably people will have to retire at a later age. In many countries the age of retirement is 65. However, this number is a relic from a hundred years ago. In those hundred years, the average life span has risen significantly and the chance of reaching age 65 has tripled, while the retirement age has remained the same.

In the past, the retirement age was not only much higher in relation to the life span but people also looked differently at retirement. At the beginning of the twentieth century, many workers were not keen to retire. It would mean that they would be no longer useful and be left to their own devices to find something to fill their day. The boss, on the other hand, would like it if his workers retired because as a result of industrialization, work had become more complex and faster. It became very difficult for an older worker with declining eyesight or trembling hands to run the complicated machines, and he could also not do it as fast as a younger person. The boss was therefore only too happy to send his older workers into retirement. Today, it is the other way around: Workers look forward to their retirement, but employers do not like to see experienced employees retire as long as they are physically and mentally still healthy and capable.

Whether we like or not, we will have to work increasingly longer. Maybe this is actually not that bad for our health. Studies show that retiring is not that healthy, either physically or mentally. People are very social beings who feel good when they have goals and belong to a group. Having a job makes you belong (to a department, your colleagues, the company, or a business group), it makes you feel useful, and it gives you a fixed routine. Furthermore, you continually interact with people, which is cognitively demanding for our brain but also keeps it healthy and sharp. People often underestimate the long-term consequences of retirement; suddenly you do not belong anywhere and have no function or task and have to fall back on yourself (and maybe your partner) to fill your day. The first few months of that may be no problem, but what about after years or decades?

Physicians have known for some time that patients who keep working past retirement age are healthier. The question is: Do people stay healthier because they continue to work or do they continue working because they are healthier? Research shows, however, that retiring can undermine one's health. A study that followed 1,000 older people shows that people who were still working after they turned 70 had a 2.5 times greater chance to be alive at age 82 than did those who did not (taking into account the health of the participants at the start of the study).[296] According to another study, which followed more than 5,000 older people, those who retired had a 40 percent greater risk of having a heart attack or stroke than did those who continued to work.[297] Another study with more than 400,000 participants found that with each year a person continued to work, the risk of dementia decreased by

3.2 percent (taking into account the health of the brain at the beginning of the study).[298] The researchers concluded: "We show strong evidence of a significant decrease in the risk of developing dementia associated with older age at retirement, in line with the 'use it or lose it' hypothesis." A job makes you use your brain more and train it and maintain it, so that the risk of Alzheimer's disease is decreased. People who continue working have better health, both mentally and physically. A headline in *The New York Times* summarized it as follows: "For a healthy retirement, keep working."

Nonetheless, there are lots of people who would really like to retire. Some people do not like their job, some find that they have worked long enough, others have a job that is mentally or physically exhausting. But is retiring the only solution? Maybe people should not necessarily stop working, but could work differently. They could find another job that is better, or less tiring, work part-time, or do volunteer work, so that they can continue to be occupied, which is healthy for body and soul.

In view of this, retirement can be made more flexible: Allow people to choose when they retire, or allow people to retire temporarily (for example, you can retire at age 65 for ten years, and at age 75 decide to return to work part-time). Another possibility is to abolish retirement altogether and give everyone over the age of eighteen a basic income. This can be an income that you get regardless of whether you are working or not or can be a basic amount of money that decreases as you earn more by working. By giving everyone a basic income, the state no longer has to pay for retirement, unemployment, illness, disability, or civil servants' salaries.

In addition to making pensions more flexible, older people could be encouraged to retrain, to learn new skills, so that after their retirement they can do something completely different, like a civil servant becoming a tour guide, librarian, translator, or salesperson. Many older people already do that, particularly in the United States, because a full pension is less guaranteed. An example is Newton Murray, a 99-year-old American who is still working. Every day, it takes him three hours to get to his job as a parking lot attendant. He does not earn a lot, but he does not want to hear talk about a regular retirement: "I really can't stay home and sit on the couch. What else can I do? Watch television all day?" It does take him a bit longer to perform maintenance work but his employer does not mind, since he is always right on time and, because of his age, he is respected by younger employees. Another example is Ted Di Nunzio, who is 100 years old. He works in a trendy clothing store in a shopping center where, dressed in a nice suit, he greets the customers. He used to be a butcher, but he likes his new job so much that he calls the store his second home. Or take Sara Dappen, a spry lady of 92 who works in a fast-food restaurant, where she cleans tables, fries hamburgers, and chats with the customers from time to time. She has worked there for five years. When she was 87, she decided to start working part-time because, she says, that is better than walking the streets or just sitting still all the time. Sitting still is not Loren Wades's cup of tea either. He is 101 years old and works in a supermarket, where on an average day he walks about three miles, going around tidying things and serving customers.

Having a job gives these people something to do, a routine, a goal, satisfaction, and social contacts. This is all very healthy for body and soul. Our brain loves goals and social contacts. In one study, older people who all had early cognitive decline (often a precursor of Alzheimer's disease), participated in a volunteer program. For six months, fifteen hours a week, they helped teaching first graders how to read. After six months, it was found that the volunteers scored much better on cognitive tests. Brain scans also showed that the thickness of their frontal cortex had increased significantly.[299] Keeping busy benefits your brain.

In the future, retirement will get a different meaning. Both pensions and jobs will become more flexible. Some people will work full- or part-time after retirement or they may do different types of work. Some scientists advocate giving older people medications and food supplements, so they can remain healthy, mentally sharp, and productive for many more years. If life span increases significantly in the future—because new technologies allow people to become 200 years old in perfect health—there will be a dramatic change in retirement. Maybe people will retire several times during their lifetime. For example, after working for 30 years, people retire for ten years, train for several years, and then work in a completely different job for a number of years, then retire again for some time, and so on.

We are already evolving toward such a world, one in which our education and retirement are no longer milestones at the beginning and the end of our life, but are woven into our life. Since knowledge is increasing so rapidly, people need to keep learning on an ongoing basis. What you learned twenty years ago may already be outdated. People will be able to take courses at any time, alternating with sabbaticals or micro-retirements—time off they can take in between various jobs, projects, and trainings.

SUMMARY

As a result of natural (evolutionary) mechanisms as well as medical, technological, and social breakthroughs, **people will** on average continue to **grow older**.

From a biological perspective there is **no ultimate age limit** for our species.

The fact that we will continue to live longer will bring about significant social and economic **changes**.

The healthiest way to **retire** is to continue working (full-time, part-time, or volunteer work).

5

Recipes

It is noteworthy that people who look younger than their age often:
- Eat little meat, particularly red meat*
- Eat lots of vegetables and often eat soup (sometimes every day)**
- Eat few grain products (bread, potatoes, pasta, rice)
- Stay away from junk food, such as hamburgers, pizza, hot dogs, chips, and cookies
- Eat more healthy fats (olive oil, nuts, avocado)

A few tips:
- Season your food with herbs and spices that have a positive effect on all kinds of aging mechanisms, such as reducing inflammation, protecting the DNA, and slowing the growth of cancer. Some examples are turmeric, basil, parsley, rosemary, dill, and oregano.
- Add flavor to vegetables with dressings and vinaigrettes (mixtures of oil with something sour, usually vinegar). A simple vinaigrette consists of 3 tablespoons olive oil, 1 tablespoon red wine vinegar, and some pepper and salt. The oil and vinegar prevent sugar peaks and contain substances that slow down aging (such as oleocanthal in olive oil).
- Prepare food to keep for several days (for example, store oatmeal and seasoned beans or vegetables in airtight containers in the refrigerator).

* Make sure you get enough protein, preferably by eating white meat (poultry), (fatty) fish, and vegetable protein sources, like legumes (beans, peas, lentils) and vegetables (kale, broccoli, spinach).
** If you do not have time to make soup, you can buy soups, gazpacho (cold tomato soup), or vegetable juice at the supermarket.

- Cook extra food in the evening, so that you can have the leftovers for breakfast ("dinner for breakfast").
- Replace sugar with natural sweeteners (such as stevia or erythritol): These have little or no effect on blood sugar levels. Stevia has a somewhat bitter aftertaste, whereas erythritol does not.
- Replace wheat flour (starch, therefore glucose) with almond flour or coconut flour: They contain much less starch.
- Replace regular salt (sodium chloride) with potassium salt (potassium chloride). (Many supermarkets carry salt that consists of 70 percent potassium chloride and 30 percent sodium chloride—100 percent potassium chloride tastes quite bitter.)
- Buy mayonnaise that is made, wholly or partially, with olive oil (available in most supermarkets, or make it yourself with 2 egg yolks, 1 cup [250 ml] olive oil, 1 teaspoon mustard, 1 tablespoon lemon juice, pepper, and salt).
- Nuts are good for satisfying hunger.
- Frozen fruit, such as frozen raspberries, blueberries, and mangoes, is much cheaper than fresh, available year-round, and also very healthy.
- Breakfast should be the most important and largest meal of the day. In the morning, the body is best able to process carbohydrates and proteins. Eat a light meal in the evening. In the West, we often do it the other way around: in the morning just a small breakfast or none at all, and in the evening a much too large and heavy meal.
- Instead of bread twice a day, you could have twice a hot or cold meal with vegetables, beans, mushrooms, white meat, or fish (See "Lunch and Dinner").
- Wash fruit and vegetables to remove pesticides and bacteria but do not peel off the edible skin because most healthy substances can be found right underneath.
- Add lemon juice to your green tea: The lemon juice stabilizes the healthy substances in the tea and ensures that they are better absorbed.
- Add black pepper and maybe a little olive oil to turmeric. These substances make the body absorb the tumeric at least twenty times better.

BREAKFAST

Some examples of a healthy breakfast:
- A bowl of almond milk with mixed nuts (hazelnuts, almonds, cashews, walnuts) and pieces of fruit (blueberries, raisins . . .)
- A bowl of chia seeds with blueberries, cherries, and pumpkin seeds.
- A smoothie: fruit and vegetables mixed in a blender, optionally with nuts, plant-based milk, or silken tofu (a softer, yogurt-like form of tofu)
- Oatmeal made with a plant-based milk (such as almond milk) and, for example, raisins, cinnamon, walnut pieces, and chopped apple (you could make enough oatmeal for three days and heat it up in the microwave every time); eat this with dark chocolate and fruit, such as blueberries.
- A bowl of soy yogurt with walnut pieces, flaxseeds, and pieces of pear and banana
- A bowl of soy yogurt with fresh fruit, flaxseeds, and avocado drizzled with olive oil and sprinkled with salt and freshly ground black pepper
- 2 eggs fried or scrambled with onion, mushrooms, spinach, or broccoli
- A few pieces of cold cooked salmon with avocado or goat cheese
- Vegetables (such as broccoli or spinach) with a fungi-based meat substitute and optional beans
- Sautéed tofu with vegetables
- Be creative: In Japan, people eat soup and natto (fermented soybeans) for breakfast; in India, lentils with spicy vegetable and fruit puree.

Breakfast Smoothie

Make a smoothie by blending the following ingredients in a blender:
- Fruit: for example, 1 banana or 1 freshly squeezed orange with pulp, 1 mango, a handful of red or blue fruit (frozen fruit is cheapest)
- Vegetables: such as kale, spinach, or broccoli (fresh or frozen)
- Nuts and seeds (walnuts, almonds, flaxseeds; optional: these give the smoothie a creamier taste)
- Plant-based milk (soy, almond, coconut milk . . .) or silken tofu: for additional vegetable protein (optional)

Fruit Breakfast with Nuts and Flaxseeds

1 pear, unpeeled
1 apple, unpeeled
1 banana
Handful of walnuts
1 tablespoon flaxseeds (or chia or pumpkin seeds)
A few tablespoons coconut milk, optional

Blend the fruit in a blender or puree with a mixer. Alternatively, cut the fruit into chunks if you would rather not have fruit puree. Add the nuts and flax-seeds. Add the coconut milk, if using.

Quick Oatmeal Cake, Pancakes, or Balls

For oatmeal cake:
¼ cup (20 g) rolled oats
1 large egg
1 ripe banana, mashed
Fruit and nuts, for serving

For oatmeal pancakes:
¼ cup (20 g) rolled oats
1 large egg
1 ripe banana, mashed
Pinch of salt
Pinch of ground cinnamon
1 tablespoon coconut oil

For coconut-oat balls:
1 cup (80 g) rolled oats
Scant ⅔ cup (50 g) coconut flakes
2 ripe bananas, mashed
Pinch of salt
1 tablespoon stevia or erythritol powder

To make the cake: Place the oats, egg, and banana in a bowl. Microwave for 3 minutes or preheat the oven to 350°F (180°C) and bake for 15 minutes. Serve with fruit and nuts.

To quickly whip up pancakes: Mix the oats (or better yet, cooked oatmeal), egg, and banana in a bowl with the salt and cinnamon. Heat a skillet and grease the bottom with the oil. Pour a small amount of the mixture into the pan so that a small pancake is formed and cook over not too high a heat, flipping to cook the other side. Repeat to make additional pancakes.

To make coconut-oat balls: Preheat the oven to 350°F (180°C). Mix together the oats, coconut, and bananas in a bowl to get a creamy mixture. Add the salt and stevia. Place tablespoon-size heaps of the mixture on a baking sheet. Bake for 20 minutes or until a toothpick inserted in the center comes out clean.

Hot Cereal with Nuts and Flaxseeds

¼ cup (35 g) almonds
¼ cup (25 g) walnuts
2 tablespoons flaxseeds
3 large eggs
½ ripe banana
¼ cup (60 ml) almond milk, plus more if needed
Pinch of ground cinnamon
Strawberries or other fruit, for serving

First, place the nuts and flaxseeds in a blender and blend until you get a thick paste. Add the remaining ingredients, except the fruit. Transfer the mixture to a saucepan and heat, stirring, over low heat until the mixture reaches your desired consistency; add more almond milk, if desired. Serve with your choice of fruit.

Goat Cheese Frittata

1 tablespoon olive oil
½ onion, finely chopped
Salt and freshly ground black pepper
5 cups (150 g) spinach, rinsed
3 large eggs, beaten
1 ounce (30 g) goat cheese
3 tablespoons (20 g) shredded Gruyère

Preheat the oven to 400°F (200°C). Meanwhile, heat an ovenproof skillet on the stove over medium-high heat. Add the oil and onion plus salt and pepper to taste. Stir-fry until the onion is translucent, about 3 minutes. Add the spinach and a little water and stir-fry until the spinach curls up, about 1 minute. Add the eggs, goat cheese, Gruyère, and additional salt and pepper. Cook for 1 to 2 minutes. Then, transfer the pan to the oven and bake for 10 minutes. Remove the pan from the oven and serve.

Omelet with Tomato and Avocado

1 teaspoon coconut oil (or heat-resistant olive oil)
1 small onion, chopped
2 large eggs, beaten
1 tomato, chopped
½ avocado, sliced
Salt and freshly ground black pepper
Ground turmeric
Olive oil, to serve

Heat the coconut oil in a skillet over medium heat. Add the onion and then the eggs and tomato. Cook for a few minutes, until the eggs are cooked through, then serve the omelet with the avocado and a little bit of salt, pepper, turmeric, and olive oil.

Variation: Make an omelet with 2 large eggs, 5 cups (150 g) spinach, and 1 boiled and chopped red beet: Heat 1 teaspoon coconut oil in a skillet, add the spinach and chopped beet, make two dents between the vegetables, and pour in the eggs so that they touch the bottom of the pan. Cook until the eggs are cooked through.

Hot Cereal with Walnuts and Coconut

2½ tablespoons walnuts, plus a few more for serving
2 tablespoons unsweetened shredded coconut
1 tablespoon almond meal
1 teaspoon ground cinnamon
1 teaspoon pumpkin seeds or flaxseeds
1 cup (240 ml) water
2 tablespoons stevia or erythritol powder, for serving
Walnuts, for serving
Sliced banana, for serving

Place all the ingredients, except the water, stevia, walnuts, and banana in a blender. Blend until the mixture is a fine powder. Bring the water to a boil and add to the mixture. Stir well. Serve topped with the stevia and a few walnuts and banana slices.

Almond Pancakes with Blueberries

¾ cup (100 g) almond meal
1 tablespoon coconut flour
3 large eggs
Scant ¼ cup (50 ml) water
⅓ cup (75 ml) prune juice
¼ teaspoon ground nutmeg
Olive oil, for the skillet
1⅓ cups (200 g) blueberries, for serving
Stevia or erythritol powder, for serving

Place the almond meal, coconut flour, eggs, and water in a mixing bowl and whisk to make a smooth batter (so that there are no clumps left). Mix in the prune juice and nutmeg. Set aside for a few minutes. Heat a nonstick skillet over medium heat until hot. Add a little oil and then 1 tablespoon of the batter to make a little pancake. Cook for 1 minute, then flip the pancake over and cook the other side for 1 to 2 minutes. Repeat to make additional pancakes. Serve with blueberries and stevia.

LUNCH AND DINNER

In the West, our meals often consist of three components: vegetables, starch (potatoes, rice, or pasta), and meat or fish. Replace the starch products with healthier alternatives: mushrooms, legumes (peas, beans, or lentils), extra vegetables (for example, cauliflower puree), or quinoa. Instead of potatoes you can make, for example, lentils or mushrooms. You can also step away from this threesome altogether. In many non-Western countries people eat a meal with only two components (such as tofu with mushrooms), or sometimes even only one component (for example, Ikarian ratatouille, which consists solely of vegetables).

Ikarian Ratatouille

This healthy recipe is from the Greek island of Ikaria, where you find many centenarians.

- 2 eggplants, coarsely chopped
- 2 zucchini, coarsely chopped
- 2 red or green bell peppers, coarsely chopped
- 3 tomatoes, coarsely chopped
- 2 onions, coarsely chopped
- ⅔ cup (150 ml) olive oil, plus more for serving
- 3 tablespoons fresh lemon juice
- 2 teaspoons crushed garlic
- 2 teaspoons dried oregano
- 2 teaspoons ground sage
- 1 teaspoon salt

Place all the ingredients in a large saucepan and simmer over low heat for about 30 minutes, stirring occasionally. To serve, drizzle with additional olive oil.

Tofu with Shiitake Mushrooms

As eaten on the Japanese island of Okinawa, home of many centenarians.

> One 16-ounce (454 g) package firm or extra-firm tofu
> 2 tablespoons olive oil
> ½ teaspoon salt
> ½ teaspoon freshly ground black pepper
> 2 shallots, chopped
> 9 ounces (250 g) shiitake mushrooms, trimmed and sliced
> 1 tablespoon sake (Japanese rice wine) or white wine
> 1 tablespoon soy sauce

Cut the tofu into slices. Heat 1 tablespoon of the oil in a skillet over medium-high heat. Add the tofu strips, together with the salt and pepper. Cook for about 4 minutes until browned on both sides. Transfer the tofu strips to a plate. Add the remaining tablespoon of oil to the pan and cook the shallots over low heat for about 1 minute. Add the mushrooms and stir-fry for 2 minutes. Add the sake and soy sauce. Serve the mushrooms with the tofu.

Seventh Day Adventists' Antipasto

As eaten by the Seventh Day Adventists, a religious sect originating in the United States, whose members place a high value on healthy eating. According to researchers, they live four to seven years longer than average. This recipe makes enough for ten portions or as a large dish to serve at a party.

> 9 ounces (250 g) cherry tomatoes (about 2 cups)
> 6 ounces (180 g) marinated artichoke hearts (about 1 small jar), drained
> 1¾ cups (180 g) walnuts
> 1¾ cups (120 g) broccoli florets
> 1½ cups (120 g) cauliflower florets

1¼ cups (120 g) mushrooms, trimmed and sliced
1 cup (120 g) olives
2 bell peppers (red, green, or yellow), cut into 2 cm–long pieces
7 scallions, chopped
⅓ cup (90 ml) olive oil
2 tablespoons balsamic vinegar
1 tablespoon finely chopped fresh oregano or basil
1½ teaspoons salt
½ teaspoon finely chopped or crushed garlic
½ teaspoon dried marjoram

Mix together all the ingredients in a large bowl. Cover with plastic wrap or a lid. Refrigerate and marinate at least 8 hours, stirring every 2 hours.

Cauliflower with Mushrooms

1 small cauliflower
2 tablespoons olive oil
Handful of pumpkin seeds
Salt and freshly ground black pepper
9 ounces (250 g) mushrooms, cut into pieces

Cut and crumble the cauliflower into small pieces. Heat 1 tablespoon of the oil in a large skillet over medium heat and add the pumpkin seeds. Add salt and pepper to taste. When the pumpkin seeds are golden brown, take them out of the pan and set them aside. Add the remaining tablespoon of olive oil to the pan and then the cauliflower and mushrooms. Season with salt and pepper. Simmer, pouring off any excess water. Serve with the toasted pumpkin seeds.

Vegetables with Salmon and Avocado

1 avocado
Fresh lemon juice
1 ounce (30 g) cooked salmon, cut into small chunks
1 shallot, finely chopped
½ apple, chopped
1 tablespoon mayonnaise (preferably made with olive oil)
Freshly ground black pepper
Finely chopped fresh parsley
2 cups (100 g) chopped lettuce rinsed (or cold, cooked cauliflower and/
or green peas)

Cut the avocado in half and scrape out the flesh. Finely chop the flesh and
sprinkle with lemon juice so it does not discolor. Mix together the avocado,
salmon, shallot, apple, and mayonnaise in a bowl. Add the pepper and parsley
to taste. Serve with the lettuce.

Quinoa with Peas and Feta

This makes enough for a few days of servings.

¾ cup (125 g) quinoa
1¾ cups (250 g) cooked green peas
4.5 ounces (125 g) feta
⅓ cup (50 g) raisins
1 teaspoon onion powder or 2 finely chopped scallions
2 tablespoons chopped fresh cilantro
Salt and freshly ground black pepper

Cook the quinoa according to the directions on the package and let cool.
Add the peas, feta, raisins, onion powder, and cilantro. Season with salt and
pepper to taste.

Walnut-Date Salad

    2 cups (100 g) chopped lettuce, rinsed
    1 orange, peeled, seeded, and thinly sliced
    ⅓ cup (30 g) walnuts
    ¼ cup (30 g) dates, pitted and chopped

For the dressing:
    1 tablespoon olive oil
    1 tablespoon fresh lemon juice
    ½ teaspoon stevia or erythritol powder
    Freshly ground black pepper

Combine the lettuce, orange slices, walnuts, and dates in a bowl. In a small bowl or cup, stir together the dressing ingredients, adding pepper to taste. Sprinkle the salad with the dressing.

Chicken with Shiitake Mushrooms and Spinach

    6 cups (1.5 L) water
    2 chicken thighs
    3.5 ounces (100 g) shiitake mushrooms, bottom part of the stems
    removed
    ½ red bell pepper, cut into strips
    6 garlic cloves, chopped
    ¼ cup (60 ml) soy sauce
    6⅔ cups (200 g) spinach leaves, rinsed
    Juice of 1 lemon

Bring the water to a boil in a large saucepan. Place all the ingredients, except the spinach and lemon juice, in the pan and simmer for 45 minutes. Add the spinach and lemon juice and simmer for 5 more minutes.

Roasted Vegetables with Pesto

1 pound 5 ounces (600 g) carrots, peeled and sliced
14 ounces (400 g) brussels sprouts
14 ounces (400 g) cauliflower florets (about 3⅓ cups)
1 small butternut or other winter squash, peeled, seeded, and cut into 4 pieces
1 red onion, peeled and cut into 4 wedges
¼ cup (60 ml) olive oil
Freshly ground black pepper
7 ounces (200 g) pesto (about ¾ cup)

Preheat the oven to 425°F (220°C). Place all the vegetables in a large baking pan, stir in the oil, and sprinkle with pepper. Roast for 40 minutes in the oven, turning the vegetables after 20 minutes. Serve with the pesto.

Quick Salmon with Broccoli and Beans

Salt or a vegetable bouillon cube
5.5 ounces (150 g) frozen broccoli florets (about ¾ cup)
One 15-ounce (425 g) can white beans (or peas), drained and rinsed
1 tablespoon mayonnaise (preferably made with olive oil)
Freshly ground black pepper
Garlic powder, ground cumin, or savory, optional
4 cups (1L) water
1 vegetable or fish bouillon cube
1 salmon fillet

Bring a saucepan of water to a boil, seasoning the water with salt or a vegetable bouillon cube, then add the broccoli and cook for 6 minutes. Alternatively, you can cook the broccoli in the microwave in a bowl covered with a plate along with a scant tablespoon of water on high for 2 to 3 minutes. Meanwhile, place the beans in a bowl and season with the mayonnaise, salt and pepper to taste, and the garlic powder, if desired. Bring the 4 cups of water to a boil in a second pan and add the fish bouillon cube, salt, and pepper. Lower the heat to low and place the salmon in the water. Poach the salmon for 5 minutes. You'll have a meal in 15 minutes. Serve with the beans and broccoli.

Acorn Squash Spaghetti

2 tablespoons olive oil
1 acorn squash, peeled, seeded, and sliced into long, thin ribbons
2 zucchini, sliced into long, thin ribbons
2 garlic cloves, crushed
6 ounces (175 g) cherry tomatoes (about 1¼ cups), halved
2 tablespoons sun-dried tomato paste
Handful of fresh basil leaves, torn
Freshly ground black pepper

Heat 1 tablespoon of the oil in a nonstick skillet over medium-high heat and stir-fry the squash for 3 minutes. Add the zucchini and stir-fry for 3 more minutes. Add the remaining tablespoon of oil and the garlic, tomatoes, and tomato paste and stir-fry for 3 minutes. Serve sprinkled with the basil and pepper.

Portobello Mushrooms with Almond Stuffing

4 large portobello mushroom caps, stems removed
½ cup (75 g) almonds
⅔ cup (75 g) almond meal
2 teaspoons fresh parsley leaves, plus more for garnish
1 garlic clove, finely chopped or crushed
3 tablespoons olive oil
Freshly ground black pepper
2½ cups (150 g) chopped lettuce, rinsed
1 lemon, cut into wedges

Preheat the oven to 450°F (240°C). Clean the mushroom caps with a paper towel (cleaning them under the tap will make them swell too much). Place the almonds, almond meal, parsley, and garlic in a blender and blend. Transfer the mixture to a bowl. Add 2 tablespoons of the oil and pepper to taste.

Stir well. Press the top side of the portobellos into the mixture and then take them out, so that a lot of the almond mixture sticks to the mushrooms. Place the portobellos on a baking sheet, top-side down. Spread the remaining almond mixture over the bottom side of the portobellos so that the entire mushroom is now covered. Sprinkle with the remaining tablespoon of oil. Bake for 15 minutes, or until the almond filling is golden brown and crispy. Serve with the lettuce and lemon wedges, sprinkled with parsley.

Spinach and Lentil Salad with Feta and Walnuts

For the dressing:
   ¼ cup (60 ml) water
   3 tablespoons olive oil
   3 tablespoons vinegar
   1 tablespoon Dijon mustard
   Salt and freshly ground black pepper

For the salad:
   8 cups (240 g) spinach leaves, rinsed
   1½ cups (300 g) lentils, cooked
   ¼ cup (25 g) walnuts, chopped
   2½ tablespoons crumbled feta

Prepare the dressing by mixing together the water, olive oil, vinegar, mustard, and salt and pepper to taste in a small bowl. Place the spinach and lentils in a large bowl. Pour on the dressing and mix well, then add the walnuts and feta.

Pizza with Pesto

For the crust:
　　¾ cup (100 g) almond meal
　　2 large eggs
　　⅓ cup (90 ml) water
　　3 tablespoons olive oil

For the pesto:
　　Scant ⅔ cup (80 g) pine nuts
　　¼ cup (60 ml) olive oil
　　Handful of fresh basil leaves
　　1 garlic clove

Preheat the oven to 375°F (190°C). Mix together the almond meal, eggs, water, and oil in a large bowl. When the mixture comes together into a dough, knead by hand until smooth (do it gently because this dough is more crumbly than regular flour dough). Make the pesto by blending the pine nuts, olive oil, basil, and garlic together in a blender. Form the dough into two small pizza crusts. Place them on a nonstick baking sheet. Spread the pesto over the dough and bake for 12 minutes or until the crusts are golden brown. Turn the oven off but leave the pizzas in for another 3 minutes.

Wheat-Free Bread

　　2 tablespoons olive oil, plus more for baking sheet
　　1½ cups (190 g) almond meal
　　Scant ½ cup (45 g) ground flaxseeds
　　1½ tablespoons coconut flour
　　2 teaspoons baking soda
　　¼ cup (60 ml) water
　　2 tablespoons vinegar
　　½ teaspoon salt
　　3 large eggs, beaten

Preheat the oven to 375°F (190°C). Grease a loaf pan. Place the almond meal, ground flaxseeds, coconut flour, and baking soda in a bowl and mix well. In a small bowl, mix together the water, 2 tablespoons of oil, and the vinegar and salt. Add this mixture to the dry ingredients and mix well. Let stand for 1 minute, then add the beaten eggs and mix well. Pour the dough into the loaf pan and bake for 15 minutes, or until golden brown. Cut the bread into slices and refrigerate.

Tip: You can also add 2 teaspoons dried rosemary, 1 teaspoon garlic powder, and 1 teaspoon dried oregano to give the bread a different flavor. You can spread the bread with any of the following: hummus, pesto, guacamole, goat cheese, sun-dried tomato, and watercress plus salt.

SOUPS

Soups can be made quickly, such as with leftover vegetables. They are an ideal way to eat lots of vegetables every day. Try making soups with the healthiest vegetables, such as broccoli, kale, and spinach. This is a quick basic recipe:

Basic Broccoli Soup

¼ cup (60 ml) olive oil
2 garlic cloves, chopped
4 cups (1 L) water
1 pound (500 g) broccoli, chopped into bite-size pieces
2 vegetable bouillon cubes
Freshly ground black pepper
Finely chopped fresh parsley

Heat the oil in a large saucepan over medium heat. Add the garlic and stir-fry for 1 to 2 minutes. Pour the water into the pan and add the broccoli, bouillon cubes, and pepper to taste. Simmer for about 40 minutes. Remove the pan from the heat and blend the broccoli with an electric mixer or immersion blender to puree. Serve with parsley.

Tip: You can also add 1 tablespoon dried basil, 1 bay leaf (removed before blending), and 1 small, chopped onion, for extra flavor. You can also make the soup thicker by using more vegetables, for example, substitute 1 pound 10 ounces (750 g) of vegetables for the water.

HEALTHY SNACKS

Does a snack always have to be cookies or chips? Here are some much healthier alternatives:
- Raw vegetables (broccoli or cauliflower florets, carrots, cherry tomatoes, red or green bell pepper strips) with hummus dip, pesto (made with pine nuts, basil, garlic, and olive oil), guacamole, vegetable pâté, or nut butter
- ½ avocado sprinkled with olive oil, salt, and freshly ground black pepper
- Olives
- Nuts (mixed) with dried fruit or olives
- Sardines with olives
- A piece of dark chocolate (minimum 70 percent cacao)
- Soy yogurt with raspberries
- Cheese
- Apple slices with cheddar
- Fruit (peach, cherries, plum, nectarine, apricot, banana, pear, apple, grapefruit, kiwi . . .)
- Tomato slices sprinkled with olive oil and crumbled feta

Kale Chips

Kale, rinsed, hard stems removed, and leaves cut into pieces
2 tablespoons olive oil, plus more for the parchment
Salt

Preheat the oven to 300°F (150°C). Mix the pieces of kale with the oil. Sprinkle with salt. Place the kale on a baking sheet lined with greased parchment paper. Bake for 15 minutes, or until the kale is crispy.

Apple Slices with Almond Butter

Apples, sliced

Fresh lemon juice

Almond butter (store-bought, or make it yourself by grinding almonds in a blender to make a paste—this can take up to 15 minutes)

Chopped almonds

Crumbled dark chocolate

Unsweetened coconut flakes

Mix the apple slices with the lemon juice (the lemon juice ensures that the apple slices do not brown so quickly). Place the apple slices on a plate and cover with almond butter. Sprinkle with the almonds, chocolate, and coconut.

Cashew-Coconut Balls

1 cup (150 g) dates, pitted and chopped

¾ cup (105 g) cashews

½ cup (40 g) shredded or grated coconut

Pinch of salt (optional)

Place all the ingredients in a blender and mix well until they turn into a dough. With the palms of your hands, roll the dough into balls. Refrigerate for 1 hour. A delicious, healthy snack.

DESSERTS

Note: Some people find that the natural sweetener stevia has a bitter after-taste; erythritol does not have that as much. Some examples of healthy desserts (which could also serve as snacks):

- 2 handfuls of red and blue fruit (blueberries, raspberries, blackberries, strawberries, cherries), with whipped cream, if you desire
- A piece of dark chocolate (minimum 70 percent cacao)
- Soy yogurt with blue fruit and flaxseeds
- 1 apple, sliced, sprinkled with stevia and ground cinnamon
- Chocolate-covered strawberries
- Mixed nuts with chopped dried fruit

Chocolate-Nut Clusters

7 ounces (200 g) dark chocolate (minimum 70 percent cacao)
9 ounces (250 g) nuts (walnuts, almonds, cashews . . .), coarsely chopped
Freshly ground black pepper

Break the chocolate into chunks, place in a saucepan, and melt over low heat (105°F/40°C is sufficient). Add the nuts. Sprinkle with a little black pepper. Drop spoonfuls of the chocolate mixture onto aluminum foil or parchment paper. Refrigerate and allow them to cool before serving.

Lemon Cake

⅓ cup (90 ml) coconut oil, plus 1 teaspoon for the pan
4 tablespoons stevia powder or erythritol powder
2 cups (185 g) almond meal
½ cup (60 g) coconut flour
4 large eggs, beaten
Grated zest and juice of 1 lemon, or 1 teaspoon lemon extract

Preheat the oven to 350°F (180°C). Grease a 9-inch (23 cm) round pie dish with 1 teaspoon of the oil. In a small saucepan over low heat, melt the remaining ⅓ cup (90 ml) oil (or microwave for 30 seconds), then add the stevia and remove from the heat. Stir together the almond meal and coconut flour in a large bowl. Add the melted oil, eggs, and lemon zest and juice. Beat until the mixture is creamy. Drop the batter into the prepared pie dish and bake for 30 minutes, or until a knife inserted into the center of the cake comes out clean.

Coconut Mousse

One 13.5-ounce can (400 ml) coconut milk (refrigerated so that the coconut milk becomes cream)
¼ cup (20 g) cacao powder
1 to 2 tablespoons stevia or erythritol powder
Unsweetened coconut flakes or ground cinnamon for serving, optional

Spoon the cooled coconut milk cream from the can into a medium bowl. With an electric mixer, beat the coconut cream until fluffy (until it is no longer a liquid). While beating, add the cacao powder and stevia until the mixture turns into a mousse. If desired, sprinkle with coconut flakes or cinnamon and serve.

Tofu-Chocolate Mousse with Raspberries

14 ounces (400 g) silken tofu
8.5 ounces (240 g) dark chocolate (minimum 70 percent cacao), melted
2 teaspoons stevia powder or erythritol powder
1 tablespoon pure vanilla extract
A pinch of ground nutmeg
2 handfuls of raspberries

Place all the ingredients, except the raspberries, in a blender and blend. Refrigerate and let set at least 2 hours. Serve with the raspberries.

Chocolate Truffles

½ cup (120 ml) heavy whipping cream
1 teaspoon vanilla extract
8.5 ounces (240 g) dark chocolate (minimum 70 percent cacao), finely chopped
Cacao powder or crushed nuts

Bring the cream to a boil in a small pan. Add the vanilla. Place the chocolate in a large bowl and pour the cream mixture over the chocolate. Stir until well mixed. Allow to cool and then refrigerate for about 2 hours. Place 1 teaspoon at a time of the mixture in the palm of your hand and quickly roll it into a ball. Place the truffles on parchment paper. Roll the truffles in the cacao powder or crushed nuts. The truffles can be kept in a tightly closed container in a cool place for up to a week.

AFTERWORD

If there is one thing multimillionaires dislike, it is having to die. For them, the most precious thing in the universe is not money, a red diamond, or a piece of a white dwarf star, but time. That is why such billionaires as Craig Venter and the founders of Google engage in all kinds of initiatives to extend life span. They found companies and institutions with the goal of prolonging human lives. Venter, one of the first pioneers who mapped the human genome (all our DNA), has founded Human Longevity Inc., a company that uses supercomputers to search for genes that play a role in aging. The founders of Google have appointed neurobiologist and investor Bill Maris as CEO of Google Ventures to invest hundreds of millions of dollars in companies and research institutes involved in research to tackle the problem of aging. According to Bill Maris, "If you ask me today if it is possible to live to be 500, the answer is yes." Google also signed a $1.5 billion contract with AbbVie, a large pharmaceutical firm. The goal of this collaboration is to develop medications and technologies to slow down aging. Meanwhile, the founder of Facebook, Mark Zuckerberg, and Jack Ma, a Chinese Internet entrepreneur, together with a few other billionaires, created the Breakthrough Prize in Life Sciences. This prize is awarded annually to top scientists for discoveries to extend the human life span. The prize is $3 million—three times as much as the Nobel Prize. These young entrepreneurs, who have already drastically changed our lives with Google, Facebook, and Android smartphones now also want to change our bodies and our life span.

Some people will argue that the desire for a longer life and immortality is nothing new. In the past, pharaohs and emperors built pyramids and tombs to achieve immortality. Today, it is billionaires who invest hundreds of millions of dollars in companies that research aging. However, there is a definite difference now. For the first time in the almost 200,000-year history of humankind, thanks to the discovery of DNA, proteins, and the development of molecular biology, we now know what life is and how it works. Life and aging are no longer a great mystery. Furthermore, we have come to the surprising conclusion that extending the life span or reversing the aging process is not as difficult as we always thought. Actually, this should not surprise us, because nature was far ahead of us in creating organisms that age very little or not at all and can even accomplish this fairly quickly, as was the case with the opossums that migrated to an island without predators and since then age more slowly.

The human species has already undergone some significant changes. We were transformed from nomadic hunter-gatherers to settled farmers and eventually inhabitants of cities—more than half of the world's population now lives in cities. Not only the way in which we live has changed drastically but also the way in which we die. In the past, most people died of infectious diseases. Children, adolescents, and adults in the prime of life succumbed to tuberculosis, cholera, plague, pneumonia, gastroenteritis, polio, diphtheria, or smallpox. As recently as the twentieth century, funeral homes had a large supply of small coffins for children and babies. Fortunately, today that is rarely the case. Now it mainly is old people who die, not of infectious diseases but of cardiovascular disease, dementia, and cancer.

However, a new change is on the horizon. People will live longer and longer. They will reach an age their ancestors would not have dreamed possible. This will be the result not only of new man-made breakthroughs but also because of natural evolutionary mechanisms. In the future, family reunions will be very large: Children, parents, grandparents, great-grandparents, and great-great-grandparents will sit down together at a very long dinner table. Old people will look much younger than their age. Some scientists predict that new technologies will allow people of 90 to look like 30-year-olds. It is important for us to prepare ourselves for such a world and plan for it. Our retirement will change, as well as our work methods, lifestyle, and diet. People will be held responsible for their own health, retirement, and care.

For many people, the most important thing is not to live as long as possible but to stay young, fit, and healthy as long as possible. As we have seen, a healthy lifestyle plays the most important role in this. It is not a coincidence that a healthy lifestyle both reduces the risk of aging-related diseases and overweight, for aging and overweight are two sides of the same coin. And for those who want to become really old, a healthy lifestyle is the best way to achieve it. They may be able to profit from LEV, longevity escape velocity, to achieve a much longer life. Each time, they will live long enough to profit from the latest life-extending technology. To put it in the words of Bill Maris, the Google investing maverick, "I just hope to live long enough not to die."

AFTERWORD TO THIS EDITION

Humankind has gone through several major revolutions, each time drastically changing our way of life. About 10,000 years ago, the *agricultural revolution* took us from a nomadic existence hunting wildlife and searching for berries to a settled life on the farm. In the eighteenth century, the *First Industrial Revolution* saw the introduction of the first efficient steam engines, which replaced human muscle power with engine power. A short time later, in the nineteenth century, this was followed by the discovery and use of electricity, which among other things paved the way for the mass production of goods, from nails and shoes to typewriters and cars (the *Second Industrial Revolution*). Around 1960, a *Third Industrial Revolution* brought us electronics in the form of computer chips, the personal computer, and the Internet, which once again transformed our society.

Some people believe that we are now at the beginning of the *Fourth Industrial Revolution*. This revolution has two pillars: the advent of intelligent machines and the advance of biotechnology. The advent of intelligent machines includes among other things artificial intelligence (AI). Artificial intelligence can learn, be creative, find solutions to complex problems, and discover new insights. It is therefore not simply old school, faster computing power. No, AI is different; working similarly to the human brain, it consists of digital nerve cells that form neural networks that can learn, see new patterns and connections, and draw original conclusions, just like humans. Such programs are already able to write original stories and poems, invent new materials and compose music that the public cannot distinguish from the work of a human composer.

Artificial intelligence will play an important role in the future of health care and medicine. AI will help physicians make diagnoses, analyze medical records, and interpret medical images, and it will help researchers develop new drugs and treatments. This brings us to the second pillar of the Fourth

Industrial Revolution: biotechnology. The coming decades will see great advances in this field—new breakthroughs that will transform medicine and health care. To begin with, for the first time in human history, physicians will be able to really cure many diseases. Currently, most diseases cannot be cured. The consequences of a heart attack or stroke cannot be reversed; the destroyed heart or brain tissue cannot be restored. We can cure almost none of the thousands of existing genetic disorders; we cannot rewrite genes to undo them. The same is true for most nerve disorders, such as multiple sclerosis (MS) and ALS; inflammatory diseases such as Crohn's disease, ulcerative colitis, rheumatoid arthritis, and lupus; lung diseases, such as emphysema; and numerous aggressive cancers. We cannot even cure the common cold. Medications mainly alleviate the symptoms, but they do not address the causes.

This is going to change. In the near future, physicians will for the first time be able to cure many of these diseases via new interventions, several of which we have discussed in this book, such as CRISPR proteins, stem cell therapy, repair of mitochondrial DNA, and blood-derived rejuvenating substances. Everyone who follows the medical literature can feel that we are at a turning point. At an unprecedented rate, we see one article after another appear about things that were considered impossible a few years ago: researchers who can dramatically reduce the consequences of a stroke, blind people who regain part of their vision, genetic diseases that are removed from embryos, stem cells that can be reprogrammed, and children who are alive today thanks to cancer therapies that did not exist a few years ago. The Fourth Revolution is gaining steam. Much of that steam originates from cross-fertilization between the two pillars of this revolution: artificial intelligence and biotechnology.

Calico, the sister company of Google, which aims to slow down the aging process, has recently hired Daphne Koller, a brilliant computer scientist who specializes in artificial intelligence. Calico wants to apply artificial intelligence to find ways to extend the human life span. It is significant that a computer company ventures onto the terrain of biotechnology and biosciences. Life is being digitalized: The human genome (all the DNA in our cells) is mapped with powerful computers and stored on them. New technologies reprogram life, such as CRISPR proteins, which can rewrite DNA, like a computer program does. Artificial intelligence analyses our health and body, because human organisms are too complex for human brains to fully understand, assess, and monitor.

Artificial intelligence and new biotechnologies will be employed not only to cure diseases but also to slow down the aging process. After all, aging is the cause of all aging-related diseases, from heart disease and Alzheimer's to eye diseases and osteoporosis. Tackling aging itself will therefore drastically change our health, since aging-related diseases can be addressed much better all together by focusing on the underlying, driving force behind all of them: aging. This approach will dramatically change medicine, our health care, and our society.

However, we do not necessarily need supercomputers, AI, DNA scanners, and other advanced technologies of the Fourth Industrial Revolution to research or slow down aging. A pen or a dog can also help. People can participate in aging research by submitting blood samples and filling in questionnaires about their dietary and lifestyle habits. This helps scientists find out why one person lives longer than another. People who have a dog can participate in the Dog Aging Project (www.dogagingproject.com), in which dogs are given rapamycin, a medication that in various studies has extended the life of lab animals. Similar projects are under way for people as well. Recently the TAME (Targeting Aging with Metformin) study was approved. This study will investigate whether a medication for the treatment of type 2 diabetes (namely, metformin) can also slow down aging. This is the first study specifically designed to test whether a medication can slow down aging; usually studies are aimed only at testing a medication for a specific disease, not for aging as a whole. This study is one example of an increasing amount of studies, projects, and companies that are investigating how people can live longer and stay healthy.

We are at the dawn of the Fourth Industrial Revolution, which for the first time will allow people to live much longer and healthier lives. Just like the previous agricultural and industrial revolutions, this Fourth Revolution will cause dramatic changes in our society. But this revolution is inherently different; this will be the first revolution that will not only change our society but also our bodies and brains. It is important to prepare ourselves for that. It is even more important that we use our new knowledge and insights responsibly, to achieve a society in which everyone can fully enjoy their full potential in terms of life and health, so that everyone can fulfill hundreds of wishes, in contrast to the one wish all sick and suffering people have: the wish to get better.

ADDITIONAL READING

What Are Proteins?

This information is for readers who want to know more about proteins; but first, we need to explain what atoms and molecules are. All our food is made up of this stuff.

All matter around us consist of *atoms*. A piece of iron consists of iron atoms; a gold ring consists of gold atoms; and a tree is a combination of carbon, hydrogen, and oxygen atoms. A diamond consists of carbon atoms that are bonded together very closely, which is what makes the diamond so hard. Graphite in a pencil consists of the same carbon atoms as the diamond, but the carbon atoms in the graphite are bonded together differently, so that graphite crumbles while the diamond is the hardest material found in nature. More complex things, such as living beings, consist of combinations of all kinds of atoms, including hydrogen, oxygen, and carbon atoms.

There are 92 types of atoms in total, including hydrogen, carbon, nitrogen, iron, and gold atoms (apart from some very rare atoms that exist briefly in nuclear reactors). All these 92 atoms are ordered according to their weight. The lightest is hydrogen (atom #1). The heaviest is uranium (atom #92). Each atom has an abbreviated name: H is a hydrogen atom; C, a carbon atom; O, an oxygen atom; N, a nitrogen atom; and so on. Atoms have a tendency to bond with other atoms. When two or more atoms are bonded together, we call it a *molecule*. The simplest molecule is dihydrogen (H_2)—two hydrogen atoms that are bonded together. Water consists of water molecules, composed of two hydrogen atoms and one oxygen atom (H_2O). Those water molecules also like to loosely stick together, and if you put many millions of billions of water molecules (H_2O) together, you get the slightly sticky conglomeration we call a drop of water.

Like everything else in the world, proteins are composed of atoms. A protein may consist of hundreds or up to hundreds of thousands of atoms. These atoms order themselves into a certain shape that determines the function and the name of the protein. Some proteins are shaped like a hollow cylinder and sit perpendicular to the cell wall. These proteins act as a kind of entry channel that allows certain substances in the cell. Other proteins are

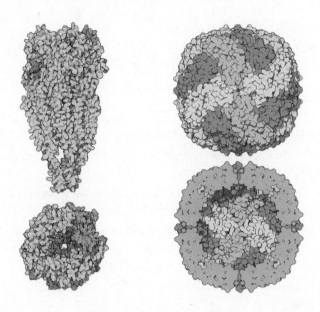

Two types of proteins: a cylinder-shaped protein and a ball-shaped protein. Each little ball represents an atom. (Source: David S. Goodsell, the Scripps Research Institute.)

shaped like a ball. If we were to cut this ball in half, we would see it is hollow. That is for a reason: This type of protein (called ferritin) stores iron atoms. Just like apples are stored in baskets, iron atoms are stored in this ball-shaped protein. When you have a blood test to check whether you have sufficient iron in your blood, it is the concentration of this type of protein in your blood that will be measured.

More specifically, proteins are composed of *amino acids*. These are groups of atoms that are always built according to a specific pattern. The *backbone* of an amino acid always has the same pattern. Different groups of atoms can attach themselves to the backbone to form different amino acids. There exist twenty types of amino acids in the body (that can form proteins), each with its own specific group of atoms.

The basic structure of all amino acids. H represents a hydrogen atom; C, a carbon atom; O, an oxygen atom; and N, a nitrogen atom. R is the functional group—this can be any one of the twenty types of small atom groups, which then determine the kind of amino acid.

Amino acids form a long string, like pearls on a necklace. Each string is a protein. The sequence of the amino acids on the string determines the type of protein. One protein may begin with, for example, glycine-arginine-tryptophan, while another protein begins with tryptophan-tryptophan-arginine, and so forth. There are numerous different combinations. The twenty types of amino acids form about 100,000 different types of proteins in our body. Some proteins consist of only several tens of amino acids; insulin, for example, is a string of 51 amino acids. Other proteins are gigantic, such as titin, an important muscle protein that consists of 30,000 amino acids.

What Are Carbohydrates?

Like proteins, carbohydrates are also composed of atoms. Carbohydrates are sugars. *Glucose* is one of the simplest carbohydrates. It can stand on its own or serve as a basic unit to form larger carbohydrates (long sugar chains). Glucose itself is composed of six atoms in the form of a hexagon, with a few atoms attached.

Glucose. C represents a carbon atom; O, an oxygen atom; and H, a hydrogen atom.

A cube of grape sugar (glucose) is composed of billions and billions of separate glucose units. *Fructose* (fruit sugar) is like glucose a basic unit, but is composed of five atoms in the form of a pentagon, with a few atoms attached.

Fructose. C is a carbon atom; O, an oxygen atom; and H, a hydrogen atom.

In the same way that amino acids can bond together in a long string to form proteins, simple sugars, such as glucose and fructose, can bond together to form sugar chains. When one glucose molecule and one fructose molecule bond together, they form *sucrose*. Sucrose is the scientific name for the sugar we regularly use in our coffee and tea.

Sucrose (white table sugar) is composed of a glucose molecule and a fructose molecule that are bonded together.

Carbohydrates can be composed of even longer chains. *Starch*, for example, is composed of many thousands of glucose molecules strung together. The starch found in bread, potatoes, rice, or pasta is thus made from glucose.

$$CH_2OH \qquad CH_2OH \qquad CH_2OH$$

Starch consists of many thousands of glucose molecules that are strung together and form long chains. (Note: At the corners where the lines cross, there is always a carbon atom [C], which, in accordance with standard scientific notation, is not included in the figure).

GLOSSARY

Adenosine triphosphate (ATP): The molecule of life that keeps everything running in the body. ATP molecules react to proteins by sticking to them. This causes those proteins to change their structure so as to perform certain specific functions. An ATP molecule may, for example, stick to a channel protein in the cell wall and open it, so that certain molecules can flow into the cell.

Alzheimer's disease: See: Dementia.

Amino acid: Amino acids are the building blocks of proteins. An amino acid is a small molecule composed of about ten atoms that always have the same basic backbone structure plus a few specific atoms that determine the type of amino acid. There are twenty types of amino acids in the body that stick together into chains that form proteins. One protein consists of tens, or up to thousands, of amino acids.

Antioxidant: A substance that readily reacts with free radicals and neutralizes them. See also: Free radicals.

Atherosclerosis: Clogging of the arteries, particularly those of the heart and the brain. When an artery in the heart becomes completely clogged, part of the heart dies from a lack of oxygen; in medical terms, this is a heart attack. When an artery in the brain becomes completely clogged, it is called a stroke.

Atom: The building block of all matter. An atom consists of a nucleus and electrons that circulate around the nucleus. The nucleus is composed of protons and neutrons. The number of protons in the nucleus determines the name of the atom. Hydrogen has one proton; iron, 26; and uranium, 92.

ATP: See: Adenosine triphosphate (ATP).

Bacteria: A one-celled organism that has neither a nucleus nor mitochondria.

Base or base molecule: A molecule such as guanine (G), cytosine (C), adenine (A), or thymine (T). Each base consists of a group of about fifteen carbon, nitrogen, hydrogen, and oxygen atoms. Two bases together form the rungs of a DNA ladder.

Billion: 1,000 million (1,000,000,000).

Brain cell: See: Neuron.

Calorie: A measure of energy. Calories provide the energy to keep our body running. Part of our food is converted to calories. Calories can represent ATP or heat. One calorie is the amount of energy necessary to heat 1 liter of water by 1°C. A human uses about 2,200 calories per day. In some countries one calorie means 1,000 calories. So in this case, a human would consume about 2,200 kilocalories per day (a kilocalorie is 1,000 calories). See also: Adenosine triphosphate (ATP).

Cancer: See: Mutation.

Carbohydrate: A carbohydrate may consist of one sugar molecule (such as glucose), or two sugar molecules (such as granulated sugar, or sucrose, which in turn consists of glucose and fructose), or many thousands of sugar molecules (such as starch, which consists of thousands of glucose molecules). See also: Glucose.

Cardiovascular disease: Most often refers to the clogging up and hardening of the blood vessels. When a blood vessel in the heart suddenly becomes completely clogged, it is called a heart attack. When a blood vessel in the brain becomes completely clogged or ruptures, it is called a stroke. See also: Heart attack and Stroke.

Cell: A minuscule sack of water containing a nucleus (harboring the DNA), a number of mitochondria, millions of proteins, and many other components. Our body is built up of cells, each with a specific form and function, such as stomach cells, liver cells, and eye cells. The average diameter of a cell is one fiftieth of one millimeter. The first primitive cell may have contained mitochondria but no cell nucleus yet (that came later).

Cell fluid: Also called cytoplasm. This is the area of the cell outside the cell nucleus. In our cells, the cell fluid consists of water, in which proteins, mitochondria, and other cell components float around.

Cell nucleus: Our cells all have a nucleus inside that contains the DNA. See also: DNA (deoxyribonucleic acid).

Cell skeleton: Also called cytoskeleton. It consists of long, interlinked tubes made of proteins. Small molecules such as ATP attach themselves to the cell skeleton, causing it to change its structure and thus the entire cell. This makes it possible for cells to become mobile, attach themselves to other cells, or capture bacteria. See: Adenosine triphosphate (ATP).

Cell wall: The cell wall, often called the membrane, consists mainly of fatty molecules. It separates the cell from the outside world.

Cortex: The outer layer of the brain. This layer is a few millimeters thick and consists of elongated pyramid cells arranged in layers; it plays an important role in consciousness. When surgeons run an electric current through the cortex during a brain operation, we may feel as if we are touched somewhere or suddenly a long-forgotten memory may resurface.

Cortisol: A hormone produced by the adrenal gland that is released during stress. See also: Hormone.

Cross-link: A connection between two proteins. This connection may be composed of a sugar molecule. Cross-links between the collagen proteins in the skin can reduce the elasticity of the skin and play a role in the formation of wrinkles.

Cytoplasm: See: Cell fluid.

Cytoskeleton: See: Cell skeleton.

Dementia: The death of brain cells, usually caused by proteins that cluster in and around the brain cells and suffocate them. In other forms of dementia, the proteins accumulate in the blood vessel walls, making them fragile and prone to breaking. Depending on the type of proteins and the areas of the brain most affected, it may be called Alzheimer's disease, Lewy body dementia, frontotemporal dementia, or vascular dementia See also: Stroke.

Diabetes: A disease in which too much sugar circulates in the bloodstream. Type 1 diabetes is caused by the immune system that mistakenly attacks the insulin-producing cells in the pancreas so that not enough insulin is produced. Without insulin, the cells cannot absorb sugar and process it, so that the sugar accumulates in the blood and damages the body. This type of diabetes often occurs in children. However, 90 percent of diabetes cases are type 2 diabetes. In this type of diabetes, mainly the liver, fat, and muscle cells no longer sufficiently react to insulin, so that these cells cannot properly absorb and process sugar. This causes the sugar to circulate in the bloodstream too long and damage other body cells, such as kidney, eye, or nerve cells. The reason why the liver, fat, and muscle cells no longer sufficiently react to insulin, is because they became resistant or "numb" to insulin because they were exposed to too much high insulin peaks for many years or decades, caused by unhealthy foods that bring about big insulin peaks because they contain too much sugars, starches, and animal protein.

DNA (deoxyribonucleic acid): A gigantic molecule in the shape of a spiral staircase. The DNA contains the instructions for building the proteins that perform virtually all tasks in the cell. The DNA contains the "letter" code (composed of the bases guanine [G], cytosine [C], adenine [A], or thymine [T]) for tens of thousands of types of protein.

Dopamine: A small molecule that acts as a neurotransmitter. It maintains communication between nerve cells, especially those involved in feelings such as addiction and reward. See also: Neurotransmitter.

Electron: A very small, negatively charged particle. Electrons and the atomic nucleus together form an atom. Electrons are the glue used by atoms to stick together to form molecules. See also: Atom.

Element: See: Atom.

Endorphin: A substance that plays a role in feelings of pleasure. When their body makes endorphins, people feel good or they become less aware of pain. There are also synthetic endorphins with a similar effect, such as heroin and morphine.

Enzyme: See: Protein.

Evolution: A change in the characteristics of organisms so that they are better adapted to their environment. This change can be the result of random mutations in their DNA, which can occasionally have positive consequences in the sense that an organism is then better able to survive and reproduce. The DNA that can mutate determines how proteins are made. Proteins in turn determine the function, form, and cooperation between cells that build up an entire organism.

Fat: A molecule that consists of a head and several tails. These tails are long chains of carbon atoms with hydrogen atoms attached. The tails are called *fatty acids*. When the fatty acid contains one or more double bonds between two carbon atoms (a *double bond* means a stronger bond), it is called an *unsaturated fat*. When the fatty acid has no double bonds, it is called a *saturated* *fat* (since the carbon chain is completely saturated with hydrogen atoms). *Trans fats* consist of unsaturated fatty acids in which two hydrogen atoms are located opposite the double bond. Due to this unusual configuration, trans fats cannot easily processed in the body. Trans fats are can be found in industrially prepared foods, such a baked goods and fast food.

Flavonoids: These are the substances that give flowers, vegetables, and fruit their red, blue, or other specific color. Flavonoids are often very healthy for the body, usually because they are mildly toxic or because they interact with certain proteins in the cell, not so much because they are antioxidants.

Free radicals: A free radical is an atom or molecule that is highly reactive. That is, a free radical very quickly involves a chemical reaction with stable molecules in the environment, such as proteins or DNA. Free radicals thus react with proteins, DNA, or molecules in the cell walls, causing them to be damaged. Free radicals arise as a by-product of cell metabolism, especially in the mitochondria. See also Oxidation and Antioxidant.

Gene: A piece of the DNA string that serves as the code for making a certain protein. Human DNA contains about 24,000 genes. See also: DNA and Protein.

Glucose: Glucose consists of a hexagon of carbon, oxygen, and hydrogen atoms. See also: Carbohydrate.

Glycemic index: A measurement to determine how fast sugars in a food end up in the blood and cause a blood sugar peak. Especially products that are composed of many simple sugars or heated starches, such as soft drinks, potatoes, and pizza dough, are rapidly broken down in the intestines so that the sugars wind up in the bloodstream quickly and cause steep sugar peaks.

Glycemic load: Measures both *how fast* the sugars in a food end up in the bloodstream *and* the *amount* of digestible carbohydrates the food contains. It is an even better measure of how healthy a food is, although for many foods the glycemic index is sufficient.

Growth hormone: See: IGF.

Growth stimulation: Stimulation of the growth and activity of cells. This happens via substances such as IGF, insulin, growth hormone, sugars, and amino acids.

Heart attack: The sudden complete closure of a blood vessel that was already narrow as a result of years of clogging. This clogging is the result of a buildup of cholesterol and inflammatory cells in the blood vessel wall.

Homo neanderthalensis: See: Neanderthal.

Homo sapiens: The human species, which originated about 180,000 years ago.

Hormesis: The phenomenon whereby mild damage can be healthy. Toxic substances, in small amounts can be healthy because they activate defense and repair mechanisms in the body.

Hormone: A hormone can be a (small) protein, or a fatty molecule, such as cortisol or testosterone. Many hormones are produced by glands, such as the thyroid or the adrenal glands, and released into the bloodstream. Then, they travel to their targets in the body, where they influence the activity of the cellular machinery: More or fewer proteins are made, so that the cell gets new functions.

IGF: Insulin-like growth factor. IGF consists of a short chain of amino acids. It stimulates cell growth. An excess of IGF increases the risk of cancer and type 2 diabetes. Growth hormone stimulates the production of IGF.

Immune cells: See: White blood cells.

Immune system: A system consisting of many billions of white blood cells circulating in the tissues and bloodstream to remove foreign substances, like bacteria and viruses, from the body. The immune system can also target cancer cells.

Insulin: See: Diabetes.

Lysosome: A little sack within the cell that breaks down debris. Lysosomes are the waste disposal incinerators of the cell.

Macular degeneration: The death of retinal cells in the back of the eye due to accumulation of debris in the cells.

Micrometer: One millionth of a meter or one thousandth of a millimeter.

Mitochondrion: A cell usually contains several hundreds of mitochondria. Mitochondria are the energy generators of the cell. They take in oxygen, fats, and sugars in order to produce energy-rich molecules, namely, ATP. These ATP molecules stick to proteins, which causes them to change structure and enables them to perform certain functions. See also: Adenosine triphosphate (ATP).

Molecule: When two or more atoms are bonded together, we call it a molecule. A water molecule consists of two hydrogen atoms (H) and one oxygen atom (O) to form H_2O. A DNA molecule consists of many millions of atoms.

mTOR: An aging switch. It is a protein inside cells that is mainly activated by amino acids (coming from the proteins we eat). Sugar can also activate mTOR. When it is activated, mTOR switches on all kinds of mechanisms that make cells "grow" (work harder) and accelerate the aging process.

Mutation: A change in the DNA of a cell. The DNA contains the building instructions for proteins. A change in DNA also involves a change in proteins, so that cells, or entire bodies, can acquire different characteristics. Mutations may be caused by small errors during the multiplying of the cells, or by radiation, for example from the sun, or by chemical substances. Sometimes mutations in a regular body cell can enable that cell to continue to divide: this is what causes cancer. Cancer cells continue to divide and ultimately spread through the entire body. See also: Protein and DNA (deoxyribonucleic acid).

Nanometer: One millionth of a millimeter.

Neanderthal: A human-like species that lived on earth about a quarter of a million until 30,000 years ago and then became extinct. The Neanderthals wore clothing, buried their dead, and made complex hunting tools.

Neuron: A brain cell or nerve cell. Neurons can send nerve signals (impulses) along their cell wall. This happens via charged atoms (ions), such as sodium, that flow into the cell through open protein channels (specific proteins). They can then also open other nearby channels that will allow more charged atoms (ions) to flow in, and so on. The nerve impulse moves along the cell membrane through opening protein channels.

Neurotransmitter: Neurotransmitters maintain the communication between nerve cells. They are molecules that are sprayed between two neurons, whereby one neuron activates the other neuron. Examples of neurotransmitters are serotonin and dopamine.

Oxidation: The process whereby an atom loses electrons. This may occur because a free radical steals an electron from the atom and thereby "damages" the atom or the molecule it is part of. See also: Antioxidant and Free radical.

Placebo: A dummy medicine. When the effectiveness of a medicine is tested in research, one group of people will receive the real medication and a second group of people (the control group) gets a placebo. This is necessary because usually people will already feel better, simply by getting medication, even if it contains no active substance (this is called the placebo effect).

Protein: An enormous molecule, often consisting of tens or thousands of amino acids and therefore of hundreds or many tens of thousands of atoms. Proteins can assume all kinds of shapes and functions and perform a great variety of jobs in our body. Implanted in cell walls (membranes), they can function as channels; in muscle cells, they can contract to make the muscle move; and in the bloodstream, they transport oxygen or attack bacteria.

Proton: The nucleus of an atom consists of neutrons and protons. Protons are relatively heavy, positively charged particles.

Saturated fat: See: Fat.

Serotonin: A neurotransmitter and also a small molecule that maintains the communication between billions of nerve cells in the brain. See also: Neurotransmitter.

Stem cell: Stem cells produce new cells to maintain or repair our tissues. When a stem cell divides, it can create two cells: a stem cell and a regular cell that builds up tissue, such as a skin cell, intestinal cell, or liver cell.

Stroke: A stroke occurs when a blood vessel in the brain tears or clogs completely, shutting off the blood supply to that part of the brain. As a result the brain cells in that area die.

Sugar: See: Carbohydrate.

Sugar peak: See: Glycemic index.

Telomere: The end piece of a DNA string. Telomeres consist of DNA. With each cell division, they become shorter. When they become too short, the DNA becomes less stable and "unravels," just like a shoelace unravels when the aglet at the end is gone.

Trans fat: See: Fat.

Unsaturated fat: See: Fat.

White blood cells: These cells are part of the immune system; they fight foreign substances, like bacteria and viruses, that have invaded the body.

REFERENCES

To prevent the list of references from being thicker than the book, this is a summary list of references. They may be a point of departure for readers who want to know more about the topics discussed in this book.

1   C. E. Finch, "Update on slow aging and negligible senescence—a mini-review." *Gerontology* 55, no. 3 (January 2009): 307–13.

2   V. Ziuganov et al., "Life span variation of the freshwater pearl shell: a model species for testing longevity mechanisms in animals." *AMBIO: A Journal of the Human Environment* 29, no. 2 (March 2000): 102.

3   K.-J. Min et al., "The lifespan of Korean eunuchs." *Current Biology* 22, no. 18 (September 2012): R792–93.

4   J. B. Hamilton et al., "Mortality and survival: comparison of eunuchs with intact men and women in a mentally retarded population." *Journal of Gerontology* 24, no. 4 (October 1969): 395–411.

5   M. S. Willis et al., "Proteotoxicity and cardiac dysfunction—Alzheimer's disease of the heart?" *New England Journal of Medicine* 368, no. 5 (January 2013): 455–64.

6   L. S. Coles et al., "Supercentenarians and transthyretin amyloidosis: the next frontier of human life extension." *Preventive Medicine* 54 Suppl (May 2012): S9–11.

7   J. Azpurua et al., "Naked mole-rat has increased translational fidelity compared with the mouse, as well as a unique 28S ribosomal RNA cleavage." *Proceedings of the National Academy of Sciences of the United States of America* 110, no. 43 (October 2013): 17350–55.

8   R. C. Grandison et al., "Amino-acid imbalance explains extension of lifespan by dietary restriction in *Drosophila*." *Nature* 462, no. 7276 (December 2009): 1061–64.

9   B. P. Yu et al., "Nutritional influences on aging of Fischer 344 rats: I. Physical, metabolic, and longevity characteristics." *Journal of Gerontology* 40, no. 6 (November 1985): 657–70.

10 S. Leto et al., "Dietary protein, life-span, and biochemical variables in female mice." *Journal of Gerontology* 31, no. 2 (March 1976): 144–48.

11 M. Ross et al., "Food preference and length of life." *Science* 190, no. 4210 (October 1975): 165–67.

12 J. P. Richie et al., "Methionine restriction increases blood glutathione and longevity in F344 rats." *FASEB Journal: Official Publication of the Federation of American Societies for Experimental Biology* 8, no. 15 (December 1994): 1302–7.

13 M. López-Torres et al., "Lowered methionine ingestion as responsible for the decrease in rodent mitochondrial oxidative stress in protein and dietary restriction possible implications for humans." *Biochimica et biophysica acta* 1780, no. 11 (November 2008): 1337–47.

14 D. Fau et al., "Effects of ingestion of high protein or excess methionine diets by rats for two years." *Journal of Nutrition* 118, no. 1 (January 1988): 128–33.

15 S. M. Solon-Biet et al., "The ratio of macronutrients, not caloric intake, dictates cardiometabolic health, aging, and longevity in ad libitum-fed mice." *Cell Metabolism* 19, no. 3 (March 2014): 418–30.

16 E. Parrella et al., "Protein restriction cycles reduce IGF-1 and phosphorylated Tau, and improve behavioral performance in an Alzheimer's disease mouse model." *Aging Cell* 12, no. 2 (April 2013): 257–68.

17 A. Pan et al., "Red meat consumption and mortality: results from 2 prospective cohort studies." *Archives of Internal Medicine* 172, no. 7 (April 2012): 555–63.

18 S. Rohrmann et al., "Meat consumption and mortality—results from the European Prospective Investigation into Cancer and Nutrition." *BMC Medicine* 11, no. 1 (January 2013): 63.

19 E. W.-T. Chong et al., "Red meat and chicken consumption and its association with age-related macular degeneration." *American Journal of Epidemiology* 169, no. 7 (April 2009): 867–76.

20 M. E. Levine et al., "Low protein intake is associated with a major reduction in IGF-1, cancer, and overall mortality in the 65 and younger but not older population." *Cell Metabolism* 19, no. 3 (March 2014): 407–17.

21 S. Zhang et al., "Dietary fat and protein in relation to risk of non-Hodgkin's lymphoma among women." *JNCI Journal of the National Cancer Institute* 91, no. 20 (October 1999): 1751–58.

22 E. Cho et al., "Red meat intake and risk of breast cancer among premenopausal women." *Archives of Internal Medicine* 166, no. 20 (November 2006): 2253–59.

23 William Manner et al., "Effects of dietary regimen and tissue site on bovine fatty acid profiles." *Journal of Animal Science* 59, no. 1 (February 1984): 109–21.

24 A. P. Simopoulos et al., "n-3 fatty acids in eggs from range-fed Greek chickens." *New England Journal of Medicine* 321, no. 20 (November 1989): 1412.

25 C. B. Hauswirth et al., "High omega-3 fatty acid content in alpine cheese: the basis for an alpine paradox." *Circulation* 109, no. 1 (January 2004): 103–7.

26 U. Ericson et al., "High intakes of protein and processed meat associate with increased incidence of type 2 diabetes." *British Journal of Nutrition* 109, no. 6 (March 2013): 1143–53.

27 T. T. Fung et al., "Low-carbohydrate diets and all-cause and cause-specific mortality: two cohort studies." *Annals of Internal Medicine* 153, no. 5 (September 2010): 289–98.

28 P. Lagiou et al., "Low carbohydrate-high protein diet and mortality in a cohort of Swedish women." *Journal of Internal Medicine* 261, no. 4 (April 2007): 366–74.

29 P. Lagiou et al., "Low carbohydrate-high protein diet and incidence of cardiovascular diseases in Swedish women: prospective cohort study." *BMJ (Clinical Research Ed.)* 344 (June 2012): e4026.

30 F. Tremblay et al., "Identification of IRS-1 Ser-1101 as a target of S6K1 in nutrient- and obesity-induced insulin resistance." *Proceedings of the National Academy of Sciences of the United States of America* 104, no. 35 (August 2007): 14056–61.

31 F. Tremblay et al., "Overactivation of S6 kinase 1 as a cause of human insulin resistance during increased amino acid availability." *Diabetes* 54, no. 9 (September 2005): 2674–84.

32 N. E. Allen et al., "The associations of diet with serum insulin-like growth factor I and its main binding proteins in 292 women meat-eaters, vegetarians, and vegans." *Cancer Epidemiology, Biomarkers and Prevention: A Publication of the American Association for Cancer Research, Cosponsored by the American Society of Preventive Oncology* 11, no. 11 (December 2002): 1441–48.

33 M. J. Orlich et al., "Vegetarian dietary patterns and mortality in Adventist Health Study 2." *JAMA Internal Medicine* 173, no. 13 (July 2013): 1230–38.

34 M. F. McCarty et al., "The low-methionine content of vegan diets may make methionine restriction feasible as a life extension strategy." *Medical Hypotheses* 72, no. 2 (February 2009): 125–28.

35 S. S. Hall, "Longevity." *National Geographic*, May 2013.

36 A. Fasano, "Surprises from celiac disease." *Scientific American* 301, no. 2 (August 2009): 54–61.

37 A. N. Pedersen et al., "Health effects of protein intake in healthy elderly populations: a systematic literature review." *Food and Nutrition Research* 58 (January 2014).

38 M. Holzenberger et al., "IGF-1 receptor regulates lifespan and resistance to oxidative stress in mice." *Nature* 421, no. 6919 (January 2003): 182–87.

39 C. Hale, "Oldest living mouse dies at home in SIUC laboratory." *Southern Illinoisan*, January 15, 2003.

40 L. Salaris et al., "Height and survival at older ages among men born in an inland village in Sardinia (Italy), 1866–2006." *Biodemography and Social Biology* 58, no. 1 (January 2012): 1–13.

41 Q. He et al., "Shorter men live longer: association of height with longevity and FOXO3 genotype in American men of Japanese ancestry." *PloS One* 9, no. 5 (January 2014): e94385.

42 J. Green et al., "Height and cancer incidence in the Million Women Study: prospective cohort, and meta-analysis of prospective studies of height and total cancer risk." *Lancet Oncology* 12, no. 8 (August 2011): 785–94.

43 J. Guevara-Aguirre et al., "Growth hormone receptor deficiency is associated with a major reduction in pro-aging signaling, cancer, and diabetes in humans." *Science Translational Medicine* 3, no. 70 (February 2011): 70ra13.

44 H. Gardener et al., "Diet soft drink consumption is associated with an increased risk of vascular events in the Northern Manhattan Study." *Journal of General Internal Medicine* 27, no. 9 (September 2012): 1120–26.

45 Q. Yang et al., "Added sugar intake and cardiovascular diseases mortality among US adults." *JAMA Internal Medicine* 174, no. 4 (April 2014): 516–24.

46 W. C. Willett et al., "Rebuilding the food pyramid." *Scientific American* 288, no. 1 (January 2003): 64–71.

47 H. Wu et al., "Association between dietary whole grain intake and risk of mortality." *JAMA Internal Medicine* 175, no. 3 (January 2015): 373–84.

48 E. W. Manheimer et al., "Paleolithic nutrition for metabolic syndrome: systematic review and meta-analysis." *American Journal of Clinical Nutrition* 102, no. 4 (October 2015): 922–32.

49 E. L. Lim et al., "Reversal of type 2 diabetes: normalisation of beta cell function in association with decreased pancreas and liver triacylglycerol." *Diabetologia* 54, no. 10 (October 2011): 2506–14.

50 "Beter eten en meer bewegen kunnen diabetes type 2 genezen" (Better nutrition and more exercise can cure type 2 diabetes). NOS News/Voeding Leeft, November 25, 2016.

51 R. D. Feinman et al., "Dietary carbohydrate restriction as the first approach in diabetes management: critical review and evidence base." *Nutrition* 31, no. 1 (July 2014): 1–13.

52 S. Liu et al., "A prospective study of dietary glycemic load, carbohydrate intake, and risk of coronary heart disease in US women." *American Journal of Clinical Nutrition* 71, no. 6 (June 2000): 1455–61.

53 J. W. J. Beulens et al., "High dietary glycemic load and glycemic index increase risk of cardiovascular disease among middle-aged women: a population-based follow-up study." *Journal of the American College of Cardiology* 50, no. 1 (July 2007): 14–21.

54 S. Sieri et al., "Dietary glycemic load and glycemic index and risk of cerebrovascular disease in the EPICOR cohort." *PloS One* 8, no. 5 (January 2013): e62625.

55 R. O. Roberts et al., "Relative intake of macronutrients impacts risk of mild cognitive impairment or dementia." *Journal of Alzheimer's Disease* 32, no. 2 (January 2012): 329–39.

56 N. Cherbuin et al., "Higher normal fasting plasma glucose is associated with hippocampal atrophy: the PATH Study." *Neurology* 79, no. 10 (September 2012): 1019–26.

57 C. Enzinger et al., "Risk factors for progression of brain atrophy in aging: six-year follow-up of normal subjects." *Neurology* 64, no. 10 (May 2005): 1704–11.

58 D. D. Perlmutter, *Grain Brain* (New York: Little, Brown, 2013).

59 S. Austad, *Why We Age* (Wiley, 1997).

60 D. Lieberman, *The Story of the Human Body* (New York: Pantheon, 2013).

61 J. Diamond, "The worst mistake in the history of the human race." discovermagazine.com, May 1, 1999.

62 R. Villegas et al., "Prospective study of dietary carbohydrates, glycemic index, glycemic load, and incidence of type 2 diabetes mellitus in middle-aged Chinese women." *Archives of Internal Medicine* 167, no. 21 (December 2007): 2310–16.

63 R. Kuipers, "Fatty acids in human evolution: contributions to evolutionary medicine." PhD diss., Rijksuniversiteit Groningen, 2012.

64 K. Rees et al., "Mediterranean diet for the prevention of cardiovascular disease." *Cochrane Database of Systematic Reviews* 8 (August 2013): CD009825.

65 R. Smith, "Are some diets 'mass murder'?" *BMJ (Clinical Research Ed.)* 349 (December 2014): g7654.

66 J. Mattei et al., "Substituting homemade fruit juice for sugar-sweetened beverages is associated with lower odds of metabolic syndrome among Hispanic adults." *Journal of Nutrition* 142, no. 6 (June 2012): 1081–87.

67 Q. Dai et al., "Fruit and vegetable juices and Alzheimer's disease: the Kame Project." *American Journal of Medicine* 119, no. 9 (September 2006): 751–59.

68 M. Aviram et al., "Pomegranate juice consumption for 3 years by patients with carotid artery stenosis reduces common carotid intima-media thickness, blood pressure and LDL oxidation." *Clinical Nutrition* 23, no. 3 (June 2004): 423–33.

69 R. Krikorian et al., "Blueberry supplementation improves memory in older adults." *Journal of Agricultural and Food Chemistry* 58, no. 7 (April 2010): 3996–4000.

70 P. Riso et al., "Effect of a wild blueberry (*Vaccinium angustifolium*) drink intervention on markers of oxidative stress, inflammation and endothelial function in humans with cardiovascular risk factors." *European Journal of Nutrition* 52, no. 3 (April 2013): 949–61.

71 A. J. Stull et al., "Bioactives in blueberries improve insulin sensitivity in obese, insulin-resistant men and women." *Journal of Nutrition* 140, no. 10 (October 2010): 1764–68.

72 R. A. Whitmer et al., "Central obesity and increased risk of dementia more than three decades later." *Neurology* 71, no. 14 (September 2008): 1057–64.

73 M. Ashwell et al., "Waist-to-height ratio is more predictive of years of life lost than body mass index." *PloS One* 9, no. 9 (January 2014): e103483.

74 L. C. Aiello et al., "Energetic consequences of being a *Homo erectus* female." *American Journal of Human Biology: The Official Journal of the Human Biology Council* 14, no. 5 (January): 551–65.

75 J. M. Seddon et al., "Cigarette smoking, fish consumption, omega-3 fatty acid intake, and associations with age-related macular degeneration: the US Twin Study of Age-Related Macular Degeneration." *Archives of Ophthalmology* 124, no. 7 (July 2006): 995–1001.

76 J. P. SanGiovanni et al., "The relationship of dietary lipid intake and age-related macular degeneration in a case-control study: AREDS Report No. 20." *Archives of Ophthalmology* 125, no. 5 (May 2007): 671–79.

77 K. M. Connor et al., "Increased dietary intake of omega-3-polyunsaturated fatty acids reduces pathological retinal angiogenesis." *Nature Medicine* 13, no. 7 (July 2007): 868–73.

78 E. Cho et al., "Prospective study of dietary fat and the risk of age-related macular degeneration." *American Journal of Clinical Nutrition* 73, no. 2 (February 2001): 209–18.

79 D. Di Giuseppe et al., "Long-term intake of dietary long-chain n-3 polyunsaturated fatty acids and risk of rheumatoid arthritis: a prospective cohort study of women." *Annals of the Rheumatic Diseases* (August 2013).

80 C. Raji et al., "Regular fish consumption is associated with larger gray matter volumes and reduced risk for cognitive decline in the cardiovascular health study." Conference paper, December 2011.

81 B. M. van Gelder et al., "Fish consumption, n-3 fatty acids, and subsequent 5-y cognitive decline in elderly men: the Zutphen Elderly Study." *American Journal of Clinical Nutrition* 85, no. 4 (April 2007): 1142–47.

82 A. Chauhan et al., "Walnuts-rich diet improves memory deficits and learning skills in transgenic mouse model of Alzheimer's disease." *Alzheimer's and Dementia* 6, no. 4 (July 2010): S69.

83 B. Muthaiyah et al., "Dietary supplementation of walnuts improves memory deficits and learning skills in transgenic mouse model of Alzheimer's disease." *Journal of Alzheimer's Disease* 42, no. 4 (January 2014): 1397–405.

84 J. O'Brien et al., "Long-term intake of nuts in relation to cognitive function in older women." *Journal of Nutrition, Health and Aging* 18, no. 5 (May 2014): 496–502.

85 P. Pribis et al., "Effects of walnut consumption on cognitive performance in young adults." *British Journal of Nutrition* 107, no. 9 (May 2012): 1393–401.

86 F. B. Hu et al., "Nut consumption and risk of coronary heart disease: a review of epidemiologic evidence." *Current Atherosclerosis Reports* 1, no. 3 (November 1999): 204–9.

87 A. Leaf, "Clinical prevention of sudden cardiac death by n-3 polyunsaturated fatty acids and mechanism of prevention of arrhythmias by n-3 fish oils." *Circulation* 107, no. 21 (June 2003): 2646–52.

88 H. Cao et al., "Omega-3 fatty acids in the prevention of atrial fibrillation recurrences after cardioversion: a meta-analysis of randomized controlled trials." *Internal Medicine* 51, no. 18 (January 2012): 2503–8.

89 H. Aarsetøy et al., "Low levels of cellular omega-3 increase the risk of ventricular fibrillation during the acute ischaemic phase of a myocardial infarction." *Resuscitation* 78, no. 3 (September 2008): 258–64.

90 R. Marchioli et al., "Early protection against sudden death by n-3 polyunsaturated fatty acids after myocardial infarction: time-course analysis of the results of the Gruppo Italiano per lo Studio della Sopravvivenza nell'Infarto Miocardico (GISSI)-Prevenzione." *Circulation* 105, no. 16 (April 2002): 1897–903.

91 C. M. Albert et al., "Blood levels of long-chain n-3 fatty acids and the risk of sudden death." *New England Journal of Medicine* 346, no. 15 (April 2002): 1113–18.

92 G. P. Amminger et al., "Long-chain omega-3 fatty acids for indicated prevention of psychotic disorders: a randomized, placebo-controlled trial." *Archives of General Psychiatry* 67, no. 2 (February 2010): 146–54.

93 E. C. Rizos et al., "Association between omega-3 fatty acid supplementation and risk of major cardiovascular disease events: a systematic review and meta-analysis." *JAMA* 308, no. 10 (September 2012): 1024–33.

94 Q. Chen et al., "Effects of omega-3 fatty acid for sudden cardiac death prevention in patients with cardiovascular disease: a contemporary meta-analysis of randomized, controlled trials." *Cardiovascular Drugs and Therapy* 25, no. 3 (June 2011): 259–65.

95 M. C. Morris et al., "Consumption of fish and n-3 fatty acids and risk of incident Alzheimer disease." *Archives of Neurology* 60, no. 7 (July 2003): 940–46.

96 E. J. Schaefer et al., "Plasma phosphatidylcholine docosahexaenoic acid content and risk of dementia and Alzheimer disease: the Framingham Heart Study." *Archives of Neurology* 63, no. 11 (November 2006): 1545–50.

97 P. Barberger-Gateau et al., "Dietary patterns and risk of dementia: the Three-City cohort study." *Neurology* 69, no. 20 (November 2007): 1921–30.

98 H. M. Krumholz et al., "Lack of association between cholesterol and coronary heart disease mortality and morbidity and all-cause mortality in persons older than 70 years." *JAMA* 272, no. 17 (November 1994): 1335–40.

99 A. C. M. Jansen et al., "The contribution of classical risk factors to cardiovascular disease in familial hypercholesterolaemia: data in 2400 patients." *Journal of Internal Medicine* 256, no. 6 (December 2004): 482–90.

100 R. Champeau, "Most heart attack patients' cholesterol levels did not indicate cardiac risk." newsroom.ucla.edu, January 12, 2009.

101 A. C. M. Jansen et al., "Genetic determinants of cardiovascular disease risk in familial hypercholesterolemia." *Arteriosclerosis, Thrombosis, and Vascular Biology* 25, no. 7 (July 2005): 1475–81.

102 P. K. Elias et al., "Serum cholesterol and cognitive performance in the Framingham Heart Study." *Psychosomatic Medicine* 67, no. 1 (January 2005): 24–30.

103 A. W. Weverling-Rijnsburger et al., "Total cholesterol and risk of mortality in the oldest old." *Lancet* 350, no. 9085 (October 1997): 1119–23.

104 Y. Takata et al., "Serum total cholesterol concentration and 10-year mortality in an 85-year-old population." *Clinical Interventions in Aging* 9 (January 2014): 293–300.

105 L. M. L. de Lau et al., "Serum cholesterol levels and the risk of Parkinson's disease." *American Journal of Epidemiology* 164, no. 10 (November 2006): 998–1002.

106 L. Dupuis et al., "Dyslipidemia is a protective factor in amyotrophic lateral sclerosis." *Neurology* 70, no. 13 (March 2008): 1004–9.

107 X. Huang et al., "Low LDL cholesterol and increased risk of Parkinson's disease: prospective results from Honolulu-Asia Aging Study." *Movement Disorders: Official Journal of the Movement Disorder Society* 23, no. 7 (May 2008): 1013–18.

108 D. S. Ng et al., "HDL—is it too big to fail?" *Nature Reviews Endocrinology* 9, no. 5 (May 2013): 308–12.

109 N. Barzilai et al., "Unique lipoprotein phenotype and genotype associated with exceptional longevity." *JAMA* 290, no. 15 (October 2003): 2030–40.

110 P. W. Siri-Tarino et al., "Meta-analysis of prospective cohort studies evaluating the association of saturated fat with cardiovascular disease." *American Journal of Clinical Nutrition* 91, no. 3 (March 2010): 535–46.

111 M. U. Jakobsen et al., "Major types of dietary fat and risk of coronary heart disease: a pooled analysis of 11 cohort studies." *American Journal of Clinical Nutrition* 89, no. 5 (May 2009): 1425–32.

112 R. P. Mensink et al., "Effects of dietary fatty acids and carbohydrates on the ratio of serum total to HDL cholesterol and on serum lipids and apolipoproteins: a meta-analysis of 60 controlled trials." *American Journal of Clinical Nutrition* 77, no. 5 (May 2003): 1146–55.

113 J. E. Hokanson et al., "Plasma triglyceride level is a risk factor for cardiovascular disease independent of high-density lipoprotein cholesterol level: a meta-analysis of population-based prospective studies." *Journal of Cardiovascular Risk* 3, no. 2 (April 1996): 213–19.

114 M. U. Jakobsen et al., "Intake of carbohydrates compared with intake of saturated fatty acids and risk of myocardial infarction: importance of the glycemic index." *American Journal of Clinical Nutrition* 91, no. 6 (June 2010): 1764–68.

115 E. E. Canfora et al., "Short-chain fatty acids in control of body weight and insulin sensitivity." *Nature Reviews Endocrinology* 11, no. 10 (August 2015): 577–91.

116 A. Andoh, "Physiological role of gut microbiota for maintaining human health." *Digestion* 93, no. 3 (February 2016): 176–81.

117 A. Menotti et al., "Food intake patterns and 25-year mortality from coronary heart disease: cross-cultural correlations in the Seven Countries Study. The Seven Countries Study Research Group." *European Journal of Epidemiology* 15, no. 6 (July 1999): 507–15.

118 C. B. Ebbeling et al., "Effects of dietary composition on energy expenditure during weight-loss maintenance." *JAMA* 307, no. 24 (June 2012): 2627–34.

119 R. Estruch et al., "Primary prevention of cardiovascular disease with a Mediterranean diet." *New England Journal of Medicine* 368, no. 14 (April 2013): 1279–90.

120 D. C. Wallace, "A mitochondrial paradigm of metabolic and degenerative diseases, aging, and cancer: a dawn for evolutionary medicine." *Annual Review of Genetics* 39 (January 2005): 359–407.

121 B. Bernardes de Jesus et al., "Telomerase gene therapy in adult and old mice delays aging and increases longevity without increasing cancer." *EMBO Molecular Medicine* 4, no. 8 (August 2012): 691–704.

122 G. Atzmon et al., "Evolution in health and medicine Sackler colloquium: genetic variation in human telomerase is associated with telomere length in Ashkenazi centenarians." *Proceedings of the National Academy of Sciences of the United States of America* 107 Suppl (January 2010): 1710–17.

123 M. Crous-Bou et al., "Mediterranean diet and telomere length in Nurses' Health Study: population based cohort study." *BMJ (Clinical Research Ed.)* 349 (January 2014): g6674.

124 P. Sjogren et al., "Stand up for health—avoiding sedentary behaviour might lengthen your telomeres: secondary outcomes from a physical activity RCT in older people." *British Journal of Sports Medicine* 48, no. 19 (September 2014): 1407–9.

125 D. Ornish et al., "Effect of comprehensive lifestyle changes on telomerase activity and telomere length in men with biopsy-proven low-risk prostate cancer: 5-year follow-up of a descriptive pilot study." *Lancet Oncology* 14, no. 11 (October 2013): 1112–20.

126 C. W. Leung et al., "Soda and cell aging: associations between sugar-sweetened beverage consumption and leukocyte telomere length in healthy adults from the National Health and Nutrition Examination Surveys." *American Journal of Public Health* 104, no. 12 (December 2014): 2425–31.

127 H. Holstege et al., "Somatic mutations found in the healthy blood compartment of a 115-yr-old woman demonstrate oligoclonal hematopoiesis." *Genome Research* 24, no. 5 (April 2014): 733–42.

128 G. Bjelakovic et al., "Mortality in randomized trials of antioxidant supplements for primary and secondary prevention: systematic review and meta-analysis." *JAMA* 297, no. 8 (February 2007): 842–57.

129 H. Macpherson et al., "Multivitamin-multimineral supplementation and mortality: a meta-analysis of randomized controlled trials." *American Journal of Clinical Nutrition* 97, no. 2 (March 2013): 437–44.

130 H. D. Sesso et al., "Multivitamins in the prevention of cardiovascular disease in men: the Physicians' Health Study II randomized controlled trial." *JAMA* 308, no. 17 (November 2012): 1751–60.

131 D. H. Baker, "Cupric oxide should not be used as a copper supplement for either animals or humans." *Journal of Nutrition* 129, no. 12 (December 1999): 2278–79.

132 G. S. Omenn, "Chemoprevention of lung cancer: the rise and demise of beta-carotene." *Annual Review of Public Health* 19 (January 1998): 73–99.

133 B. K. Dunn et al., "A nutrient approach to prostate cancer prevention: The Selenium and Vitamin E Cancer Prevention Trial (SELECT)." *Nutrition and Cancer* 62, no. 7 (January 2010): 896–918.

134 L. C. Clark et al., "Effects of selenium supplementation for cancer prevention in patients with carcinoma of the skin. A randomized controlled trial. Nutritional Prevention of Cancer Study Group." *JAMA* 276, no. 24 (December 1996): 1957–63.

135 A. Vogiatzoglou et al., "Vitamin B_{12} status and rate of brain volume loss in community-dwelling elderly." *Neurology* 71, no. 11 (September 2008): 826–32.

136 G. Douaud et al., "Preventing Alzheimer's disease-related gray matter atrophy by B-vitamin treatment." *Proceedings of the National Academy of Sciences of the United States of America* 110, no. 23 (June 2013): 9523–28.

137 N. L. van der Zwaluw et al., "Results of 2-year vitamin B treatment on cognitive performance: secondary data from an RCT." *Neurology* 83, no. 23 (December 2014): 2158–66.

138 J. G. Walker et al., "Oral folic acid and vitamin B-12 supplementation to prevent cognitive decline in community-dwelling older adults with depressive symptoms—the Beyond Ageing Project: a randomized controlled trial." *American Journal of Clinical Nutrition* 95, no. 1 (January 2012): 194–203.

139 A. D. Smith et al., "Homocysteine-lowering by B vitamins slows the rate of accelerated brain atrophy in mild cognitive impairment: a randomized controlled trial." *PloS One* 5, no. 9 (January 2010): e12244.

140 "Three of the B vitamins: folate, vitamin B6 and vitamin B12." Harvard School of Public Health, The Nutrition Source, 2012.

141 W. C. Willett, *Eat, Drink, and Be Healthy* (New York: Free Press, 2005).

142 Y. Song et al., "Effects of oral magnesium supplementation on glycaemic control in type 2 diabetes: a meta-analysis of randomized double-blind controlled trials." *Diabetic Medicine: A Journal of the British Diabetic Association* 23, no. 10 (October 2006): 1050–56.

143 F. Guerrero-Romero et al., "Oral magnesium supplementation improves insulin sensitivity in non-diabetic subjects with insulin resistance. A double-blind placebo-controlled randomized trial." *Diabetes and Metabolism* 30, no. 3 (June 2004): 253–58.

144 F. C. Mooren et al., "Oral magnesium supplementation reduces insulin resistance in non-diabetic subjects—a double-blind, placebo-controlled, randomized trial." *Diabetes, Obesity and Metabolism* 13, no. 3 (March 2011): 281–84.

145 L. Kass et al., "Effect of magnesium supplementation on blood pressure: a meta-analysis." *European Journal of Clinical Nutrition* 66, no. 4 (April 2012): 411–18.

146 O. Onalan et al., "Meta-analysis of magnesium therapy for the acute management of rapid atrial fibrillation." *American Journal of Cardiology* 99, no. 12 (June 2007): 1726–32.

147 Y. Bashir et al., "Effects of long-term oral magnesium chloride replacement in congestive heart failure secondary to coronary artery disease." *American Journal of Cardiology* 72, no. 15 (November 1993): 1156–62.

148 W. Zhang et al., "Associations of dietary magnesium intake with mortality from cardiovascular disease: the JACC study." *Atherosclerosis* 221, no. 2 (April 2012): 587–95.

149 E. Giovannucci et al., "25-hydroxyvitamin D and risk of myocardial infarction in men: a prospective study." *Archives of Internal Medicine* 168, no. 11 (June 2008): 1174–80.

150 H. Dobnig et al., "Independent association of low serum 25-hydroxyvitamin D and 1,25-dihydroxyvitamin D levels with all-cause and cardiovascular mortality." *Archives of Internal Medicine* 168, no. 12 (June 2008): 1340–49.

151 J. A. Ford et al., "Cardiovascular disease and vitamin D supplementation: trial analysis, systematic review, and meta-analysis." *American Journal of Clinical Nutrition* 100, no. 3 (September 2014): 746–55.

152 G. Bjelakovic et al., "Vitamin D supplementation for prevention of mortality in adults." *Cochrane Database of Systematic Reviews* 1 (January 2014): CD007470.

153 Y. Zheng et al., "Meta-analysis of long-term vitamin D supplementation on overall mortality." *PloS One* 8, no. 12 (January 2013): e82109.

154 P. Autier et al., "Vitamin D status and ill health: a systematic review." *Lancet Diabetes and Endocrinology* 2, no. 1 (January 2014): 76–89.

155 K. M. Sanders et al., "Annual high-dose oral vitamin D and falls and fractures in older women: a randomized controlled trial." *JAMA* 303, no. 18 (May 2010): 1815–22.

156 C. Annweiler et al., "Higher vitamin D dietary intake is associated with lower risk of Alzheimer's disease: a 7-year follow-up." *Journals of Gerontology. Series A, Biological Sciences and Medical Sciences* 67, no. 11 (November 2012): 1205–11.

157 S. Cockayne et al., "Vitamin K and the prevention of fractures: systematic review and meta-analysis of randomized controlled trials." *Archives of Internal Medicine* 166, no. 12 (June 2006): 1256–61.

158 K. M. McCabe et al., "Dietary vitamin K and therapeutic warfarin alter the susceptibility to vascular calcification in experimental chronic kidney disease." *Kidney International* 83, no. 5 (May 2013): 835–44.

159 J. W. J. Beulens et al., "High dietary menaquinone intake is associated with reduced coronary calcification." *Atherosclerosis* 203, no. 2 (April 2009): 489–93.

160 L. J. Schurgers et al., "Oral anticoagulant treatment: friend or foe in cardiovascular disease?" *Blood* 104, no. 10 (November 2004): 3231–32.

161 L. J. Schurgers et al., "Regression of warfarin-induced medial elastocalcinosis by high intake of vitamin K in rats." *Blood* 109, no. 7 (April 2007): 2823–31.

162 J. Uitto et al., "Pseudoxanthoma elasticum: progress in research toward treatment: summary of the 2012 PXE international research meeting." *Journal of Investigative Dermatology* 133, no. 6 (June 2013): 1444–49.

163 M. Vos et al., "Vitamin K2 is a mitochondrial electron carrier that rescues pink1 deficiency." *Science* 336, no. 6086 (June 2012): 1306–10.

164 J. W. J. Beulens et al., "Dietary phylloquinone and menaquinones intakes and risk of type 2 diabetes." *Diabetes Care* 33, no. 8 (August 2010): 1699–705.

165 G. Ferland, "Vitamin K, an emerging nutrient in brain function." *BioFactors* 38, no. 2 (January): 151–57.

166 G. C. M. Gast et al., "A high menaquinone intake reduces the incidence of coronary heart disease." *Nutrition, Metabolism, and Cardiovascular Diseases* 19, no. 7 (September 2009): 504–10.

167 J. M. Geleijnse et al., "Dietary intake of menaquinone is associated with a reduced risk of coronary heart disease: the Rotterdam Study." *Journal of Nutrition* 134, no. 11 (November 2004): 3100–3105.

168 D. Feskanich et al., "Vitamin K intake and hip fractures in women: a prospective study." *American Journal of Clinical Nutrition* 69, no. 1 (January 1999): 74–79.

169 Y. Ikeda et al., "Intake of fermented soybeans, natto, is associated with reduced bone loss in postmenopausal women: Japanese Population-Based Osteoporosis (JPOS) Study." *Journal of Nutrition* 136, no. 5 (May 2006): 1323–28.

170 M. L. L. Chatrou et al., "Vascular calcification: the price to pay for anticoagulation therapy with vitamin K-antagonists." *Blood Reviews* 26, no. 4 (July 2012): 155–66.

171 R. C. Morris et al., "Relationship and interaction between sodium and potassium." *Journal of the American College of Nutrition* 25, no. 3 Suppl (June 2006): 262S–70S.

172 N. J. Aburto et al., "Effect of increased potassium intake on cardiovascular risk factors and disease: systematic review and meta-analyses." *BMJ (Clinical Research Ed.)* 346 (January 2013): f1378.

173 S. C. Larsson et al., "Dietary potassium intake and risk of stroke: a dose-response meta-analysis of prospective studies." *Stroke: A Journal of Cerebral Circulation* 42, no. 10 (October 2011): 2746–50.

174 Richard D. Moore et al., *The Salt Solution* (Avery, 2001).

175 F. Forouzandeh et al., "Metformin beyond diabetes: pleiotropic benefits of metformin in attenuation of atherosclerosis." *Journal of the American Heart Association* 3, no. 6 (December 2014): e001202.

176 M. L. Wahlqvist et al., "Metformin-inclusive sulfonylurea therapy reduces the risk of Parkinson's disease occurring with type 2 diabetes in a Taiwanese population cohort." *Parkinsonism and Related Disorders* 18, no. 6 (July 2012): 753–58.

177 C. A. Bannister et al., "Can people with type 2 diabetes live longer than those without? A comparison of mortality in people initiated with metformin or sulphonylurea monotherapy and matched, non-diabetic controls." *Diabetes, Obesity and Metabolism* 16, no. 11 (November 2014): 1165–73.

178 R. I. Misbin, "The phantom of lactic acidosis due to metformin in patients with diabetes." *Diabetes Care* 27, no. 7 (July 2004): 1791–93.

179 S. R. Salpeter et al., "Risk of fatal and nonfatal lactic acidosis with metformin use in type 2 diabetes mellitus." *Cochrane Database of Systematic Reviews* 1 (January 2010): CD002967.

180 M. S. HOOD et al., "Low-volume interval training improves muscle oxidative capacity in sedentary adults." *Medicine and Science in Sports and Exercise* 43, no. 10 (October 2011): 1849–56.

181 J. P. Little et al., "A practical model of low-volume high-intensity interval training induces mitochondrial biogenesis in human skeletal muscle: potential mechanisms." *Journal of Physiology* 588, no. 6 (March 2010): 1011–22.

182 S. Rovio et al., "Leisure-time physical activity at midlife and the risk of dementia and Alzheimer's disease." *Lancet Neurology* 4, no. 11 (November 2005): 705–11.

183 K. I. Erickson et al., "Aerobic fitness is associated with hippocampal volume in elderly humans." *Hippocampus* 19, no. 10 (October 2009): 1030–39.

184 P. Sarup et al., "The long-term effects of a life-prolonging heat treatment on the *Drosophila melanogaster* transcriptome suggest that heat shock proteins extend lifespan." *Experimental Gerontology* 50 (March 2014): 34–39.

185 M. Mattson et al., "Best in small doses." *New Scientist* 199, no. 2668 (August 2008): 36–39.

186 J. R. Cameron, "Moderate dose rate ionizing radiation increases longevity." *British Journal of Radiology* 78, no. 925 (January 2005): 11–13.

187 D. B. Panagiotakos et al., "Sociodemographic and lifestyle statistics of oldest old people (>80 years) living in Ikaria Island: the Ikaria study." *Cardiology Research and Practice* 2011 (January 2011): 679187.

188 C. Chrysohoou et al., "Exposure to low environmental radiation and longevity. Insights from the Ikaria Study." *International Journal of Cardiology* 169, no. 6 (November 2013): e97–98.

189 M. Ristow et al., "Antioxidants prevent health-promoting effects of physical exercise in humans." *Proceedings of the National Academy of Sciences of the United States of America* 106, no. 21 (May 2009): 8665–70.

190 V. I. Sayin et al., "Antioxidants accelerate lung cancer progression in mice." *Science Translational Medicine* 6, no. 221 (January 2014): 221ra15.

191 W. Yang et al., "A mitochondrial superoxide signal triggers increased longevity in *Caenorhabditis elegans*." *PLoS Biology* 8, no. 12 (January 2010): e1000556.

192 M. H. Eskelinen et al., "Midlife coffee and tea drinking and the risk of late-life dementia: a population-based CAIDE study." *Journal of Alzheimer's Disease* 16, no. 1 (January 2009): 85–91.

193 G. W. Ross et al., "Association of coffee and caffeine intake with the risk of Parkinson disease." *JAMA* 283, no. 20 (May 2000): 2674–79.

194 E. Salazar-Martinez et al., "Coffee consumption and risk for type 2 diabetes mellitus." *Annals of Internal Medicine* 140, no. 1 (January 2004): 1–8.

195 M. S. Butt et al., "Coffee and its consumption: benefits and risks." *Critical Reviews in Food Science and Nutrition* 51, no. 4 (April 2011): 363–73.

196 U. Boettler et al., "Coffee constituents as modulators of Nrf2 nuclear translocation and ARE (EpRE)-dependent gene expression." *Journal of Nutritional Biochemistry* 22, no. 5 (May 2011): 426–40.

197 K. Trinh et al., "Induction of the phase II detoxification pathway suppresses neuron loss in *Drosophila* models of Parkinson's disease." *Journal of Neuroscience: The Official Journal of the Society for Neuroscience* 28, no. 2 (January 2008): 465–72.

198 M. J. Steinbaugh et al., "Activation of genes involved in xenobiotic metabolism is a shared signature of mouse models with extended lifespan." *American Journal of Physiology Endocrinology and Metabolism* 303, no. 4 (August 2012): E488–95.

199 S. Ayyadevara et al., "Lifespan and stress resistance of *Caenorhabditis elegans* are increased by expression of glutathione transferases capable of metabolizing the lipid peroxidation product 4-hydroxynonenal." *Aging Cell* 4, no. 5 (October 2005): 257–71.

200 A. A. Powolny et al., "The garlic constituent diallyl trisulfide increases the lifespan of *C. elegans* via skn-1 activation." *Experimental Gerontology* 46, no. 6 (June 2011): 441–52.

201 K. Canene-Adams et al., "Combinations of tomato and broccoli enhance anti-tumor activity in dunning r3327-h prostate adenocarcinomas." *Cancer Research* 67, no. 2 (January 2007): 836–43.

202 L. Tang et al., "Intake of cruciferous vegetables modifies bladder cancer survival." *Cancer Epidemiology, Biomarkers and Prevention: A Publication of the American Association for Cancer Research* 19, no. 7 (July 2010): 1806–11.

203 C. B. Ambrosone et al., "Breast cancer risk in premenopausal women is inversely associated with consumption of broccoli, a source of isothiocyanates, but is not modified by GST genotype." *Journal of Nutrition* 134, no. 5 (May 2004): 1134–38.

204 P. Riso et al., "DNA damage and repair activity after broccoli intake in young healthy smokers." *Mutagenesis* 25, no. 6 (November 2010): 595–602.

205 C. L. Saw et al., "Impact of Nrf2 on UVB-induced skin inflammation/photoprotection and photoprotective effect of sulforaphane." *Molecular Carcinogenesis* 50, no. 6 (June 2011): 479–86.

206 L. Arab et al., "Green and black tea consumption and risk of stroke: a meta-analysis." *Stroke: A Journal of Cerebral Circulation* 40, no. 5 (May 2009): 1786–92.

207 S. Bettuzzi et al., "Chemoprevention of human prostate cancer by oral administration of green tea catechins in volunteers with high-grade prostate intraepithelial neoplasia: a preliminary report from a one-year proof-of-principle study." *Cancer Research* 66, no. 2 (January 2006): 1234–40.

208 A. Buitrago-Lopez et al., "Chocolate consumption and cardiometabolic disorders: systematic review and meta-analysis." *BMJ (Clinical Research Ed.)* 343 (January 2011): d4488.

209 G. Desideri et al., "Benefits in cognitive function, blood pressure, and insulin resistance through cocoa flavanol consumption in elderly subjects with mild cognitive impairment: the Cocoa, Cognition, and Aging (CoCoA) study." *Hypertension* 60, no. 3 (September 2012): 794–801.

210 B. Buijsse et al., "Cocoa intake, blood pressure, and cardiovascular mortality: the Zutphen Elderly Study." *Archives of Internal Medicine* 166, no. 4 (March 2006): 411–17.

211 I. Muraki et al., "Fruit consumption and risk of type 2 diabetes: results from three prospective longitudinal cohort studies." *BMJ (Clinical Research Ed.)* 347 (January 2013): f5001.

212 E. E. Devore et al., "Dietary intakes of berries and flavonoids in relation to cognitive decline." *Annals of Neurology* 72, no. 1 (July 2012): 135–43.

213 L. Dauchet et al., "Fruit and vegetable consumption and risk of coronary heart disease: a meta-analysis of cohort studies." *Journal of Nutrition* 136, no. 10 (October 2006): 2588–93.

214 O. Oyebode et al., "Fruit and vegetable consumption and all-cause, cancer and CVD mortality: analysis of Health Survey for England data." *Journal of Epidemiology and Community Health* 68, no. 9 (September 2014): 856–62.

215 C. S. Fuchs et al., "Alcohol consumption and mortality among women." *New England Journal of Medicine* 332, no. 19 (May 1995): 1245–50.

216 G. Taubes, *Why We Get Fat* (New York: Alfred A. Knopf, 2011).

217 A. Stunkard et al., "The results of treatment for obesity: a review of the literature and report of a series." *A.M.A. Archives of Internal Medicine* 103, no. 1 (January 1959): 79–85.

218 M. L. Dansinger et al., "Meta-analysis: the effect of dietary counseling for weight loss." *Annals of Internal Medicine* 147, no. 1 (July 2007): 41–50.

219 W. L. Haskell et al., "Physical activity and public health: updated recommendation for adults from the American College of Sports Medicine and the American Heart Association." *Circulation* 116, no. 9 (August 2007): 1081–93.

220 M. Fogelholm et al., "Does physical activity prevent weight gain—a systematic review." *Obesity Reviews: An Official Journal of the International Association for the Study of Obesity* 1, no. 2 (October 2000): 95–111.

221 I.-M. Lee et al., "Physical activity and weight gain prevention." *JAMA* 303, no. 12 (March 2010): 1173–79.

222 P. T. Williams et al., "The effects of changing exercise levels on weight and age-related weight gain." *International Journal of Obesity* 30, no. 3 (March 2006): 543–51.

223 R. Dunn, "Everything you know about calories is wrong." *Scientific American* 309, no. 3 (September 2013): 56–59.

224 R. U. Almario et al., "Effects of walnut consumption on plasma fatty acids and lipoproteins in combined hyperlipidemia." *American Journal of Clinical Nutrition* 74, no. 1 (July 2001): 72–79.

225 M. A. Martínez-González et al., "Nut consumption, weight gain and obesity: epidemiological evidence." *Nutrition, Metabolism, and Cardiovascular Diseases* 21 Suppl 1 (June 2011): S40–45.

226 S. Natoli et al., "A review of the evidence: nuts and body weight." *Asia Pacific Journal of Clinical Nutrition* 16, no. 4 (January 2007): 588–97.

227 K. K. Ryan et al., "Physiology. Food as a hormone." *Science* 339, no. 6122 (March 2013): 918–19.

228 I. A. Munro et al., "Prior supplementation with long chain omega-3 polyunsaturated fatty acids promotes weight loss in obese adults: a double-blinded randomised controlled trial." *Food and Function* 4, no. 4 (April 2013): 650–58.

229 F. Bäckhed et al., "The gut microbiota as an environmental factor that regulates fat storage." *Proceedings of the National Academy of Sciences of the United States of America* 101, no. 44 (November 2004): 15718–23.

230 N. Alang et al., "Weight gain after fecal microbiota transplantation." *Open Forum Infectious Diseases* 2, no. 1 (February 2015): ofv004.

231 D. S. Ludwig et al., "High glycemic index foods, overeating, and obesity." *Pediatrics* 103, no. 3 (March 1999): E26.

232 D. B. Pawlak et al., "Effects of dietary glycaemic index on adiposity, glucose homoeostasis, and plasma lipids in animals." *Lancet* 364, no. 9436 (January): 778–85.

233 D. S. Ludwig et al., "Increasing adiposity: consequence or cause of overeating?" *JAMA* 311, no. 21 (June 2014): 2167–68.

234 A. N. Gearhardt et al., "Preliminary validation of the Yale Food Addiction Scale." *Appetite* 52, no. 2 (April 2009): 430–36.

235 B. V Howard et al., "Low-fat dietary pattern and weight change over 7 years: the Women's Health Initiative Dietary Modification Trial." *JAMA* 295, no. 1 (January 2006): 39–49.

236 D. E. Thomas et al., "Low glycaemic index or low glycaemic load diets for overweight and obesity." *Cochrane Database of Systematic Reviews* 3 (January 2007): CD005105.

237 A. Kekwick et al., "Calorie intake in relation to body-weight changes in the obese." *Lancet* 271, no. 6935 (July 1956): 155–61.

238 J. H. Jaap Seidell, *Tegenwicht* (Bert Bakker, 2011).

239 P. Curtis, "Researchers see bias in private-funded studies." *Guardian*, January 8, 2007.

240 W. Willett, "The case for banning trans fats. The FDA's new policy on these deadly artificial fatty acids is long overdue." *Scientific American* 310, no. 3 (March 2014): 13.

241 M. de Lorgeril et al., "Mediterranean alpha-linolenic acid-rich diet in secondary prevention of coronary heart disease." *Lancet* 343, no. 8911 (June 1994): 1454–59.

242 S. C. Johnson et al., "mTOR is a key modulator of ageing and age-related disease." *Nature* 493, no. 7432 (January 2013): 338–45.

243 A. Bruning, "Inhibition of mTOR signaling by quercetin in cancer treatment and prevention." *Anti-Cancer Agents in Medicinal Chemistry* 13, no. 7 (September 2013): 1025–31.

244 A. Reinke et al., "Caffeine targets TOR complex I and provides evidence for a regulatory link between the FRB and kinase domains of Tor1p." *Journal of Biological Chemistry* 281, no. 42 (October 2006): 31616–26.

245 G. S. Van Aller et al., "Epigallocatechin gallate (EGCG), a major component of green tea, is a dual phosphoinositide-3-kinase/mTOR inhibitor." *Biochemical and Biophysical Research Communications* 406, no. 2 (March 2011): 194–99.

246 Y. Kokubo et al., "The impact of green tea and coffee consumption on the reduced risk of stroke incidence in Japanese population: the Japan public health center-based study cohort." *Stroke: A Journal of Cerebral Circulation* 44, no. 5 (May 2013): 1369–74.

247 C. Laurent et al., "Beneficial effects of caffeine in a transgenic model of Alzheimer's disease-like tau pathology." *Neurobiology of Aging* 35, no. 9 (September 2014): 2079–90.

248 F. Yang et al., "Curcumin inhibits formation of amyloid beta oligomers and fibrils, binds plaques, and reduces amyloid in vivo." *Journal of Biological Chemistry* 280, no. 7 (February 2005): 5892–901.

249 K. Ono et al., "Curcumin has potent anti-amyloidogenic effects for Alzheimer's beta-amyloid fibrils in vitro." *Journal of Neuroscience Research* 75, no. 6 (March 2004): 742–50.

250 G. P. Lim et al., "The curry spice curcumin reduces oxidative damage and amyloid pathology in an Alzheimer transgenic mouse." *Journal of Neuroscience: The Official Journal of the Society for Neuroscience* 21, no. 21 (November 2001): 8370–77.

251 M. C. Monti et al., "New insights on the interaction mechanism between tau protein and oleocanthal, an extra-virgin olive-oil bioactive component." *Food and Function* 2, no. 7 (July 2011): 423–28.

252 A. H. Abuznait et al., "Olive-oil-derived oleocanthal enhances β-amyloid clearance as a potential neuroprotective mechanism against Alzheimer's disease: in vitro and in vivo studies." *ACS Chemical Neuroscience* 4, no. 6 (June 2013): 973–82.

253 A. Frydman-Marom et al., "Orally administrated cinnamon extract reduces β-amyloid oligomerization and corrects cognitive impairment in Alzheimer's disease animal models." *PloS One* 6, no. 1 (January 2011): e16564.

254 T. Lu et al., "Cinnamon extract improves fasting blood glucose and glycosylated hemoglobin level in Chinese patients with type 2 diabetes." *Nutrition Research* 32, no. 6 (June 2012): 408–12.

255 F. Brighenti et al., "Effect of neutralized and native vinegar on blood glucose and acetate responses to a mixed meal in healthy subjects." *European Journal of Clinical Nutrition* 49, no. 4 (April 1995): 242–47.

256 E. Ostman et al., "Vinegar supplementation lowers glucose and insulin responses and increases satiety after a bread meal in healthy subjects." *European Journal of Clinical Nutrition* 59, no. 9 (September 2005): 983–88.

257 L. Fontana et al., "Long-term calorie restriction is highly effective in reducing the risk for atherosclerosis in humans." *Proceedings of the National Academy of Sciences of the United States of America* 101, no. 17 (April 2004): 6659–63.

258 T. E. Meyer et al., "Long-term caloric restriction ameliorates the decline in diastolic function in humans." *Journal of the American College of Cardiology* 47, no. 2 (January 2006): 398–402.

259 L. K. Heilbronn et al., "Effect of 6-month calorie restriction on biomarkers of longevity, metabolic adaptation, and oxidative stress in overweight individuals: a randomized controlled trial." *JAMA* 295, no. 13 (April 2006): 1539–48.

260 K. A. Varady et al., "Short-term modified alternate-day fasting: a novel dietary strategy for weight loss and cardioprotection in obese adults." *American Journal of Clinical Nutrition* 90, no. 5 (November 2009): 1138–43.

261 N. Halberg et al., "Effect of intermittent fasting and refeeding on insulin action in healthy men." *Journal of Applied Physiology* 99, no. 6 (December 2005): 2128–36.

262 E. Patterson et al., "Association between dairy food consumption and risk of myocardial infarction in women differs by type of dairy food." *Journal of Nutrition* 143, no. 1 (January 2013): 74–79.

263 G. Stix, "Got (skim) milk?: maybe a recipe for obesity and cancer." *Talking Back* (blog), *Scientific American*, July 3, 2013.

264 X. Song et al., "Advanced glycation in D-galactose induced mouse aging model." *Mechanisms of Ageing and Development* 108, no. 3 (May 1999): 239–51.

265 X. Cui et al., "Chronic systemic D-galactose exposure induces memory loss, neurodegeneration, and oxidative damage in mice: protective effects of R-α-lipoic acid" *Journal of Neuroscience Research* 83, no. 8 (June 2006): 1584–90.

266 X. Cui et al., "D-Galactose-caused life shortening in *Drosophila melanogaster* and *Musca domestica* is associated with oxidative stress." *Biogerontology* 5, no. 5 (October 2004): 317–26.

267 K. Michaëlsson et al., "Milk intake and risk of mortality and fractures in women and men: cohort studies." *BMJ (Clinical Research Ed.)* 349 (January 2014): g6015.

268 J. M. Chan et al., "Dairy products, calcium, and prostate cancer risk in the Physicians' Health Study." *American Journal of Clinical Nutrition* 74, no. 4 (October 2001): 549–54.

269 L.-Q. Qin et al., "Milk consumption and circulating insulin-like growth factor-I level: a systematic literature review." *International Journal of Food Sciences and Nutrition* 60 Suppl 7 (January 2009): 330–40.

270 M. Park et al., "Consumption of milk and calcium in midlife and the future risk of Parkinson disease." *Neurology* 64, no. 6 (March 2005): 1047–51.

271 C. Rodriguez et al., "Calcium, dairy products, and risk of prostate cancer in a prospective cohort of United States men." *Cancer Epidemiology Biomarkers and Prevention* 12, no. 7 (July 2003): 597–603.

272 H. A. Bischoff-Ferrari et al., "Milk intake and risk of hip fracture in men and women: a meta-analysis of prospective cohort studies." *Journal of Bone and Mineral Research* 26, no. 4 (April 2011): 833–39.

273 J. J. B. Anderson et al., "Calcium intake from diet and supplements and the risk of coronary artery calcification and its progression among older adults: 10-year follow-up of the multi-ethnic study of atherosclerosis (MESA)." *Journal of the American Heart Association* 5, no. 10 (October 2016): e003815.

274 K. Verburgh, "Nutrigerontology: why we need a new scientific discipline to develop diets and guidelines to reduce the risk of aging-related diseases." *Aging Cell* (December 2014).

275 B. Vellas et al., "Long-term follow-up of patients immunized with AN1792: reduced functional decline in antibody responders." *Current Alzheimer Research* 6, no. 2 (April 2009): 144–51.

276 M. Asif et al., "An advanced glycation endproduct cross-link breaker can reverse age-related increases in myocardial stiffness." *Proceedings of the National Academy of Sciences of the United States of America* 97, no. 6 (March 2000): 2809–13.

277 P. V Vaitkevicius et al., "A cross-link breaker has sustained effects on arterial and ventricular properties in older rhesus monkeys." *Proceedings of the National Academy of Sciences of the United States of America* 98, no. 3 (January 2001): 1171–75.

278 D. A. Kass et al., "Improved arterial compliance by a novel advanced glycation end-product crosslink breaker." *Circulation* 104, no. 13 (September 2001): 1464–70.

279 W. C. Little et al., "The effect of alagebrium chloride (ALT-711), a novel glucose cross-link breaker, in the treatment of elderly patients with diastolic heart failure." *Journal of Cardiac Failure* 11, no. 3 (April 2005): 191–95.

280 P. M. Keeney et al., "Mitochondrial gene therapy augments mitochondrial physiology in a Parkinson's disease cell model." *Human Gene Therapy* 20, no. 8 (August 2009): 897–907.

281 S. Ellouze et al., "Optimized allotopic expression of the human mitochondrial ND4 prevents blindness in a rat model of mitochondrial dysfunction." *American Journal of Human Genetics* 83, no. 3 (September 2008): 373–87.

282 R. R. Thomas et al., "RhTFAM treatment stimulates mitochondrial oxidative metabolism and improves memory in aged mice." *Aging* 4, no. 9 (September 2012): 620–35.

283 T.-Y. Lu et al., "Repopulation of decellularized mouse heart with human induced pluripotent stem cell-derived cardiovascular progenitor cells." *Nature Communications* 4 (January 2013): 2307.

284 I. M. Conboy et al., "Rejuvenation of aged progenitor cells by exposure to a young systemic environment." *Nature* 433, no. 7027 (February 2005): 760–64.

285 S. A. Villeda et al., "Young blood reverses age-related impairments in cognitive function and synaptic plasticity in mice." *Nature Medicine* 20, no. 6 (June 2014): 659–63.

286 A. Ocampo et al., "In vivo amelioration of age-associated hallmarks by partial reprogramming." *Cell* 167, no. 7 (December 2016): 1719–33.e12.

287 A. Akesson et al., "Low-risk diet and lifestyle habits in the primary prevention of myocardial infarction in men: a population-based prospective cohort study." *Journal of the American College of Cardiology* 64, no. 13 (September 2014): 1299–306.

288 E. S. Ford et al., "Healthy living is the best revenge: findings from the European Prospective Investigation into Cancer and Nutrition-Potsdam study." *Archives of Internal Medicine* 169, no. 15 (August 2009): 1355–62.

289 E. S. Ford et al., "Low-risk lifestyle behaviors and all-cause mortality: findings from the National Health and Nutrition Examination Survey III Mortality Study." *American Journal of Public Health* 101, no. 10 (October 2011): 1922–29.

290 S. Yusuf et al., "Effect of potentially modifiable risk factors associated with myocardial infarction in 52 countries (the INTERHEART study): case-control study." *Lancet* 364, no. 9438 (January): 937–52.

291 S. E. Chiuve et al., "Adherence to a low-risk, healthy lifestyle and risk of sudden cardiac death among women." *JAMA* 306, no. 1 (July 2011): 62–69.

292 A. M. Herskind et al., "The heritability of human longevity: a population-based study of 2872 Danish twin pairs born 1870–1900." *Human Genetics* 97, no. 3 (March 1996): 319–23.

293 S. Moalem, *Het nut van ziekte* (De Bezige Bij, 2007).

294 N. Barzilai et al., "The rationale for delaying aging and the prevention of age-related diseases." *Rambam Maimonides Medical Journal* 3, no. 4 (October 2012): e0020.

295 L. A. Gavrilov et al., "Demographic consequences of defeating aging." *Rejuvenation Research* 13, no. 2–3 (January): 329–34.

296 T. Parker-Pope, "For a healthy retirement, keep working." *The New York Times*, October 19, 2009.

297 "Health and retirement study." University of Michigan, hrsonline.isr.umich.edu.

298 C. Dufouil et al., "Older age at retirement is associated with decreased risk of dementia." *European Journal of Epidemiology* 29, no. 5 (May 2014): 353–61.

299 M. C. Carlson et al., "Evidence for neurocognitive plasticity in at-risk older adults: the experience corps program." *Journals of Gerontology Series A, Biological Sciences and Medical Sciences* 64, no. 12 (December 2009): 1275–82.

INDEX

billion, defined, 264

biotechnology, future of, 255–57

birds, 2, 8

birth rate, worldwide decline in, 221–24

bladder, carbohydrates and, 60

Blanding's turtles, 6

blood rejuvenation, 198–201, *200*

blood sugar leval, 66–67

blood thinners, 130–32

blueberries, 146

"blue zones," 46

bone health
  carbohydrates and, 68
  vitamin K for, 130

brain
  carbohydrates and, 60, 66–67
  cholesterol for, 89–90
  cortex, 265
  fats for, 82–83
  Huntington's disease, 13–14
  neurons, defined, 269
  neurotransmitters, 269
  proteins and effect on, 34–40, *35, 39*
  quality of life *vs.* long life of, 219
  stroke, 60, 270
  vitamin B12 for, 126
  See also micronutrients; nutrition

Brandt's bats, 11

Brazil nuts, selenium in, 128

breakfast recipes
  Almond Pancakes with Blueberries, 236–37
  Breakfast Smoothie, 232
  Fruit Breakfast with Nuts and Flaxseeds, 233
  Goat Cheese Frittata, 235
  Hot Cereal with Nuts and Flaxseeds, 234

Hot Cereal with Walnuts and Coconut, 236
  Omelet with Tomato and Avocado, 235–36
  overview, 232
  Quick Oatmeal Cake, Pancakes, or Balls, 233–34

Breakthrough Prize in Life Sciences, 252

British Medical Journal, 172

broccoli
  Basic Broccoli Soup, 246–47
  hormesis and, 144–45, *148*

Brundtland, Gro Harlem, 169

butter, 184

butyrate, 91

B vitamins
  from animal-based proteins, 49
  micronutrients in, 126–27

C

cacao, 145–46

calcium, dairy intake and, 184

Calico, 217, 256

Calment, Jeanne, 10–11

calories
  defined, 264
  growth stimulation and, 153–61
  restricting, 180
  from sugar, 61–62

cancer
  Alzheimer's disease and, 15
  from animal-based proteins, 43–44, *44*
  cancer cells as immortal, 23–25
  free radicals, 267
  growth hormone and, 56
  immortal cells of, 23–24
  telomeres and, 115

flavonoids, 267

flight, life span and, 8

flow, happiness as, 220–21

folic acid, 126

Food Hourglass, The (Verburgh), 72, 185

food hourglass concept, 180–82, *181*

food industry
    food addiction and, 165–66
    industrialization of food, 122–23
    influence of, 168–69

Fourth Industrial Revolution, 255–57

Framingham Heart Study, 88

free radicals
    antioxidants and, 141–43, 263
    defined, 267
    DNA damage and, 111
    free radical theory, 30
    mitochondria and, 104
    oxidation, 269
    See also antioxidants

freshwater polyps, 21–22

frontotemporal dementia, 36–37

fructose, 157–58

fruit
    Fruit Breakfast with Nuts and
        Flaxseeds, 233
    fruit juices, 74–75
    hormesis and, 146
    See also recipes

fruit flies, reproduction and aging of, 17

G

galactose, 183

Gaucher's disease, 191–92

Gems, David, 199, 215–16

genetics
    DNA and cancer cells, 8

genes, defined, 267
    life span and sex hormones, 20
    mitochondrial DNA, 96, *97, 98*, 105
        (*See also* mitochondria)
    mutations, positive consequences of, 4
    mutations that accelerate aging
        process, 12–15
    telomeres, 270
    See also DNA

glossary terms, 263–70

glucose
    defined, 267
    as fast carbohydrates, 52–53
    growth stimulation from, 151–52
    weight gain from, 157–58
    See also carbohydrates

glycation, 66–67

glycemic index
    defined, 267
    low carbohydrate diet and, 71
    low-fat diets and, 166–67
    of oatmeal, 73

glycemic load
    carbohydrates, 66
    defined, 267
    low-fat diets and, 167
    of oatmeal, 73

Goat Cheese Frittata, 235

Google, 217, 252, 256

government recommendations on
    nutrition, 173–74

grain-fed *vs.* grass-fed animal food
    sources, 44–45

grains, agriculture history and, 67–69

grandparents, life span of humans and,
    20–21

green tea, 145

growth hormone (GH)
  growth stimulation from, 151–52
  overview, 55–59
  See also IGF

growth stimulation reduction, 151–86
  caloric intake and, 153–61
  dieting and, 152–53
  growth-stimulating substances, 151–52
  growth stimulation, defined, 267
  longevity staircase, overview, 121, *122*
  public health and nutrition
    information, 168–75
  specific nutrition for, 178–86, *181*
  weight gain causes, 161–68, *163*

guilt, weight gain and, 164–65

gut bacteria, 159–61

H

hair, melanocytes in, 119

happiness, 220–21

Harman, Denham, 30, 141–42

Harvard University, 94, 146, 155,
  164–65, 182, 201–2, 204–5

Haslam, David, 158

HbA1c, 66–67

HDL cholesterol, 89–90

healthy snack recipes
  Apple Slices with Almond Butter, 248
  Cashew-Coconut Balls, 248
  Kale Chips, 247
  overview, 247

healthy substitutions
  for animal-based proteins, 49–50
  for carbohydrates, 71–75

heart
  carbohydrates and, 60
  cardiovascular disease, defined, 264
  cholesterol and, 87–90 (*See also* fats)

heart attack, 267
  magnesium for, 127–28
  stem call techniques, 198
  See also micronutrients; nutrition

heat. *See* temperature

heredity. *See* DNA; genetics

heterochronic parabiosis, 199–201, *200*

high blood pressure
  carbohydrates and, 60
  potassium for, 133

high-intensity interval training (HIIT),
  139

HIV, mitochondria and, 106–7

homo neanderthalensis. See Neanderthals

homo sapiens. See humans

hormesis stimulation, 137–51
  antioxidants and free radicals, 141–43
  detoxification and, 143–50, *147, 148*
  exercise for, 138–40
  longevity staircase, overview, 121, *122*
  metformin example, 137–38
  radioactivity and, 140–41

hormones
  cortisol, 16, 265
  defined, 268
  estrogen, 20
  IGF, 54–55
  insulin, 54
  testosterone, 17–18, 19, 20, 151–52
  See also growth hormone (GH);
    testosterone

Hot Cereal with Nuts and Flaxseeds, 234

Hot Cereal with Walnuts and Coconut,
  236

Hoyeraal-Hreidarsson disease, 116

Human Longevity Inc., 252

humans
  average life span of, 11

macular degeneration (AMD)
animal-based protein and, 43
defined, 268
fats in diet and, 84

magnesium, 127–28

malocclusion (teeth), 205

Mann, George, 88

Maris, Bill, 252

medical profession, nutrition knowledge
of, 174, 175

Mediterranean diet
life span and, 70
public information and
recommendations, 173

melanocytes, 119

MELAS (encephalopathy, lactate
acidosis, and stroke-like episodes),
105–6

menopause, 20

metabolism
defined, 1–2
hormesis and, 142
weight gain and, 161–62
MAIN:metformin, 137–38

methionine, 41, 46

mice
experiments on (*See* aging causes;
scientific studies)
life span of, 1–2, 4–5, 11
reproduction and aging of, 16–17

microbiome, 159–61

micrometer, 268

micronutrients, 122–37
B vitamins, 126–27
copper, 124
deficiencies and food industrialization,
122–23
defined, 122

dietary supplement industry and,
123–25
from diet *vs.* supplements, 134
iodine, 133
longevity staircase, overview, 121, *122*
magnesium, 127–28
potassium, 132–33
selenium, 128
vitamin D, 128–30
vitamin K, 130–32

micro-retirement concept, 226–28

milk (dairy), cheese compared to,
183–84

milk drinks, from nuts, 184

minerals
carbohydrates and, 69
copper, 124
iodine, 133
magnesium, 127–28
potassium, 132–33
selenium, 128
See also micronutrients

Ming (mollusk), 7

Mini-Mental State Examination, 126

mitochondria, 95–110
aging-related and affluence-related
diseases and, 107–9
aging reversal and repairing, 194–96,
195
ATP and, 98–101, *99*, *100*, *101*
as bacteria, 97–98, 102
cell skeletons of, *102*, 102–3, *103*, 265
defined, 268
disease of, 105–7
energy generated from, 104–5
evolution and, 102–4
free radical theory and, 30
mitochondrial DNA, 96, *97*, *98*, 105
overview, 95–98, *96*

opossums, 11

overpopulation, perception of, 221–24

oxidation
  antioxidants and, 141–42, 263
  defined, 269
  See also free radicals

P

paleo diet, 48–49

parasites, 10

Parkinson's disease, 36, 89–90, 144

pear shape body, 80

persistence hunting, 83

Peto's paradox, 8

pharmaceuticals
  blood thinners, 130–32
  HIV drugs, 106–7
  statins, 90

Philip Morris, 168

pigment, 119

Pizza with Pesto, 245

placebo, 269

plant-based diet
  animal-based proteins *vs.*, 46–47
  reducing growth stimulation with, 178–79

polio vaccine, 188

porcupines, 7

portion size, 163–64

Portobello Mushrooms with Almond Stuffing, 243–44

potassium, 132–33

potatoes, 62–63

poverty, weight gain and, 154–55

predators
  fat in diet for, 82–83

life span and, 6–11

progeria, 111–13, *112*

prostate, hormesis and, 145

pro-sugar campaign, 169

proteins, 31–51
  agglomeration of, 34–41, *35, 39,* 60–61, 178–79, 187–92, *188, 190*
  amino acids in, 32–33 (*See also* amino acids)
  ATP function and, 101, *101*
  as building blocks and workhorses of cells, 32, 33
  burning calories and, 159
  cross-links, 265
  defined, 270
  as macronutrients, 30
  nutrition and, 41–51, *44*
  overview, 31, *31, 32*

protons, 270

puberty, as start of aging process, 18, 19

pulmonary fibrosis, 115–16

Q

quality of life, long life *vs.*, 218–24, 252–54

quercetin, 179

Quick Oatmeal Cake, Pancakes, or Balls, 233–34

Quick Salmon with Broccoli and Beans, 242–43

Quinoa with Peas and Feta, 240

R

radioactivity, 140–41

rapamycin, 257

Ravussin, Eric, 155

recipes, 230–51
  Acorn Squash Spaghetti, 243

dieting and problems of, 152–53
high-protein diets and, 47–48
Weismann, August, 2–3
whales, 7–8
Wheat-Free Bread, 245–46
white blood cells
antibodies and, 187–88, *188*
defined, 270
telomerase and, 115
white meat, red meat *vs.*, 44
whole grains
oatmeal *vs.* whole wheat bread, 73–74
overview, 63–65
See also carbohydrates

Willett, Walter, 182, 203
Williams, Bernard, 221
Williams, George, 12–13
wisdom teeth, 205
World Health Organization, 61, 153, 169

Y

Yale University, 165–66
Yamanaka, Shinya, 197

Z

Zuckerberg, Mark, 252

ABOUT THE AUTHOR

KRIS VERBURGH, MD, is a researcher at the Center Leo Apostel for Interdisciplinary Studies at the Free University of Brussels and is on the faculty of Singularity University, a Silicon Valley think tank devoted to tackling the world's biggest challenges with emerging technology. Dr. Verburgh researches interventions that can extend healthy life span and combat aging-related diseases through nutrition and state-of-the-art biotechnology. He has established a new scientific discipline, nutrigerontology, which researches diets and guidelines to slow down aging and reduce the risk of aging-related diseases. Dr. Verburgh is frequently invited to speak at venues all around the world about new developments and paradigm shifts in medicine, health care, the science of aging, and more.

krisverburgh.com